AN ACCIDENTAL HISTORY OF CANADA

McGill-Queen's/AMS Healthcare Studies in the History of Medicine, Health, and Society

SERIES EDITORS: J.T.H. CONNOR AND ERIKA DYCK

This series presents books in the history of medicine, health studies, and social policy, exploring interactions between the institutions, ideas, and practices of medicine and those of society as a whole. To begin to understand these complex relationships and their history is a vital step to ensuring the protection of a fundamental human right: the right to health. Volumes in this series have received financial support to assist publication from Associated Medical Services, Inc. (AMS), a Canadian charitable organization with an impressive history as a catalyst for change in Canadian healthcare. For eighty years, AMS has had a profound impact through its support of the history of medicine and the education of healthcare professionals, and by making strategic investments to address critical issues in our healthcare system. AMS has funded eight chairs in the history of medicine across Canada, is a primary sponsor of many of the country's history of medicine and nursing organizations, and offers fellowships and grants through the AMS History of Medicine and Healthcare Program (www.amshealthcare.ca).

AN
ACCIDENTAL
HISTORY
OF CANADA

Edited by
**MEGAN J. DAVIES AND
GEOFFREY L. HUDSON**

MCGILL-QUEEN'S UNIVERSITY PRESS
Montreal & Kingston • London • Chicago

ISBN 978-0-2280-2115-5 (cloth)
ISBN 978-0-2280-2116-2 (paper)
ISBN 978-0-2280-2171-1 (ePDF)
ISBN 978-0-2280-2347-0 (ePUB)

Legal deposit second quarter 2024
Bibliothèque nationale du Québec

Printed in Canada on acid-free paper that is 100% ancient forest free
(100% post-consumer recycled), processed chlorine free

This book has been published with the help of a grant from the Canadian
Federation for the Humanities and Social Sciences, through the Awards to
Scholarly Publications Program, using funds provided by the Social Sciences
and Humanities Research Council of Canada.

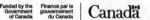 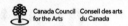

We acknowledge the support of the Canada Council for the Arts.
Nous remercions le Conseil des arts du Canada de son soutien.

McGill-Queen's University Press in Montreal is on land which long served
as a site of meeting and exchange amongst Indigenous Peoples, including the
Haudenosaunee and Anishinabeg nations. In Kingston it is situated on the
territory of the Haudenosaunee and Anishinaabek. We acknowledge and
thank the diverse Indigenous Peoples whose footsteps have marked these
territories on which peoples of the world now gather.

LIBRARY AND ARCHIVES CANADA CATALOGUING IN PUBLICATION

Title: An accidental history of Canada / edited by Megan J. Davies
    and Geoffrey L. Hudson.
Names: Davies, Megan Jean, 1959– editor. | Hudson, Geoffrey L.
    (Geoffrey Lewis), editor.
Description: Series statement: McGill-Queen's/AMS Healthcare studies in
    the history of medicine, health, and society ; 64 | Includes bibliographical
    references and index.
Identifiers: Canadiana (print) 20240306066 | Canadiana (ebook) 20240306074 |
    ISBN 9780228021155 (cloth) | ISBN 9780228021162 (paper) |
    ISBN 9780228021711 (ePDF) | ISBN 9780228023470 (ePUB)
Subjects: LCSH: Accidents—Canada—History.
Classification: LCC HB1323.A22 C3 2024 | DDC 363.100971—dc23

This collection is dedicated to all those
confronted by the immediate or long-term
physical, emotional, and financial impacts
of accidents, large and "small."

CONTENTS

FIGURES

ACKNOWLEDGMENTS

The editors thank the contributors for the excellent scholarship and the sustained professionalism they brought to our collaboration, including responding diligently to multiple rounds of peer review and editorial suggestions. It has been a joy working with them.

We are very appreciative of the support and generosity of the staff at McGill-Queen's University Press including our editor, Kyla Madden, who provided enthusiastic and effective guidance from the first stages of this accidental endeavour. We also thank the press's anonymous reviewers for their insightful and helpful suggestions, as well as J.T.H. Connor and Erika Dyck, the co-editors of the press's McGill-Queen's/AMS Healthcare Studies in the History of Medicine, Health, and Society series.

MEGAN J. DAVIES
GEOFFREY L. HUDSON

AN ACCIDENTAL HISTORY OF CANADA

INTRODUCTION

Framing an Accidental Past

John Douglas Belshaw, Megan J. Davies,
Geoffrey L. Hudson, and Sasha Mullally

The unforeseen has had devastating effects
on ordinary people and whole societies.

JOHN BURNHAM[1]

Around 9 a.m. on 6 December 1917, two naval supply vessels – one French, one Norwegian – collided in Halifax Harbour.[2] When one of the ships caught fire, many Haligonians went to their windows to watch the huge plume of black smoke rising into the sky. Moments later, the ss *Mont Blanc*'s cargo erupted, and shards of glass penetrated hundreds of eyes.[3] Almost immediately, sixteen hundred individuals were dead; that number would climb to nearly two thousand. Vastly more were injured, of course, and a huge part of the city was destroyed. Medical responses were mobilized from as far afield as Boston, with expressions of sympathy, state concern, and material support coming in from the four corners of the British Empire.[4]

Few other "accidents" loom so large in Canadian history as the Halifax Explosion, but it has a staggering amount of company. Histories of accidents and natural disasters cast the precarity of Canadian life into sharp relief. Barely a year before Halifax, a fire in Ontario's Clay Belt claimed at least two hundred lives at and around the village of Matheson. Farmers' efforts at land clearing had provided stores of kindling everywhere, and the fires attacked the hamlet from all sides.⁵ Another community was eviscerated on 29 April 1903 when a flank of Turtle Mountain sheared off into the town of Frank, Alberta, killing more than ninety people. More than a century later, an unattended freight car carrying crude oil trundled into the sleeping town of Lac-Mégantic, Quebec, and derailed. The resulting explosion laid waste to half of the town's centre, killing forty-seven people and causing extensive and costly soil and water contamination.⁶

Connecting Canadians through vast transportation networks invited accidental death. The Quebec Bridge on the lower St Lawrence River was under construction in 1907 when it gave way; only eleven of eight-six workers survived. The failure of a replacement centre span in 1916 killed another thirteen men. Incompetent engineering and supervision, along with attempts to cut costs with cheap steel, were blamed for both Quebec Bridge disasters, as well as for the collapse of the Second Narrows Bridge in Vancouver forty-two years later, with the loss of nineteen lives.⁷ Other infrastructure construction projects were also marked by dramatic accidents.⁸ By contrast, the death of as many as four thousand Chinese railway workers along the main line of the Canadian Pacific Railway in the early 1880s is not a singular momentous event, but neither is it a series of singular and unrelated tragedies: it is a drawn-out cascade of related accidents unfolding relentlessly over many months.⁹

The arrival of the internal combustion engine in the late nineteenth century and the rise of automobility created entirely new categories of risk. Accidents involving motorized transportation, of course, are typically more personal and smaller in scale, though not necessarily less tragic. Motor vehicles were the leading cause of accidental death among men and women through most of the twentieth century, killing nearly six thousand in Canada in 1979 alone.¹⁰ In 2014, *Maclean's* magazine reported that the decade from 1999 to 2008 saw "28,000 dead and 186,000 drivers, passengers, pedestrians and cyclists hospitalized" as a result of motor vehicle "accidents."¹¹ The largest single Canadian automobile accident – in terms of fatalities and injuries – occurred in September 1999, when thick fog on Highway 401 in Ontario between Tilbury and Windsor led to an eighty-seven-car pile-up causing eight deaths. An event on the roads claiming more lives involved a bus carrying the Humboldt Broncos junior hockey team, which collided with a westbound semi on 6 April 2018; sixteen people died, and another thirteen were injured, most of them young men in their teens. While accidental deaths on land and sea are an ancient phenomenon modified by technology, the coming of air travel brought entirely new dangers. Before 9 December 1956, aircraft crashes in Canada had been small events, but on that day sixty-two people, including five Canadian Football League players, died when Flight 810 from Vancouver to Calgary slammed into the side of Mount Slesse near Chilliwack.[12]

Canada has no shortage of accident and disaster stories, catastrophic for individuals and communities and laying bare the risks of life. Taken individually, they inspire awe and grief; taken collectively, they reveal much more. Economic order, changing technologies, the relative isolation of resource-extraction communities, vulnerabilities of travel and trade, childhood games, gendered workplaces, and the agendas of colonization, militarism, imperialism, and globalization all contribute to a compelling yet hazardous narrative. As a lightly populated colonial construct spanning a continent, Canada as a concept invites certain risks; this country has more road, river, and rail than most on which to falter and die.

Disaster becomes a narrative trope, part of local lore, and even an identity in some circumstances. Take the community of Fernie in British Columbia's southeast corner:

After the turn of the twentieth century, residents of Fernie experienced an alarming sequence of events that drastically shaped historical consciousness into the present ... In 1897, 1902, 1916, 1923, and 1948, rising river levels caused severe floods. Mud slides have always plagued the rough roads along the Crowsnest Pass. Outbreaks of typhoid (1897 and 1902), smallpox (1902), scarlet fever, measles, chicken pox, and influenza (1918) took many lives. Between 1902 and 1967, 226 men were killed in the mines at Coal Creek, Morrissey, and Michel-Natal. In 1904 and 1908 fires ripped through the town. Residents of Fernie risked starvation in 1911 after a heavy snowfall cut off railway transport. The following year a rock slide killed six men at Coal Creek.[13]

Historian Leslie Robertson observes that these stories – individually, ag-glomerated, and combined – "continue to circulate through reminiscences and media."[14] Disasters become foundational to the community's mythos and character. As with a small, remote town in one corner of Canada, so with the country as a whole. Often defined as natural events such as droughts, epidemics, and earthquakes that affect entire societies, disaster stories loom large as gothic horrors and as heroic tales.[15]

As compared to natural disasters, accidents are often tied to notions of human agency. Historians have found the distinctions between accidents and disasters slippery, and this imprecision has limited systematic exam-ination of "the accident" as a feature of life in the past. Do accidents weigh on the collective mind as heavily as disasters? Are they less monumental and more easily overlooked but also part of the fibre of society and com-munity? The difference between accident and disaster cannot be decided with any finality, and we do not intend to do so. Nevertheless, some useful distinctions can be made.

An Accidental History of Canada does not examine disasters that affect entire societies but instead focuses on accidents that affect groups and in-dividuals within a society.[16] As a collective of historians intrigued by the accident in the past, we are concerned with mishaps resulting in injury and sometimes death. We are not concerned with the accidental encounter, nor with the unforeseen event that might have turned out badly but did not. In a recent dissection of the fatal "accident" in contemporary America, journalist Jesse Singer also defines an accident by what it is not: "not a dis-ease like cancer, not an act of God like the weather, not an act of inten-tion like murder." We place greater stock in the environmental accident – Singer's "act of God" – but we would agree with her to ignore another category: "'Accident' can be an excuse, an explanation, a *mea culpa*, or a crime." Accidents can be distinguished from disasters by scale; as Singer writes, "When we die by accident, we die in ones and twos."[17] Similarly, Roger Cooter and Bill Luckin, editors of the groundbreaking 1997 collec-tion *Accidents in History*, argued that an accident becomes a disaster when lives are altered on a grand scale. That is, in order to qualify as a disaster, the numbers impacted generally have to be larger or the effects more con-sequential.[18] The injury and the death of smaller numbers is experienced differently and narrativized differently, and to different ends. So, it is the small accident, the intimate catastrophe, the personal disaster that may become a matter of public interest that mostly concerns us here.

This volume argues that accidents occur within particular circumstances of vulnerability, that efforts to avoid and prevent accidents are themselves histories of accidents, and that the story of the accident and the work of the storytelling deserve particular scrutiny. In this regard, we depart from earlier scholarly understandings of accidents. Sociologist Judith Green, for example, interprets accidents as blameless misfortunes that are evaluated retrospectively in terms of the damage sustained or the causal sequence of events that led to the incident. This view is a kind of reverse-engineering designed to find inherent flaws. Although Green argues that society's shrinking appetite for the unpredictable makes "accidents" problematic, her writing places greater emphasis on immediate consequences than on longer-term outcomes, not least cultural outcomes.[19] Blameworthiness is often an important part of the storytelling of accidents in the past and merits its own historicizing, which we do here. What is more, the longer-term consequences of a singular unanticipated event – some of which play out over decades or even a century – are precisely what make accident histories worthy of further work.

Embedded in studies of accidents in the past is a metaphysical element that needs to be laid bare. Cooter and Luckin, for example, note the challenge that accidents pose to notions of progress.[20] That is to say, if repeatedly and in ways that are easy to document, we do not learn from our mistakes, then the whole concept of "progress" is undermined. Contemporaries sought to control accidents insofar as they posed a threat to that modernist foundational belief. Earlier generations put more faith – literally – in notions of predetermination and divine involvement. As one study of accidents in early modern England puts it, "A falling object ... could kill someone who was unfortunate enough to be standing where it fell. Death in such cases could be explained entirely with reference to natural causes: heavy objects fall, the vital spirits are stilled by a sudden blow to the head. But if that person happened to be a murderer, the accident might seem to come about for a reason, perhaps as a kind of divine justice."[21] Even in the modern era, this moral geometry is often invoked in the event of a fatal accident: did the victim have it coming? Providence or fate may not be invoked, let alone involved, but some tipping of scales may yet be central to the storyline that emerges. This survival of morality in accident storylines is another way in which the secular motif of "progress" gets undermined. What further dents it is the strong evidence, offered up in this volume, that accidents do not just *occur* to the vulnerable: they reveal and define vulnerability. Inequality begets accidents, and precarity localizes them. While progress may be busy lifting the whole of society, the less well off are losing fingers and limbs. Accidents are not inevitable any more than they are pre-ordained, but the odds are clearly stacked.

In the early 1990s, Ulrich Beck and Anthony Giddens connected the concept of "risk" to the rise of industrial capitalism and a growing faith in expert use of science and technology to predict and control risk, and hence accidents.[22] While Beck's and Giddens's sociological framing underpins the analysis in much historical literature on the accident, historians have also contributed rich empirical studies of how people experienced accidents at different times and in different places, exploring factors such as locality, labour, capital, the state, and notions of specific vulnerabilities. Risk historicized is more nuanced, and players in the drama of the accident have their agency acknowledged through the power of the story. John Burnham's 2009 study of the psychological concept of "accident proneness," for example, historicizes the notion that some accidents are inevitable and linked to personality. Burnham points to shifting psychological perspectives and changes in the American workplace and the insurance industry to explain how the notion of the "accident-prone worker" fell by the wayside.[23] Likewise, Craig Spence details precautionary steps taken in the city of London over the eighteenth century, actions that eased the collective anxieties of urban life in an increasingly secular society, while Paul Fyfe sets out the case for the metropolis as "ground zero for some of the most important interdisciplinary thinking about causation in the nineteenth century."[24] The connection between "risk," "accidents," and modern industrial capitalism looms large in the studies by social scientists.

A historical approach to accidents is sensitive to context: location and shared beliefs clearly count. Two studies of workplace accidents in the railway sectors of, respectively, the United States and the United Kingdom in the pre–World War I era reveal a tolerance of risk in the former and

in the latter a shift in worker and public perception from fatalistic acceptance to a push for state intervention.[25] It was not until the mid-twentieth
century that Americans pivoted from a notion of individual to collective
responsibility, particularly in the field of toxic "accidents" like the Love
Canal fiasco.[26] Even so, as Derek S. Oden argues in an important 2017
book on accidents in Midwest family farms, larger machinery and dangerous chemicals inevitably increased serious mishaps, yet most entrepreneurial owner-operators rejected safety regulations in favour of "personal
caution" in avoiding injury.[27] Examining railway, gun, and amusement-park
accidents in the United States over the past two and a half centuries, historian of technology Arwen Mohun argues that the notion of collective responsibility for managing risk is constantly undermined by the American
nation's need to uphold individual freedom. The current handgun debate,
she notes, is a perfect illustration of this conundrum and the way in which
many Americans disengage from the dominant ethos of the modern "risk
society," a term coined by Beck and Giddens.[28]

Jamie Bronstein argues that in the United States and Britain, the past
century witnessed an increasing tendency to look to the state and its agents
to regulate risk.[29] European historian Julia Moses links the adoption of
workers' compensation legislation in Britain, Germany, and Italy to a bas-
ket of emerging concepts, including occupational risk, and to increasingly
sophisticated state utilization of statistics, arguing that accident compensation laws were "the first pieces of modern social legislation that set out,
through national policy, to redistribute individual risks ... systematically
to a wider community."[30] But the pattern is not uniform, nor is it universal.
As regards the risks posed by automobiles, Tamara Myers has shown how
North American police post–World War II used shocking images and
stories of childhood death in an effort to mold safety-savvy citizens who
would check the rising rate of automobile accidents through individual
rather than collective effort, let alone regulation of manufacturers.[31] While
the modern welfare state in its multiple manifestations loomed on the hori-
zon, the notion of individual responsibility was nevertheless preserved.

Canadian scholars intersect with these international works as public-
health researchers, labour historians, and cultural-history scholars interro-
gating the workings of gender and emotions. Simon P. Thomas and Steve

E. Hrudey's 1997 book *Risk of Death in Canada: What We Know and How We Know It* is a work of contemporary epidemiology and public health in keeping with the Beck and Giddens literature. Using a wide range of data, the authors present and discuss the nature of accidental death in late twentieth-century Canada.[32] But this is not historical work, and for that we look to journal articles and book chapters by a handful of Canadian historians who have worked on the period from 1900 to 1950, situating the accident in the spheres of work, community, and family. Eric Tucker's influential 1992 neo-Marxist study of the early history of occupational health and safety regulation in Ontario, along with subsequent publications, has challenged the notion of a benevolent, impartial state that watched over worker well-being.[33] Robert Storey's research on the late twentieth-century battle for adequate compensation and improved health and safety legislation demonstrates how it took the combined efforts of labour organizations, middle-class activists, militant workers, and progressive physicians to make workplaces safer and hold capital accountable.[34] In 2005, Mona Gleason's important article on children and accidents in English Canada built on the notion of precaution and the rise of the "public child."[35] Myers's 2015 article, mentioned above, discussed police use of cautionary tales of childhood death to arrest the rising rate of automobile accidents.[36] In 2010, John Belshaw and Diane Purvey explored another aspect of automobile accidents and memory in *Private Grief, Public Mourning*, a study of the narrative uses of roadside shrines in the Far West.[37] A 2011 book chapter by Megan Davies established that precautionary practices and caring for accident victims was part of the broader mother-work of settler women in northern British Columbia.[38] Some of those themes echo Nancy Forestell's 2006 work on disability and gender in Canadian mining communities, which provides groundbreaking insights into the physical and emotional work of women in tending to husbands injured and disabled on the job.[39]

Quebec historian Magda Fahrni has contributed much to the building of a specific and coherent body of research and analysis on the accident in Canadian history. In a series of studies starting in 2012, she explored accidents in the context of industrial modernity in Quebec, concluding that accidents were increasingly understood as avoidable. Employers, unions, physicians, insurance companies, and others used science, technology, and statistics to explain, predict, and prevent accidents. Religious and providential explanations for accidents persisted but waned. Fahrni examines the history of accidents in different venues: on the road, in a burning cinema, and the workplace. In the 1920s, safety advocates wrestled with new dangers constituted by automobiles and the enhanced value placed on the category of "the child." Fahrni finds that responsibility for accidents is ultimately assigned to the individual and most often to the victim. Safety education, she demonstrates, is directed at children and parents and workers and less so to business owners, drivers, or factory managers. Fahrni contends that the emerging paradigm is consistent with the liberal vision of the individual in industrial capitalism.[40]

Other good work examines accidents in the context of other historical topics. For example, the pioneering work of Catherine Cournoyer uses coroners' reports in a study of Montreal children's accidents in the early twentieth century.[41] Christopher Dummitt's *The Manly Modern: Masculinity in Postwar Canada* investigates traffic, recreational, and workplace accidents and discusses risk management and the development of masculine expertise. Like Fahrni, Dummitt is inspired by Beck and Giddens, examining how modern ideas of risk influenced gender in postwar Canada, this time with a focus on Vancouver. He compares and contrasts middle-class and working-class men, acknowledging that, while working men confront accidents every day at work, middle-class men manage risk and also voluntarily risk accidents in recreational activities.[42]

An Accidental History of Canada both builds on and departs from these earlier studies of misfortune north of the forty-ninth parallel. Our authors understand the accident as a contested and evolving public-private category of misfortune where notions of responsibility and meaning play out in an emerging and evolving nation. Like other historians, we are interested in work, gender, children, risk, the state, and legal and medical professionals as they relate to the accident, but our focus is on smaller accidents and unexplored aspects of accidents that have a public face, and our view is most often from the periphery. Thus, a central purpose of this volume is to draw back the curtain on accidents in the past to show the shifting workings of social power in both private and public realms. Human life is unpredictable and "accidents happen," but this does not mean that accidents have no social, cultural, or political meaning. The book's chapters are grouped into topical sections that highlight different aspects of this framing; we consider accident as events that reveal fundamental inequities in Canadian society, as maps delineating the progress or process of the notion of precaution, and as rich storylines that frame significant events and establish shared meaning.

As the first set of chapters establishes, equity counts in the realm of the accident. Risk is almost always mediated by wealth, power, and social position or, conversely, exacerbated by poverty, poor housing, and unsafe working conditions, yet the workings of privilege are often hidden from the public eye and their impacts felt in private pain. Samira Saramo draws from the public forums of community newspapers and histories to show how Finnish migrant socialists explained accidents through the lens of class, while John Belshaw's account of the media's treatment of cyclist accidents over three periods is punctuated by privilege and marginality. Expanding on existing work on injury and death in the Ontario mining industry, John Sandlos finds that smaller fatal accidents were handled so as to attribute injury to worker error, obscuring the role of capital's relentless thirst for profit. The inadequacies of the state and the courts at safeguarding the less privileged are illuminated most clearly in Sandlos's contribution and Blake Brown's chapter on medical malpractice but form a backdrop to Belshaw's piece as well.

The next group of chapters focuses on the notion of precaution, exploring ways in which Canadian workers, charity, capital, and the state have attempted to mitigate risk. Reading against the provenance of extant records from the construction of Montreal's Victoria Bridge, which obscure the term "accident," Anh-Dao Bui Tran hypothesizes that both labourers and contractors sought to maintain the health and productivity of workers. Turning to a period roughly half a century later, John Matchim finds that missionaries on the remote coasts of Newfoundland employed the concept of risk to reform the domestic and working arrangements of Labrador people. Taking this notion of precautionary practice into the twentieth century, Ceilidh Auger-Day maps the emergence of a collective state response to workplace injury, and Cameron Baldassarra delineates how risk became a personal responsibility in the emerging forum of wilderness recreation. Ultimately, precaution in Canada emerges as a hybrid of public and private responses, with the state and the individual both taking a role in managing risk.

The final cluster of chapters considers how stories are constructed in the aftermath of the accident and the multiple purposes these narratives can serve. Here we give particular consideration to what comprises a public accident. Colin Coates argues that contemporary narratives and ex-votos paintings depicting shipwrecks in New France helped explain and memorialize these rare but significant events and also constructed a public narrative of survival in a strange and sometimes dangerous land. Using a "Two Eyed Seeing" framework to compare how accidents are recalled and understood in Indigenous communities and settler communities, Geoffrey Hudson and Darrel Manitowabi deploy this Mi'kmaw concept to reflect on the distance between settler and Indigenous understandings of Canada and its past. Megan Davies and Tamara Myers demonstrate the importance of an accident's very public afterlife, linking the tale of a young girl's fall on a remote island to settler colonialism, maternalism, and the emerging category of disability. Sasha Mullally returns to a famous episode of rural kitchen-table surgery following a farm accident to consider the story that was left untold.

The three sections of this book are organized to highlight specific themes over others but do not compartmentalize them. They spill out and across one another, inviting the reader to look everywhere for evidence of inequity, the role of precaution, and the centrality of storytelling in order to construct an intersectional picture of accidents in history, particularly Canadian history. Thus, class clearly underpins Matchim's and Baldassarra's contributions. Inequity runs rampant through Hudson and Manitowabi's chapter. And Brown's courtroom drama and Saramo's tale of the tragic fire at a Finnish-Canadian utopian settlement could easily be read as cautionary storylines. Taken together, these chapters work from the margins inward to give collective and personal misfortune a firm location in Canada's historiographical landscape, demonstrating that accidents are malleable, multi-faceted, and often deeply significant past-present events.

Examining experiences of Canadian risk and calamity, we delve into the individual and collective management of precarity in a particular set of geographies, climates, economies, and social orders, gaining insight into the colonial power relations laid bare by the accidental moment. In addition to the history of colonialism, this book draws from fields of history taken up in the twenty-plus years since Cooter and Luckin's path-breaking *Accidents in History* appeared: Indigenous history, environmental history, the history of childhood, disability history, the history of the body, and the history of emotions. The twelve chapters that make up this volume take the reader from the 1630s to the 1980s, covering a wide swath of Canadian accidents, locations, and perspectives. Two chapters deal with accidents and the state, three chapters with workplace accidents. A further three chapters focus on the urban setting, and four are set in rural locales. Two chapters explore the all-too-common childhood accident. The sweep of Atlantic Canada, Central Canada, the Prairies, the Near North, and British Columbia are all represented here. Importantly, the authors foreground gendered experiences of both accident and aftermath throughout. All reveal important unequal experiences of precarity and the differential risk absorbed by those lives harmed or ended by accidental events. This collection, then, contributes a specific history of accidents in Canada, arguing that the national context matters at several levels.

CANADA'S ACCIDENTAL PAST

While Canada today is one of the most urban societies in the world, in the past (and even now beyond the current network of major cities) sparse numbers scattered over a vast geography was typical. Some Indigenous nations tended towards more concentrated domains; Wabanakiak, Wendake Ehen, and Haida Gwaii offer examples. Others, such as the Inuit and Nehiyawak, sprawled across huge spaces. Imperial European ambitions, even in the era of New France, inclined towards enormity. The sea itself was part of these spaces, as were the long and often treacherous waterways that functioned as the principal highways of the northern half of North America until the twentieth century. As a series of colonial and mercantile enterprises, the European settlements that became Canada were oriented for administrative and commercial purposes to the Atlantic and Pacific oceans and to Europe. Hugging several coastlines, the settler population regarded and then mythologized the "interior" as a place of wilderness and danger. Settler tales of "exploration" inevitably include hazards associated with climatic extremes – scalding summers and unforgiving winters – and the unlikelihood of getting help in the event of a tragic misstep.[43] Writing fifty years ago about what distinguishes Canadian literature, Margaret Atwood boiled it down to "death by nature."[44]

This landscape had both an affective and an economic value. From Confederation in 1867 through the first decades of the twentieth century, Canada's colonial economies reoriented from an initial emphasis on oceanic trade networks to a focus on interior continental expansion and consolidation. This process of nation building launched and accelerated a "great land rush," its goal to establish settler farmers on the Great Plains, beyond established agriculture in the Maritimes and the Canadas.[45] The political project of Confederation and capitalist expansion required the management of these colonial precarities. There was risk from American expansionism, risk from potential objections raised and obstacles posed by Indigenous peoples, and risks implied in isolation from markets in the more populated and wealthier jurisdictions in the eastern provinces as well as Europe and China. These risks were mitigated by activities such as the negotiation of the treaties with First Nations, the construction of the Canadian Pacific Railway, and the project of recruiting and managing the mass immigration of many central and eastern Europeans to the Prairie West.[46] The elites who were invested in the colonial enterprise offered opportunities to railway construction workers and settlers carving out lives in remote places, but such endeavours also required that these bit players in the game of nation building assume personal risk and exposure to accidents.

Canada's resource extraction sector – always the bedrock of national economic development – requires close investigation. Resource extraction activities entail risk for those who fish the oceans, harvest the forests, grow food in the soil, and claw minerals from the earth. We see evidence in the language used by Canadian economic historians who extend the use of the word "mining" to include the once-widespread harvest of furs and the large-scale production of grain for export. Even though more than half the population has lived in urban settings since 1921, the economic order continues to rely on the extraction of resources like fish, pelts, wheat, coal, nickel and other metals, oil, and uranium in a seasonally inhospitable environment.

It is rare to find these resources near to metropolises; places like Ontario's Sudbury, Nova Scotia's Sydney, and BC's Tumbler Ridge – mining towns with significant populations – exemplify the Canadian experience of sizable resource-extraction communities located hundreds of kilometres from local metropolitan hubs. Distance does not exert the same kind of tyranny in American and British mining districts (though it may be the case in Australia). In Canada, distance matters: distance from hospitals and seats of power accentuates the dangers that settlers faced in localized experiences of catastrophe, such as at Crowsnest Pass and the outports of Newfoundland.

That image of Canada as a nation in which the "natural" environment looms large often obscures the role of industries linked to these primary-resource activities. Modern Canada, the setting for most of these studies, was also shaped by industrial enterprises and state-supported infrastructures that enabled them. From the textile centres of Montreal to the steelworks of Hamilton, work and life in urban centres of Canada also drove the economy and carried a quantum of risk. Moving goods and people on the country's railways and highways and through its canals and ports meant that the modern infrastructures of urban life also created sites of accidents.

This is not to say that Canadian accidents are always or fundamentally unique. As this volume makes clear, many accidents take place in globally familiar domestic settings, the professional sphere, and the world of leisure. That domesticity is crafted in ways that would be familiar around much of the Atlantic basin, or that professions are recognizable from one country to another, or that leisure time is spent in ways that one could find in many countries, are historic facts that arise because of colonialism, continentalism, and globalism. In short, and as Craig Spence argues in *Accidents and Violent Death in Early Modern London, 1670–1750*, accidents are "communally constructed events contingent upon social structures and cultural configurations within which they take place."[47] Some of those cultural configurations can be global in their reach. The socio-cultural context of accidents is always significant, even as Canadians across time, place, and privilege experience different environments in which accidents occur and different precipitating factors. Taken together, the studies in this collection demonstrate the connectedness of seemingly disparate events through common themes and often very Canadian conditions.

RISK ON THE MARGINS

While this book interrogates risk along the lines of race, region, gender, ability, and class, and looks closely at the social and cultural history of accidental moments that cast unequal risk into sharp intersectional relief, the colonial enterprise figures prominently. The historical actors described in this volume knew that the task of making settler Canada was risky business. Coates's chapter on New France shows that people travelling to and from the colony were aware that a deadly shipwreck was a real possibility. The dangers faced by settlers are also visible in Matchim's study of the medical work of the Grenfell mission and Saramo's exploration of accidents and the Finnish diaspora across North America. To early twentieth-century Finnish and other immigrants, fire was both necessary and deadly: land must be cleared and homes heated, but the end result might be the charred remains of settlers' dreams.[48] Even the bucolic red fields of the Prince Edward Island farmstead turned lethal with the introduction of mechanized equipment, as Mullally's chapter shows.

This linkage between the accident and settler colonialism is brought to its logical conclusion with Hudson and Manitowabi's dissection of accidents on Manitoulin Island. Anishinaabek and settler residents shared risky experiences of the island: drowning on the water, perishing in fires, being shot while hunting, and encountering injury and death while farming, fishing, or lumbering. However, Indigenous peoples and settlers had vastly differing understandings of the meaning and significance of those experiences. By contrast, the story of Othoa Scott from Hornby Island, BC, begins as a tale of risk at the margins and becomes a vehicle for promoting colonial well-being, because she met white settler standards of purity and aesthetics. She was an ideal public poster child for disability fundraising, precisely because she was white and cute in a fashion idealized for twentieth-century youth.

Other chapters that explore state interventions into compensation for injuries, the workplace, healthcare, and engineering projects implicitly or explicitly contextualize their research in settler colonialism and the advent of the modern state. The emergent power and reach of the state is particularly well articulated and challenged in Brown's chapter on medical malpractice in 1960s Toronto, a tale that exposes the multiple layers of settler authority. Auger-Day shows how the 1908 Alberta Workmen's Compensation Act served to justify a patriarchal family structure, as was the case with many other welfare state programs. The organization of streets by Vancouver elites in the service of cycling as described by Belshaw likewise involves imposing a new set of values on a landscape in which Indigenous narratives were rendered invisible.

Inequity creates risks if those holding economic and social power do not prioritize safety, and several authors describe ruthlessly exploitive workplaces in which danger was a common feature. In his study of nautical disasters, Coates shows how the sea functions as a dangerous environment; accidents occurred with such frightening regularity that officials in New France had to find ways to understand them and did so by invoking environmental risks, the role of providence, and reassuring tales of survival. Bui Tran speculates that contractors of the Victoria Bridge put workers at risk by their system of giving bonuses for the speedy completion of a job. Grenfell mission's medical staff in Matchim's study appeared unconcerned about risking the lives of the local people they tasked with taking them on dangerous and sometimes unnecessary voyages. The Finnish immigrants who are the focus of Saramo's chapter believed that poorly built worker housing where fire could easily find a foothold was a form of class warfare. This theme of wilful neglect by authorities and employers is most clearly expressed in Sandlos's chapter on the 124,854 Ontario miners involved in accidents between 1927 and 1971. Mineworkers operated with a significant amount of autonomy, yet their safety underground was jeopardized by limited job training and supervision and a corporate focus on productivity. Brown's study, too, focuses on the ways in which "patient safety" was understood, protected, or undermined by elites.

Many of these chapters also demonstrate that to be a man in Canada was in itself a risk. Historically and today, work in Canadian resource extraction and transportation industries is gendered towards male engagement and female exclusion. Whether in mines or on the high seas, as police or as physicians, the principal roles have gone to men. "Men's work" was often dangerous and men's leisure activities equally so. The mine worksites that Saramo and Sandlos both reference are characteristically masculine and inherently dangerous, but Sandlos nuances this picture by focusing attention away from large accidents to everyday fatalities and injuries. As Bui Tran observes, nineteenth-century bridge workers were not passive victims, but a culture of masculinity, shared by management and labour, contributed to the normalization of workplace danger. Baldassarra's history of canoeing on Algonquin Park's Petawawa River showcases drowning accidents of both working men of the region and elite male writers and politicians who came to canoe these storied waters. The early twentieth-century "scorcher" and the 1970s "biketivist" in Belshaw's history of cycling accidents are mostly male. And as Auger-Day points out, the "risky" gender and the industrial accident were central to early Canadian workman's compensation legislation, with coverage centred on the male family wage-earner.

Yet gender appears in many of these studies in ways that need to be read subtly and intentionally. Matchim describes how women performed risky waged work that unsettled the Grenfell mission staff's gendered understanding of acceptable risk. Mullally's contribution, situating mother-work as central to surgical survival and recovery from accidental injury, offers one poignant example of this reclaimed space. The consequences of accidental injury or death among men are very often principally borne by women. The economic responsibilities, the healing work, and the emotional labour after the accident in many cases are picked up by women. Whether as widows or caregivers (personal, private, or professional), as advocates, or as an organized cadre of the local Women's Institute, throughout these chapters women are present and their gendered roles are explored.

To be a child meant to be at risk. Across the twentieth century, as infant and childhood mortality rates associated with illness fell, the statistical weight shifted to fatal accidents among children, with those under ten forming the most at-risk demographic. Whether it is the stories of Othoa Scott or A.J. MacCormack – two children involved in individual accidents – or the several children who died together in a conflagration on Malcolm Island, isolation often informs their experiences. Add in the stories of the many, many children injured or even killed while cycling in Vancouver, and we see another common feature: elaborate attempts by contemporaries to make sense of unexpected childhood accidents and premature death and to find meaning in random tragedies. In doing so, contemporaneous commentators often expressed their understanding of the nature of accidents and risks – very often within what they saw as explicitly Canadian ways. The history of accidents is thus, in part, historic understandings of mishap and misadventure.

Management of precarity often involves creating cultures of mitigation and precaution, another overarching theme in this volume. Each contribution here contains at least a nod to the notion of accident prevention or interrogates its absence. In some instances, this framing takes the form of cautionary tales, a narrativized map for safe living. The Anishinaabe of Manitoulin Island, for example, hold mythic stories of the Wolf who drowns after disregarding the advice of his uncle Nanabushu. Shipwrecks were the eighteenth-century archetype of a disaster, and while written and artistic memorials from New France sent out clear messages about the importance of divine intervention and the frailty of human life, they also emphasized nautical skills and a practical understanding of life at sea. Alberta politicians and reporters presented tales of families wrecked by the loss of a male wage earner to underscore the value of their new workman's compensation policy. At the same time, some stories have become darts to deflate hubris among engineers and contractors. Whole mining communities can recite stories – including lists of names of the dead – when it comes to underground disasters. The infamous Hollinger Gold Mine fire of 1928, referenced in both the Saramo and Sandlos chapters, demonstrates the failure of capital and the state to safeguard the well-being of workers on a notoriously dangerous worksite, a situation where precaution was known and understood but not pursued.

Provincial authorities and the judicial system get mixed reviews in terms of precaution and mitigation. Sandlos's detailed analysis shows a consistent pattern of provincial inspectors and the courts dismissing mining accidents as no-fault events. Miners took from this the message that they needed to carefully assess and respond to risk on the job. Safety training for cyclists – something that many Canadians are familiar with today – is historicized in Belshaw's chapter. Recreational accidents on the Petawawa River resulted in attempts by recreational governing bodies to improve the training and risk-management abilities of canoeists and campers, yet the safety of labouring men on the Petawawa was never a concern of community groups or of government.

The Canadian state and court system have also sought to mitigate accidents and risks. Several authors here note that progress was typically slow and incomplete in this regard. It is clear that Ontario legislators – or indeed their counterparts in Alberta, Nova Scotia, and British Columbia – did little to advocate for the safety of mineworkers until the later twentieth century. Similarly, as Brown explains in his chapter, even when an activist coroner attempted to improve patient safety in the 1960s, the Ontario courts chose stasis over progress by endorsing elite health professionals. Overall, however, the collection demonstrates an expanding role for both the provincial and the municipal state in responding to accidents from the late nineteenth century onwards. As fatalism loses its purchase and new statistical tools become available, ideas about risk and the possibility of mitigating its worst effects have gained ground. If accidents could not be prevented, at least their consequences could be allayed. In the first decade of the twentieth century, for example, we see attempts to extend the state's role in protecting the financial security of injured working men in Alberta. Two decades later, British Columbia became a partner in an institutionalized response to the needs of disabled youth. Police forces – and the insurance industry – show up alongside municipal authorities to reduce risks and the number of accidents among cyclists. In analyzing these responses to accidents – that ripple effect – we realize that the strategies put in place are not always sound; they often avoid addressing more thorny factors that lead to accident and injury, and they reflect the values of an emergent settler state. Modernist state interventions are made, but with very mixed and incomplete outcomes.

Cultures of precaution extend into cultures of care and remedy. Remediation might include plans for repairing broken bodies so that they could be rendered functional again, an "industrial logic of pathology" explored in disability histories. We see this in accounts published in the Grenfell mission magazine of injured or disabled coastal men who were made productive workers again through proper medical treatment, in the repair of a boy's limbs in 1910 Prince Edward Island, and in the ways in which the story of Othoa Scott became a tale of rehabilitation. That theme of physical recovery coupled to economic productivity can be seen, too, in the actions of Victoria Bridge contractors who funded beds at a local hospital.

Many of the contributors have observed how certain accidents become significant events of memory, though their meaning, narrative, and use may shift as they become collective events. Many of the accidents addressed in this book take place in private; others were entirely or eventually public accidents. Small or large, they either became renowned at the moment they took place or subsequently attained notoriety. Taken as whole, the research done by our authors suggests three typologies in these collective narratives: the public accident as a miracle, the public accident as a cautionary tale, and the public accident as a crusade.

The clearest articulation of the accident as occasion for "miraculous" or heroic intervention is the emergency surgery that Mullally describes, performed in 1910 by PEI physician Dr Gus MacDonald. That successful kitchen-table surgery became the stuff of local legend when it resurfaced in the 1960s. Narratives of this kind involve the erasure of the less miraculous and even mundane nursing work at the time by the patient's mother. The theme of "miraculous" responses can be found, too, in the 1908 Alberta legislation that provided a pre-emptive recovery plan for working people because it in effect transformed the lives of families left without the support of a male wage earner.

Yet the miracle narratives tend to lose their lustre quickly, another pattern discerned in these studies. Othoa "Polly" Scott's successful recovery at Victoria's new Queen Alexandra Solarium was moved from "miracle" to "motivation" for progressive rehabilitation therapy across the province. Barely a generation had passed since Dr Gus's surgical gymnastics before medical achievement became understood as a product and measure of science and efficiency. In Newfoundland and Labrador, the accident and recovery stories of ordinary women and men became fundraising fodder for the Grenfell medical mission. Even there – at a site explicitly associated with spiritual redemption and divine intervention – providential disasters had to make way for banal forces like ignorance and unhealthy living. Similarly, by the 1960s, Canadian leisure canoeists had eschewed miracles as a safety measure and left behind the persona of the risk-taking gentleman adventurer in favour of safety education and calculated-risk strategies.

Perhaps accidents left behind by history are the most telling because they speak to the continued ambiguities of tragic events. This book offers a number of illustrations. Victoria Bridge employer records rarely explicitly referenced accidents, a fact that Bui Tran interprets as evidence of a pre-modern understanding of the accident. Matchim notes that the accident accounts set out in the pages of the Grenfell mission's official magazine were frequently embellished to promote the institution's work, obscuring the real struggles of ordinary people of Newfoundland and Labrador.

There is, too, a general silence on the subject of emotions in the history of the accident.[49] The archives offer us little on this score: we are left to assume that tragedy begets sadness, but we have to guess at other emotions. This recognition of absence is, in itself, a finding. Two authors do an excellent job of illuminating the contours of grief and heart response. Mullally restores to her story the role and feeling of the patient's mother as something much more than a side note. Similarly, Saramo evokes *vahinko*, the Finnish word for accident, to express the depth of feeling after the tragic fire that killed eight children and three adults at the utopian community of Sointula in 1903 and to understand the historical silence on emotions in this regard. Finding these few examples hint at how much more emotion is hidden and how complex this history must be.

SUMMARY

The accidents investigated in this volume reflect and advance international scholarship on the dangers of the workplace, the home, and the road. Cooter and Luckins' *Accidents in History* presented a series of snapshots of how the accident could be understood historically; we take this two steps further, offering the accident as a dynamic tool for reconsideration of not just health history but also histories of labour, recreation, disability, and memory work. Coal mines everywhere were dangerous, farming always carried with it certain hazards, cars hit bicycles on every continent, and the sea could be merciless in any hemisphere. That said, some of these Canadian accidents could happen nowhere but Canada; the convergence of physical isolation, harshly unrelenting climatic conditions, immigrant experience, and settler colonialism creates the distinctly Canadian interpretations of the history of accident set out in this volume. Clearly, this is a place where working from the margins towards the centre makes sense.

The location and circumstances of accidents, the ways in which they are (mis)managed, and the responses that come after or separate from the immediate crisis signal a distinctively Canadian context and advance our understanding of the "accident" as an event with consequences both public and personal. This is a context of precarity dissimilar to that in Britain; American and Antipodean colonial enterprises might occur against a similar backdrop, but it seems fair to say that in these Canadian studies, colonialism is in the foreground. The conscious mapping out of spaces by settler societies – for planting, resource mining, city streets, institutions, and other purposes – did violence to Indigenous homelands and ways of living. The kind of order that the state and various agencies sought to bring to day-to-day settler life – through hospitals and solaria, medical practice, insurance, and infrastructure – was also colonialism. And the state itself, with its many agencies devoted to managing, reducing, preventing, forgiving, and ignoring risk and accidents, grew in the performance of these tasks.

An understanding of some of these elements allows us to probe the question of what constitutes an "accident" in Canadian history, as we consider the broad themes of equity, precaution, and storylines set against the backdrop of Canada's particular colonial past. Focusing on accidents allows us to consider changes in common understandings of state policy, medical practice, workplace organization, political authority, and the role of individuals and organizations in securing their own safety. It can be employed as a lens for understanding the harsh personal and community realities of Canadian socioeconomic life and the ways in which social capital and political structures have worked to contain or exacerbate catastrophe and the experience of accidents. Taken together, the chapters in this volume place the accident in wider historiographical and national contexts, including Canada's urban and rural development, the role of settlement and resource extraction, the importance of transportation, the changing nature of recreation, and the emergence of the health and welfare state. The authors make significant historiographical contributions to the analysis of gender, class, disability, settler-colonialism, and Indigenous history.

As these studies make clear, accidents are open to interpretation. Whether understood as an intervention by Providence, a miscalculation, inevitability in the face of bad odds, or the consequence of observable and empirically verifiable and mitigable risks, accidents in Canada are explained by Canadians in ways that reveal our collective values and perceived realities. And in the field of Canada history, as is demonstrated by our authors, the accident can drive analysis in a host of fields of inquiry: health history, labour history, legal history, the history of emotions, immigrant history, gender history, disability history, and the history of settler colonialism. This collection marks a beginning to this program of scholarly activity.

NOTES

1 Burnham, "Review: Accidents in History."
2 Armstrong with Granatstein, *Halifax Explosion*, 40–2.
3 McAlister, Marble, and Murray, "1917 Halifax Explosion," 374.
4 Jacob Remes chronicles and maps this far-flung affective and material impact of the Halifax Explosion in *Disaster Citizenship*, arguing that the economic and social impact was felt in Canada, northeast United States, Britain, and the West Indies.
5 Pyne, *Awful Splendour*, 423–44.
6 Campbell, *Lac-Mégantic Rail Disaster*.
7 Jamieson, *Tragedy at Second Narrows*, 176–92.
8 Connecting distant communities across dodgy infrastructure is a common theme in Canadian history. A recent account of the stagecoaches that plied the Cariboo Wagon Road in the 1860s, for example, devotes a whole chapter to "Holdups and Accidents." Mather, *Stagecoach North*, 211–32.
9 "Remembering the Chinese Railway Workers," Toronto Railway Museum, accessed 26 July 2021, https://torontorailwaymuseum.com/?p=1152.
10 Statistics Canada, "Number and Rates (Crude and Age-Standardized) of Motor Vehicle Accident Deaths, by Sex, Canada, 1979 to 2004," accessed 22 September 2022, https://www150.statcan.gc.ca/n1/pub/82-003-x/2008003/article/10648/t/5202443-eng.htm accessed 22 September 2022.
11 Brian Bethune, "Cars vs. people," *Maclean's*, 10 June 2014, https://www.macleans.ca/news/canada/the-cure-for-killer-cars/.
12 Echoes of Flight 810 reverberated a year later when an aircraft carrying Manchester United players crashed on takeoff in Munich. Twenty lives were lost, a much smaller total, but again made famous by the presence of celebrated athletes.
13 Robertson, *Imagining Difference*, 70.

14   Ibid.

15   Van Bavel et. al., *Disasters and History*, 1–15.

16   Ibid., passim.

17   Singer, *There Are No Accidents*, 1–2.

18   Cooter and Luckin, "Accidents in History: An Introduction," 2–3.

19   Green, "Accidents," 35–7. See also Green, "Some Problems in the Development of a Sociology of Accidents," 19–31; Green, *Risk and Misfortune*, 1–13.

20   Cooter and Luckin, "Accidents in History: An Introduction," 1–16.

21   Witmore, *Culture of Accidents*, 6.

22   Beck, *Risk Society*; Giddens, *Consequences of Modernity*.

23   Burnham, *Accident Prone*.

24   Spence, *Accidents and Violent Death in Early Modern London*, 237; Fyfe, *By Accident or Design*, 3.

25   Aldrich, *Death Rode the Rails*; Bronstein, *Caught in the Machinery*. For a legal and literary exploration of how Americans accepted individual responsibility – and hence accidents – as a necessary component of the industrial expansion that drove American development in that era, see Goodman, *Shifting the Blame*.

26   Love Canal was not in any manner of speaking an "accident," but the term was used at the time and after to deflect responsibility. See Goodman, *Shifting the Blame*, 159–70.

27   Oden, *Harvest of Hazards*, 183.

28   Mohun, *Risk: Negotiating Safety*, 212.

29   Bronstein, *Caught in the Machinery*, 169–75.

30   Moses, *First Modern Risk*, 3.

31   Myers, "Didactic Sudden Death," 451–75.

32   Thomas and Hrudey, *Risk of Death in Canada*.

33   Tucker, *Administering Danger in the Workplace*; Tucker, *Working Disasters*; Tucker, "Giving Voice to the Precariously Employed?"

34   See, for example, Storey, "'They Have All Been Faithful Workers'"; Storey, "Activism and the Making of Occupational Health and Safety Law in Ontario."

35   Gleason, "From 'Disgraceful Carelessness' to 'Intelligent Precaution.'"

36   Myers, "Didactic Sudden Death."

37   Belshaw and Purvey, *Private Grief, Public Mourning*.

38   Davies, "Mother's Medicine."

39   Forestell, "'And I Feel Like I'm Dying from Mining for Gold'"; see also Forestell, "Bachelors, Boarding Houses, and Blind Pigs"; Forestell, "The Miner's Wife."

40   Fahrni, "Glimpsing Working-Class Childhood through the Laurier Palace Fire of 1927"; Fahrni, "Accident Prevention in Early Twentieth-Century Québec"; Fahrni, "'La lutte contre l'accident.'"

41   Cournoyer, "Les accidents impliquant des enfants et l'attitude envers l'enfance à Montréal."

42   Dummitt, *Manly Modern Masculinity*, 125–50.

43 A noteworthy medical tragedy with important technological and financial consequences occurred in 1934 when the Bombardier family was snowed in and appen-
dicitis struck one of the children. When they were unable to get medical help, the
two-year-old died. These events spurred the child's father to develop a motorized
mode of winter transport. This was the origin of the snowmobile.

44 Atwood, *Survival*, 54.

45 The phenomenon of North American continental expansion is masterfully examined
in John Weaver's later chapters in *Great Land Rush*.

46 The literature on the numbered treaties is vast, but for a relevant analysis of the whol-
ly unaccidental impact on the First Nations of what is now Canada, see Daschuk,
Clearing the Plains.

47 Spence, *Accidents and Violent Death*, 1.

48 The literature on fire as disaster and energy in Canadian history is growing rapidly,
fuelled (pun intended) in part by fears of climate change and the reality of succes-
sive summers of wildfires. On wildfires, see, for example, Pyne, *Awful Splendour*;
Tymstra, *Chinchaga Firestorm*.

49 An important exception is Nancy Forestell's 2006 article, which provides groundbreaking insights into the physical and emotional work of women in tending to husbands injured and disabled at mining jobs. Forestell, "'And I Feel Like I'm Dying from
Mining for Gold.'"

BIBLIOGRAPHY

Periodicals

Among the Deep Sea Fishers
Maclean's

Other Works

Aldrich, Mark. *Death Rode the Rails: American Railroad Accidents and Safety,
1825–1965*. Baltimore: Johns Hopkins University Press, 2006.
Armstrong, John Griffith, with J.L. Granatstein. *The Halifax Explosion and the
Royal Canadian Navy*. Vancouver: University of British Columbia, 2002.
Atwood, Margaret. *Survival: A Thematic Guide to Canadian Literature*. Toronto:
Anansi, 1972.
Beck, Ulrich. *Risk Society: Towards A New Modernity*. London: Sage, 1992.
Belshaw, John, and Diane Purvey. *Private Grief, Public Mourning: The Rise of the
Roadside Shrine in British Columbia*. Vancouver: Anvil Press, 2010.

Bronstein, Jamie L. *Caught in the Machinery: Workplace Accidents and Injured Workers in Nineteenth-Century Britain*. Palo Alto, CA: Stanford University Press, 2008.

Burnham, John. *Accident Prone: A History of Technology, Psychology and Misfits of the Machine Age*. Chicago: University of Chicago Press, 2009.

– "Review: Accidents in History: Injuries, Fatalities and Social Relations by Roger Cooter and Bill Luckin." *Journal of Social History* 32, no. 2 (Winter 1998): 423–5.

Campbell, Bruce. *The Lac-Mégantic Rail Disaster: Public Betrayal, Justice Denied*. Toronto: James Lorimer, 2018.

Cooter, Roger, and Bill Luckin. *Accidents in History: Injuries, Fatalities and Social Relations*. Amsterdam: Rodopi Press, 1997.

Cournoyer, Catherine. "Les accidents impliquant des enfants et l'attitude envers l'enfance à Montréal, 1900–1945." Master's thesis, Université de Montréal, 1999.

Crook, Tom, and Mike Esbester, eds. *Governing Risks in Modern Britain: Danger, Safety and Accidents, c. 1800–2000*. London: Palgrave Macmillan, 2016.

Daschuk, James. *Clearing the Plains: Disease, Politics of Starvation, and the Loss of Indigenous Life*. Regina: University of Regina Press, 2013.

Davies Megan J. "Mother's Medicine: Women, Home and Health in BC's Peace River Region, 1920–1940." In *Medicine in the Remote and Rural North*, edited by J.T.H. Conner and S. Curtis, 199–214. London: Pickering and Chatto, 2011.

Dummitt, Christopher. *The Manly Modern Masculinity in Postwar Canada*. Vancouver: University of British Columbia Press, 2007.

Fahrni, Magda. "Accident Prevention in Early Twentieth-Century Québec and the Emergence of Masculine Technical Expertise." In *Making Men, Making History: Canadian Masculinities across Time and Place*, edited by Peter Gossage and Robert Rutherdale, 46–63. Vancouver: University of British Columbia Press, 2018.

– "Glimpsing Working-Class Childhood through the Laurier Palace Fire of 1927: The Ordinary, the Tragic, and the Historian's Gaze." *Journal of the History of Childhood and Youth* 8, no. 3 (Autumn 2015): 426–50.

– "'La lutte contre l'accident': Risque et accidents dans un contexte de modernité industrielle." In *Pour une histoire du risque: Québec, France, Belgique*, edited by David Niget and Martin Petitclerc, 171–91. Quebec: Presses de l'Université du Québec, 2012.

Forestall, Nancy. "'And I Feel Like I'm Dying from Mining for Gold': Disability, Gender, and the Mining Community, 1920–1950." *Labour: Studies in Working Class History of the Americas* 3, no. 3 (2006): 73–93.

– "Bachelors, Boarding Houses, and Blind Pigs: Gender Construction in a Multi-Ethnic Mining Camp, 1909–1920." In *A Nation of Immigrants: Women, Workers, and Communities in Canadian History, 1840s–1960s*, edited by Franca Iacovetta, Paula Draper, and Robert Ventresca, 251–90. Toronto: University of Toronto Press, 1998.

– "The Miner's Wife: Working-Class Femininity in a Masculine Context, 1920–1950." In *Gendered Pasts: Historical Essays in Femininity and Masculinity in Canada*, edited by Kathryn McPherson, Cecilia Morgan, and Nancy Forestell, 139–57. Toronto: University of Oxford Press, 1999.

Fyfe, Paul. *By Accident or Design: Writing the Victorian Metropolis*. Oxford: Oxford University Press, 2015.

Giddens, Anthony. *The Consequences of Modernity*. Stanford: Stanford University Press, 1990.

– "Risk and Responsibility." *Modern Law Review* 62, no. 1 (1999).

Gleason, Mona. "From 'Disgraceful Carelessness' to 'Intelligent Precaution': Accidents and the Public Child in English Canada, 1900–1950." *Journal of Family History* 30, no. 2 (April 2005): 230–41.

Goodman, Nan. *Shifting the Blame: Literature, Law and the Theory of Accidents in Nineteenth-Century America*. New York: Routledge, 1998.

Green, Judith. "Accidents: The Remnants of a Modern Classification System." In Cooter and Luckin, *Accidents in History*, 35–58.

– *Risk and Misfortune: The Social Construction of Accident*. London: UCL Press, 1997.

– "Some Problems in the Development of a Sociology of Accidents." In *Private Risks and Public Dangers*, edited by Sue Scott, 19–33. Abingdon, Oxford: Routledge, 2018.

Jamieson, Eric. *Tragedy at Second Narrows*. Madeira Park: Harbour Publishing, 2008.

Mather, Ken. *Stagecoach North: A History of Barnard's Express*. Victoria: Heritage House Publishing, 2020.

McAlister, Chryssa N., Allan E. Marble, and T. Jock Murray. "The 1917 Halifax Explosion: The First Coordinated Local Civilian Response to Medical Response in Canada." *Canadian Journal of Surgery* 60, no. 6 (December 2017): 374.

Mohun, Arwen. *Risk: Negotiating Safety in American Society*. Baltimore: Johns Hopkins University Press, 2013.

Moses, Julia. *The First Modern Risk: Workplace Accidents and the Origins of European Social States*. Cambridge: Cambridge University Press, 2018.

Myers, Tamara. "Didactic Sudden Death: Children, Police, and Teaching Citizenship in the Age of Automobility." *Journal of the History of Childhood and Youth* 8, no. 3 (Fall 2015): 451–75.

Oden, Derek S. *Harvest of Hazards: Family Farming, Accidents and Expertise in the Corn Belt, 1940–1975*. Iowa City: University of Iowa Press, 2017.

Pyne, Stephen J. *Awful Splendour: A Fire History of Canada*. Vancouver: University of British Columbia Press, 2007.

Remes, Jacob. *Disaster Citizenship: Survivors, Solidarity and Power in the Progressive Era*. Urbana: University of Illinois Press, 2016.

Robertson, Leslie. *Imagining Difference: Legend, Curse, and Spectacle in a Canadian Mining Town*. Vancouver: University of British Columbia Press, 2005.

Singer, Jesse. *There Are No Accidents: The Deadly Rise of Injury and Disaster – Who Profits and Who Pays the Price*. Toronto: Simon & Schuster, 2022.

Spence, Craig. *Accidents and Violent Death in Early Modern London, 1650–1750*. Woodbridge, UK: Boydell, 2016.

Storey, Robert. "Activism and the Making of Occupational Health and Safety Law in Ontario, 1960s –1980." *Policy and Practice in Occupational Health and Safety* 1 (2005): 41–68.

– "They Have All Been Faithful Workers: Injured Workers, Truth, and the Workers' Compensation System in Ontario, 1970–2008." *Journal of Canadian Studies* 43, no. 1 (2009): 154–85.

Thomas, Simon P., and Steve E. Hrudey. *Risk of Death in Canada: What We Know and How We Know It*. Edmonton: University of Alberta Press, 1997.

Tucker, Eric, ed. *Working Disasters: The Politics of Recognition and Response*. Amityville, NY: Baywood Publishing, 2006.

Tucker, Eric. *Administering Danger in the Workplace: The Law and Politics of Occupational Health and Safety Regulation in Ontario, 1850–1914*. Toronto: University of Toronto Press, 1992.

– "Giving Voice to the Precariously Employed? Mapping and Exploring Channels of Worker Voice in Occupational Health and Safety Regulation." Research Paper no. 14, Osgoode Hall Law School of York University Research Paper Series, 2013. https://digitalcommons.osgoode.yorku.ca/clpe/263/.

Tymstra, Cordy. *The Chinchaga Firestorm: When the Moon and Sun Turned Blue*. Edmonton: University of Alberta Press, 2015.

Van Bavel, Bas, Daniel R. Curtis, Jessica Dijkman, Matthew Hannaford, Maïka de Keyzer, Eline van Onacker, and Tim Soens, eds. *Disasters and History: The Vulnerability and Resilience of Past Societies*. Cambridge, UK: Cambridge University Press, 2020.

Weaver, John. *The Great Land Rush and the Making of the Modern World, 1650–1900*. Montreal and Kingston: McGill-Queen's University Press, 2006.

Witmore, Michael. *Culture of Accidents: Unexpected Knowledges in Early Modern England*. Stanford: Stanford University Press, 2002.

PART ONE | EQUITY

1

"Vahinko!"

Finnish Canadian Socialists Making Sense of Accidental Fire

Samira Saramo

"My last letter ended with fires and now in the same way, and perhaps like this for as long as there are wooden buildings," wrote M. North from Blairmore, Alberta, in *Toveritar* on 21 February 1922.[1] Readers' letters, like North's, published in the Finnish North American women's socialist newspaper, provide a view of how frequent accidental fires marked the lives of Finnish migrant-settlers in Canada in the early twentieth century.[2] While North reported rather matter-of-factly on local structural blazes, others wrote more evocatively of fire-caused destitution or injury, or the activation of community mutual aid structures. Such accounts demonstrate the contradictory nature of fire, both mundane in its prevalence but also shocking for its destructive power. By reading the Finnish Canadian experience through narrations of fire in community newspapers and histories, we gain new insights on how the pervasiveness and language of accidents shaped communities and worldviews.

This chapter analyzes the Finnish-language socialist press, community histories, and life-writing sources in order to better understand the sense-making, emotions, and everyday implications of accidental fire for Finnish Canadian migrants and their communities. After examining how different types of fires (homes, barns, halls, schools, industrial, etc.) were written about in the newspapers *Toveritar* and *Vapaus*, I focus in on a particularly significant and deadly fire in Finnish Canadian history, the Sointula community fire of 1903, to further analyze understandings of the "accidental" in the contexts of class and community. Through analysis of the newspapers, we learn that Finnish migrant socialists explained accidents through the lens of class; fire was yet another way that the working class was kept impoverished and oppressed. Fire was a concrete marker of the dangerous precarity in which workers lived. However, when fire devastated the Sointula community, at a distance from the capitalist world, its meaning was not – and perhaps could not be – expressed in the same way as in classed society. Accidental fire required people, adults and children alike, to work through ambivalent feelings on place and belonging, guided by their socialist worldviews but ultimately in personal ways.

Language provides a unique frame to reflect on how accidents were made sense of in the context of migrant experiences. For this chapter, I have primarily utilized Finnish-language sources produced by Finnish migrant-settlers. The Finnish word for "accident," *onnettomuus*, can be thought of as a state of being without luck/happiness; as such, it translates quite well to the English *misfortune*. More often in the sources analyzed, however, *vahinko* was used in reference to accidents, providing a more complicated and layered concept of the "accidental."[3] *Vahinko* refers to the accident itself, but also to damage and injury, whether the result of an "accident" or not. When something (even mildly) unfortunate occurs, *vahinko* can convey pity or disappointment. *Vahinko* marks error and harm. In the context of the Finnish migrant socialist press, as we will see, notions of the "accidental" as expressed in *vahinko* and *onnettomuus* were more typically rejected in favour of emphasizing the damage and injury inherently caused by the capitalist socioeconomic structure. Through close attention to the language of accidents and careful explicit translation, this chapter contributes new layers to our understanding of the histories of accidents, fire, and Canada.

Despite the pervasiveness of fires in the early twentieth century, social and cultural historians have yet had rather little to say on the topic. Fortunately, a foundation laid by key environmental histories sets us up for further exploring the history of fire. Stephen Pyne's *Awful Splendour:*

A Fire History of Canada stands as the most wide-ranging work on the subject, offering "the story of Canada as viewed by fire," from before the Little Ice Age to contemporary climate change.[4] Pyne compellingly demonstrates how settler colonialism and industrialization altered and accelerated long-standing fire cycles; though Pyne does not specifically refer to Finnish migrants in these processes, they are implicated in them. Alan MacEachern's *The Miramichi Fire: A History* provides an in-depth study of the devastating fire(s) of 1825 that centred on the Miramichi region of New Brunswick.[5] MacEachern's analysis of social memory – and more specifically, forgetting – contributes a useful way to think through the legacies of fire.

Pyne's and MacEachern's fire histories of Canada focus on conflagrations that ignited outside – forest fires/"wild" fires – and have rather little to say about what happens when fire originates and consumes from the indoors outward. Both works make clear that the ways fire is understood and approached changes over time or, as Pyne argues, "the prism for interpreting those flames evolve[s] with economies, sciences, and heavy technology."[6] Magda Fahrni, contributing rare social historical analysis of fire in Canada, rightly argues that the consequences of Montreal's 1927 Laurier Palace Fire were shaped by the age, class, and gender of those affected.[7] Together, these works make clear that fires have histories, shaped by environmental, social, and cultural factors. As the contributions of this collection demonstrate, notions of human agency, progress, and responsibility are at the core of making sense of accidents. Here I seek to further build our understanding of the history of fire in Canada through a humanist, social-historical inquiry that attends to the everyday as well as to the complicated tensions wrapped up in the "accidental."

Finnish Canadian migrant-settlers and their communities provide a useful micro-historical lens through which to analyze accidental structural fires and the ways in which their causes and consequences were made sense of, represented, and further understood through the perspective of class. My time period, roughly covering 1903 to 1929, marks an explosion in the number of Finns arriving in Canada, from 2,502 recorded in the 1901 census to 43,885 in 1931, with more settling in this country in the 1920s than in any period before or since.[8] Though this period is remarkable in the history of Finnish settlement in Canada, Finns, admittedly, were a small percentage of the total migrant mass settlement of the era. Despite their small overall numbers, however, Finns disproportionately shaped the development of Canadian socialist politics and have produced a substantial archival record of this period.[9] Their socialist worldview expanded beyond an interest in the living conditions of fellow Finns and centred on understanding and elevating the lives of all workers. While drawing on Finnish culture and language, these migrant-settler socialists drew heavily on the rhetoric and repertoire of broader socialist discourses and practices of the early twentieth century.[10] An examination of Finnish Canadian experiences with accidental fire, then, allows us to better comprehend the challenges, strategies, and networks operating among migrant communities more broadly in the early phases of settler colonial community building. In turn, migrant-settler perspectives enrich our view of the history of accidents in Canada.

NEWSPAPERS ON FIRE

The early "ethnic press" in Canada has been thought of as "a guide, an interpreter, a teacher, and an intimate friend."[11] As was the case for other migrant linguistic groups, the Finnish-language press helped newly arrived migrants navigate local and Canadian issues and happenings. However, equally importantly, and increasingly as time went on, the newspapers were tools to build the Finnish community and to preserve and develop the Finnish language of migrant-settlers and their children. Migrants established and maintained expansive transnational newspaper networks that connected Finns across Canada and the United States with each other and with Finland and beyond. For migrant socialists, Finnish-language newspapers further served to recruit and educate members and to solidify their commitment to the cause. The publications emotively portrayed the dangers and injustices facing migrant workers – Finns and others – in their uphill battle against capitalism and highlighted the promises of revolutionary life.[12] These functions of the North American Finnish-language socialist press are readily evident in *Toveritar* and *Vapaus*.

Toveritar ("Comradess" or "Woman Comrade") was published in Astoria, Oregon, from 1911 to 1930.[13] As the only Finnish-language newspaper in

North America written and edited by women specifically for women, it had broad readership across the United States and Canada. At its peak in the early 1920s, the paper had approximately twelve thousand subscribers.[14] Finnish migrant women and their families eagerly awaited its weekly arrival, scanning its pages for educational articles and editorials on crucial issues for socialist women, household and childrearing advice columns, poems, fiction, and sections specifically for children and youth.[15] *Toveritar* particularly encouraged correspondence from its readers, and the resulting pages of published letters from women, children, and youth provide unique perspectives on Finnish migrant (socialist) communities. Such reader contributions strengthened the newspaper's role as an "intimate friend" and further connected readers with each other's daily lives. Through the pages of reader letters and reports, Finnish migrant women, youth, and children forged networks of shared working-class hardships, small joys, and efforts to grow the movement. While I have paid particular attention to reports of fires by Canadian readers, gaining an understanding of all the ways and places that fire featured in *Toveritar* allows us to better appreciate the prevalence of accidental fires and the ways that the experiences and emotional responses of Finnish Canadians linked with the broader network of Finnish migrant "toveritars."

Vapaus (Liberty) was the largest and longest-running Finnish Canadian socialist newspaper. It was the organ of the Finnish (Socialist) Organization of Canada (FOC), published from 1917 to 1974 in Sudbury, Ontario (and appearing under different names from Toronto until 1990).[16] *Vapaus*'s ideological positioning moved along with that of the FOC, shifting from the Social Democratic Party of Canada to the One Big Union to the Communist Party of Canada by the mid-1920s.[17] The paper was particularly important for Canadian Finnish leftists in its early period, as major Finnish-language socialist papers from the United States, such as *Toveritar*, *Työmies*, and *Industrialisti*, could not get past the postal censor during World War I. In its first years, the paper was constantly embroiled in challenges from the Canadian chief press censor and was banned from October 1918 to April 1919.[18] By the 1920s, the pages of *Vapaus* had regained their radical boldness. In the face of direct competition from US Finnish newspapers again coming across the border, subscriptions did not exceed 3,500 until the 1930s.[19]

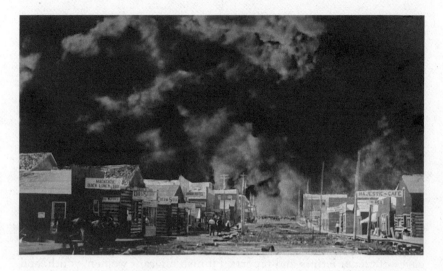

Fig. 1.1 *South Porcupine Burning.*

In its coverage of national and international daily news, substantial and deadly industrial and structural fires regularly appeared on the front page of *Vapaus* and in the section on news from Finland. Though it printed fewer reader letters and contributions than *Toveritar*, *Vapaus* featured short local reports from FOC members and branches across the country, offering additional views of accidental fires.

Together, *Toveritar* and *Vapaus* provide us with glimpses of a spectrum of community spaces on fire, including homes, farms, shops, Finnish halls (*haali*), local schools, industrial and worksite fires, vehicle fires, and the creeping, dangerous encroachment of forest fires. Reports were rarely limited to a single fire. Instead, the description of the latest fire would regularly be accompanied by a brief note about other recent local fires. For example, the article on a damaging and injurious fire at a Finnish widow's boarding house in Rosegrove, Ontario, informed readers that this was the fourth recent fire in the area and the home of another Finn had been lost about a month prior.[20] News stories and reader reports typically noted the speed with which fire "destroyed all of the working family's worldly possessions," as it had for the Byforss family in Silver Centre, Ontario, in 1928.[21] In the pages of the newspapers, fires consumed buildings "down to the foundations," destroying "beds, clothes, stoves, dishes and cookware, books, tools, etc."[22] In the worst cases, fire killed babies, sleeping families, the elderly, pets, and livestock.[23] It left survivors in the rubble, trying to figure out how to move forward from the devastation.

FIERY CLASS WAR

While causes and types may have varied, fires were nonetheless a decidedly classed issue for the Finnish migrant socialist press and its readers. Migrant-settler workers in Canada, as Finnish readers well knew, lived and worked in precarious and dangerous conditions that little resembled the narrative of progress espoused by the nation's leaders and capitalists. The editorial team of *Toveritar* utilized the familiar threat of fire for educational purposes. When urging readers to do their part to awaken fellow working women to the cause, *Toveritar* emphasized the hazards of working-class life and the "difficulties and dangers – for example of fire – that are always on offer" in substandard housing.[24] The threat of workplace fires was also ever present, framed particularly as the fault of greedy bosses and their disregard for worker lives. For example, in a short story, "The Knight of Labour on Vacation," a greedy factory owner realizes his fire-insurance policy is worth more than the factory and so decides to let it get into a state of disrepair.[25] When fire ultimately breaks out (the writer strongly hints at arson), destroying the factory and leaving "tens of workers injured and killed in the fire," the owner does not care. He simply "had a new factory built and everything was again as it should have been." Stories such as these had strong resonance for readers with first-hand knowledge of the dangers of working life.[26]

On 10 February 1928, a fire 550 feet below ground level at Hollinger Gold Mine in Timmins, Ontario, resulted in the deaths of thirty-nine workers, eight of them Finnish. From its first reports of the fire breaking out, *Vapaus* did not accept that an accident had occurred.[27] Instead, it presented the fire as a preventable yet inherent consequence of labour under capitalism: the company's failure to establish a safety plan or invest in safety equipment, coupled with the mine inspector's willingness to look the other way, had caused the fire and the deaths.[28] The socialist press's position, as John Sandlos argues in this collection, stood in stark contrast to the justice system's regular conclusion that workplace accidents were an unfortunate by-product of industrial labour and no one's fault, or to employers' tendency to place the blame and responsibility on workers, as I have demonstrated elsewhere.[29] Over the days and weeks of coverage of the tragedy, the paper emphasized that "harsh blame" should be aimed "against the mining company, which with its carelessness murders workers with extreme rapacious lust."[30] The deadly fire was announced to readers through the headline "Shocking Industrial Murder at Hollinger Gold Mine."[31] The newspaper consistently framed the deaths as "mass murder," and Hollinger mine became a "murder cave."[32]

The youth section of *Toveritar* relied on similar histrionic language and did not spare its young readers an education regarding the cruelty of the capitalist world. In the fictionalized "A picture of Class War," published in April 1919, the eighteen-year-old protagonist Sadie pauses to remember the 1911 Triangle Shirtwaist Factory fire. Her older sister and cousin were among the "147 working-class girls who burned locked inside the factory or were crushed to death on the street escaping the fire."[33] In the aftermath of the "slaughter," Sadie's sister Rachel was an unrecognizable "burnt crumb" and all that remained of cousin Emily, who had tried to escape by jumping out of a window, was "a shapeless pile of broken bones and mashed meat." The moral of the story was clear: the memory of the fire "martyrs' bodies" must push young readers to "our final victory in the class war." *Vahinko*, as presented by the editorial staff of *Toveritar* and *Vapaus*, emphasized damage and injury while adamantly arguing that the costs of capitalism endured by the working class were no accident.

COMMUNAL CARETAKING

While far less graphic in their depictions, readers' contributions also made direct links between fires and the oppression of the working class. After detailing a fire that for days had been ravaging her hometown of Weed, California, Helmi Laine concluded, "That's life for the worker. Just when they are encountering a brighter future, then it is suddenly torn away."[34] Similarly, Olga Ikäheimo observed of a local Finnish family whose farm burned, "It's no wonder they're depressed. When you get over one accident/damage/injury [*vahinko*], the next is in front of you."³⁵ After losing his house and belongings to fire in Kaministiquia, Ontario, in 1925, Aku Päiviö declared, "It feels a little gloomy to go on with life – destroyed, penniless, and, most damningly, lacking credit."³⁶

Caretaking systems were quickly activated when fire struck the home of a community member. When John Henrickson and his family lost their home and belongings to fire in the early morning of 30 March 1918, in Rossland, BC, the local Finnish community responded the next day by collecting donations amounting to $27.50 – "Even that is help in an emergency."³⁷ It was also common to organize *iltamat* (evening programs), featuring speeches, poetry, theatrical performances, and music, on behalf of a family who had been struck by fire.³⁸ In her July 1917 letter to the children's section of *Toveritar*, Sylvia Matson noted that she had recently attended a "field party" in Cromwell, Minnesota, likely with sporting events, musical performances, and a dance, organized for the benefit of the Väin Koski family after their home was destroyed by fire.³⁹

Rarer in newspapers were direct appeals for assistance from a victim, as was the case when Aku Päiviö's family of eight lost their home and belongings to fire. Päiviö, as a leading FOC member and well-regarded socialist poet, was given front-page space in *Vapaus* to share the story of his misfortune. "It seems I must, for the sake of these innocent fledgling persons [i.e., children]," Päiviö wrote, "resort to asking for help from the nearest branches [of the FOC] through a collection, of course, as bitter as being in need of assistance is. In case some comrade would like to encourage a labour poet experienced in hardship, we mention that comrade A. Päiviö's address is ..."⁴⁰

While membership in early-twentieth-century Finnish Canadian organizations typically included enrolment in a modest death and sickness fund, newspaper accounts suggest that many Finns had either inadequate or no insurance policies for their homes or belongings⁴¹ – despite the booming growth of the insurance industry at the time.⁴² Writing to *Toveritar*, someone with the pen name "R-a" explained that the fire at M. Talso's house in Cobalt, Ontario, "was a considerable accident/damage when the possessions weren't insured."⁴³ After a rented dwelling housing nearly twenty workers burned in Rosegrove, Ontario, the men were left with nothing but their underclothes "and some even without footwear."[44] The men had no insurance for their belongings, nor did the Finnish owner have insurance for the building. Newspaper coverage assumed homes were "likely insured for an insignificant amount, which makes the loss even heavier."[45] Even with more adequate insurance, families faced hardship. When the Henricksons' home burned in Rossland, BC, *Toveritar* contributor Mary understood that "even though the house was insured, it still results in damage for a worker with a large family."[46]

CHILDREN MAKING SENSE OF FIRE

Fire also strongly affected the lives of children. Many Finnish migrant children and youth were victims of fire, but they also witnessed or heard about them on the local level, and read about the experiences of fellow little comrades in the children's section of *Toveritar*. When the Great Fire of 1918 struck northern Minnesota, women and children shared their experiences in *Toveritar* in chilling detail. Young Mary Libeck described her home, belongings, and livestock burning, and her family's heroic four-mile escape through flame-enveloped bush roads.[47] Three years later, Aune Hendrickson, by then aged twelve, remembered being surrounded by deadly fire for days. "It was not fun to look death in the eyes," she told her young readers.[48]

Children's-section contributors fostered comradeship by linking personal experiences to shared frames of reference, such as attending socialist Sunday school and participating in Finnish (socialist) drama or athletics clubs at their local *haali* (figure 1.2). As such, readers would have been horrified to learn in 1917 that the Finnish socialist hall in Sand Coulee, Montana, had caught fire in the midst of Christmas Eve celebrations, preventing Joulupukki (Santa Claus) from coming. To their relief, they were told that "the Christmas gifts were saved."[49] The letter writer, William Hill, regretted that he and his friends were unable to perform their long-rehearsed Christmas play *Santa Claus on Strike* because of the fire. Hill's description of the celebrations and the hall could easily have been of another Finnish migrant community, and comrades-in-training reading his words surely imagined their own beloved *haali* consumed by flames.

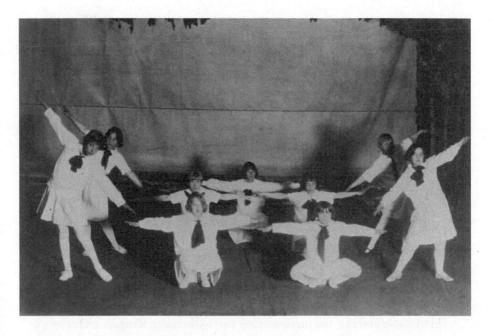

Fig. 1.2 Nahjus Athletic Club girls practice at the Finnish Labour Temple, Port Arthur, ON, 1920s.

Children's reporting on fire demonstrates the influence of adult concerns but also reveals how they interpreted fire through their developing worldviews. In the 19 February 1918 issue of *Toveritar*, young Sulo Johnson from Emo, Ontario, shared his recent tragedy: "When I last wrote to *Toveritar* I could not have guessed what harsh misfortune was coming. On December 8th our homestead burned all the way to its foundation. I was with my sister and brother at school and upon returning in the evening, our home was ash. It was a hard hit because everything was uninsured … My father made our home last autumn and we didn't get to live there for more than a few months before the accident/damage."[50] Finnish children learned about insurance and the costs of fire damage at a young age, from adult conversations, their engagement in children's socialist activities, and direct experience, but they also felt the loss of their personal belongings and the associated loss of self and place in a youth-centred fashion. Sulo grieved his home library: "I also incurred a lot of damage. I had a really good start of a library, with all kinds of Finnish and English [books], many years of

Lasten Kevät and *Lasten Joulu* [annually published children's May Day and Christmas specials by *Toveritar*]. Just last autumn I ordered from *Appeal to Reason* a three-dollar set. The library was worth close to twenty dollars, to say nothing of the other things." To readers of *Toveritar*, younger and older, the library would have marked Sulo as a good socialist youth, having invested his (and likely his family's) hard-to-come-by dollars in proper socialist educational literature.[51] His account of destruction of the library, in turn, evoked empathy and solidarity.

EVERYDAY RISKS

The steady presence of fire in newspaper pages drove home the significant risk for readers. Mrs Puurunen's house and belongings burned, the family's pet dog died, and her son suffered serious burns to his face and body from lighting the morning stove fire with gas.[52] The death of seventy-two-year-old Mrs Bey and the destruction of her cottage home in Kingston, Ontario, was the result of a spark from the wood stove setting the wallpaper on fire.[53] Drinking and horseplay presumably led to a hayloft fire in Iroquois Falls, Ontario.[54] Mary Ranta from Sicamous, BC, wrote about warding off fire from her house as her neighbour's home burned. She warned readers, "You must be careful with fire here, especially those with just a tin stovepipe."[55] Such repeated and familiar causes of fire written about in *Vapaus* and *Toveritar* resonated for Finnish Canadian readers living in similar conditions and served as important warnings to be wary of their behaviour with fire at home and elsewhere.

Despite the risk, fire was an essential part of Canadian daily life in the early twentieth century. It went hand-in-hand with the taking of land and the re/making of place in the project of "migrant settlerhood."[56] Land was quickly cleared through burning. In settlers' wooden homes, wood was by far the most prevalent fuel for heating and cooking well into the twentieth century.[57] Like everyone, Finnish migrant-settlers – women in particular – had to continuously assess potential danger and take calculated risks.[58] Those who had previously experienced a fire firsthand often feared the possibility of another.[59] Yet, as Olga Ikäheimo poignantly observed, "You have to light wood to burn, even when your heart is full of fear."[60]

The pages of *Vapaus* and *Toveritar* provide important windows onto accidental fire, as experienced and understood by Finnish migrant socialists in Canada. Through a careful reading of the language of *vahinko* and *onnettomuus*, we can consider the ways that notions of the accidental were wrapped up in Finnish migrants' socialist worldviews and daily realities. By bringing these insights to an examination of the Sointula community fire of 1903, we can gain further understanding of how Finnish Canadians practically and psychologically navigated the risks and consequences of fire. The case of the Sointula fire provides concrete insights on what a community was left with, materially, emotionally, and collectively, in the ashes of a devastating accidental fire.

SOINTULA, 1903

In 1901, under the leadership of Matti Kurikka and his particular brand of socialist theosophical ethnonationalism, a small group of Finns from the Nanaimo area and elsewhere in Canada and the United States set out to build a utopian cooperative community. Sointula was established on traditional Kwakwaka'wakw territory on Malcolm Island, off the north end of Vancouver Island. Fuelled by a desire to be freed from "wage slavery" and the drudgery of the mines, but lacking the necessary money, tools, or skills to build a new society out of the wilderness, the idealistic Kalevan Kansa project was quickly mired in debt, shortages, and significant challenges. Sointula's early settler history as a failed utopia has led to numerous studies of its leadership, politics, and economics.[61] Yet, a fire in January 1903 that killed eleven, injured sixteen, and destroyed the communal residence, settlers' supplies, and company records has resulted in little more than passing mention.[62] Here, I centre the fire in putting together a view of what happened, how it has been represented, and how it linked to broader life events and attitudes towards accidental fire, as seen in Finnish migrant-settler socialist newspapers.

After securing a land-grant agreement with the government of British Columbia, the first task for the Kalevan Kansa Colonization Company settlers was to quickly clear the forested land with axes and fire and to hew wood for building and heating. While meals were taken at the communal dining hall, many slept in crude tents. Lack of money along with other practical obstacles slowed progress, but by the fall of 1902, with approximately two hundred people living in Sointula and more coming, including many women and children,[63] the construction of a communal residential building had become urgent. In November, the community built a three-storey structure that housed the company office, twenty-eight family sleeping rooms on the first two floors, and a large meeting room that doubled as a tailor's shop on the third floor. The facility was hastily constructed of freshly cut green boards that left gaps in the floors and walls as they dried. Sound passed easily though the building, earning it the name Melula (Noisy Place).[64] Heat from a large wood-fired oven at the end of the first floor hallway was distributed throughout the building by a system of wooden and metal ducts.[65]

On the evening of Thursday, 29 January 1903, most of the adults of the community were gathered in the third-floor meeting room, engaged in a tense discussion about the dire state of colony finances. Children had been tucked into bed in the residential rooms below. "And then suddenly," according to early Sointula resident Aili Anderson, "someone screamed 'fire.'"[66] The narrow staircase to the third floor was filled with smoke, and flames were already beginning to come up through the thin, gapped floors and walls. Some forced their way down the stairs and others jumped out of the windows. Parents rushed to save their children. Many babies and children were tossed out of windows in desperation to the hopeful safety of the arms of those already outside. Within minutes, "the interior of *Melula* was red with flame and filled with a heat so intense that it blistered the skin from a distance of four and a half metres."[67] Out of the 137 people who had been in the building when the fire ignited,[68] eleven died and sixteen were injured. Eight of the dead were children between four months and eight years of age, along with two women and a man.

RESPECTABLE VICTIMS

There is no known Finnish North American newspaper coverage of the fire. Unfortunately, the Kalevan Kansa's own *Aika*, the first Finnish-language paper in Canada, was on hiatus at the time of the accident. The fire was, however, extensively reported on in the province's newspapers and picked up by the Associated Press.[69] The news quickly travelled as far as the *Hawaiian Gazette*.[70] On 2 February 1903, the *Vancouver Daily Province* devoted its entire front page to the fire, with startling headlines such as "Scenes at the Hell of Flame" and subheads including "Children were dropped into outspread arms below, while men hurled themselves from death amid the flames – heartrending scenes enacted."[71]

The press conveyed sympathy for the Sointula community, framing the accident as bad luck. The *Delta News* observed, "The demon of hard luck seems to pursue the Finnish colony."[72] The *Daily News* from Nelson, BC, in turn reported, "Relentless fate seems to pursue the Finnish colony of political refugees that is trying to establish a foothold in British Columbia, on Malcolm Island ... On Thursday night last the worst in a long series of calamities befell them."[73] The press's early support of the Kalevan Kansa's efforts to get a land grant had been instrumental in speeding up and ultimately securing the contract with the government, and newspapers had regularly reported on the happenings and financial disasters of the colony.[74] Readers, then, may have been able to place the fire within the context of Sointula's previous tumults.

The Finns were presented positively and their actions during the fire were depicted as respectable. The *Vancouver Daily Province* proclaimed they had "accepted the disaster with rare stoicism."[75] Nelson's *Daily News* claimed (with embellishment) that mothers were found burned to death curled around their living children, announcing to readers "Brave Women's Lives Sacrificed to Save Loved Ones."[76] "Injured men worked heroically" to rescue others from the flames.[77] The survivors' respectability was further extended through the English-language press's gendered portrayals. Women and children were appropriately domesticated and passive, being "left with nothing but their night garments," while the men's position as breadwinners was contrasted with statements noting that "many of the men lost all their working clothes" – notwithstanding that such stark gender roles were contrary to the ideals of the utopian community.[78]

"PITIABLE IN THE EXTREME"

As respectable victims of misfortune, the Finnish community of Sointula was also worthy of charity. Survivors of the fire were now homeless; they had lost personal belongings as well as "thirteen tons" of colony supplies.[79] The *Nelson Daily News* summed up: "The condition of some 30 women and 80 children, facing especially rigorous weather, virtually unclothed and lacking either medicines or physicians' skill, is pitiable in the extreme."[80] In its breaking front-page coverage on 2 February, the *Vancouver Daily Province* juxtaposed the victims' "despair of utter hopelessness" with calls to "Assist the Sufferers," "Clothing needed for women and children," and reports of "First Assistance To-night."[81] Aid campaigns were quickly started, and five days after the fire a steamer docked at Malcolm Island with donated food, clothing, and other supplies, including "brandy and lint bandages for the injured as well as two nurses."[82] The scarcity of available sources makes it impossible to know whether Finnish communities on Vancouver Island or elsewhere in Canada and the United States activated their own caretaking structures to aid the fire victims, though given the prevalence of such practices at this time, it was likely.

The Sointula community was praised for the gracious "surprise, overmastered by heartfelt gratefulness," expressed for the donations, as the "colonists were not expecting any aid in their distress."[83] The *Province* reported "a number of women, who when informed of the measures of relief sent to them, could not contain their feelings, but indulged in a good cry right there, after which they thanked the officers of the *Cassiar* and with the men of the colony forwarded their thanks and gratitude to the people of Vancouver."[84] Such depictions reinforced the view of the Finns at Sointula as "deserving poor," but they also provide a glimpse of the community's emotions in the immediate aftermath of the fire.

While the *Province* concluded that, with the arrival of the first shipment of aid, "the people have taken heart again," a 24 February 1903 letter from Provincial Constable Walter Wollacott to the attorney general of British Columbia indicates that the need of the community continued to be great.[85] Wollacott acknowledged that the provincial government's contribution of bedding and clothing along with the public donations had "place[d] the sufferers in a fairly comfortable condition." Nonetheless, he noted how much the community lost and how it was "not in very good condition; in fact, before the fire they were 'hard-up.'" While his letter's tone suggests that the burden of dealing with the fire's damage should rest with Kurikka and the Kalevan Kansa, Wollacott did recommend the government supply the colony with fifteen new sewing machines to replace those lost. The Sointula community's own views on the state of their hardship and the aid received is unknown.

LOOKING FOR A COMMUNITY IN MOURNING

The Finnish settlers of Sointula had no choice but to immediately set out to build new homes and to see to the basic needs of its devastated members amidst the shock of grief for their small, tight-knit community. They had just lost a significant proportion of beloved members – children no less – and witnessed a symbol and the tools of their shared dream go up in flames. As families searched for loved ones in the chaos of the fire and realized their loss, some mothers reportedly "piteously cried: 'Baby, Baby,' and covered their faces in an awful grief too deep for words."[86] Yet, in stark contrast to the rich archival record of Finnish North American death and mourning practices otherwise accessible for this period, the available sources leave little trace of the Sointula community engaged in the work of grief and mourning.[87] Remarkably, I have yet to find any mention of funerals or burials of fire victims.[88]

A.B. Mäkelä, the colony's other leading man, was burned so badly it was thought he would never see again. Yet the Melula fire was reduced to a brief footnote in his memoir *Muistoja "Malkosaarelta"*: "In Sointula's first communal building's fire, 11 burned in the flame and many, ex. me, were seriously injured." He adds a joke about how others had to hold his pipe for him as he recovered.[89] Matti Halminen's 1936 memoir *Sointula – Kalevan Kansan ja Kanadan suomalaisten historiaa* is the closest we are able to get to the feelings and actions of those who survived the fire. Halminen had been away from Sointula on the night of the fire. Returning in the morning from the other side of the island, the smoke immediately alerted him to tragedy. He recalled: "Eleven! I will not try to describe the affects of that blow, but will only say that I lost the vigour in my legs, staggered, and collapsed

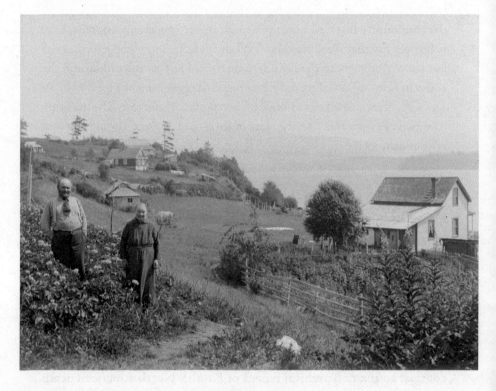

Fig. 1.3 Matti Halminen outside his Sointula home on Malcolm Island, BC, 1927.

onto a chair. To think that eleven people, who are to me like brothers and sisters burned at the same time! I heard the names of the burned, and after a moment, I was dying to go the fire site. There, those corpses, some wreckage, crawling on the fire site, and in cabins and tents cried those who had burns and were otherwise injured, among them my own daughter."[90] When police, a priest, and a justice of the peace arrived from nearby Alert Bay, an inquiry was quickly held, recording the casualties and pronouncing the cause of the fire as accidental. Halminen wrote, "I had to be part of it too, even though my heart was totally sick with grief."[91] Allowing the fact of the tragedy to speak for itself, he asked, "Does it even need to be described the feelings/atmosphere in which the aftermath of that shocking incident was lived?"[92] Nonetheless, again without detailing the community's period of grief or his own feelings, Halminen let the reader know that "those weeks and months I would not at any cost relive, if I have permission here to speak of my own feelings/moods."[93]

Not uncommonly for those working through traumatic experience, Matti Halminen tried in retrospect to find a premonition of the fire.[94] Writing about Melula's construction, he begins, "In my memory from these moments has stayed one event, which seems negligible, but I will tell it."[95] He shares a memory of finding Mäkelä and Kurikka investigating a warm-air pipe coming out of a fire pit. When Halminen realized the men were testing a potential heating system for the new residence, he "notified Kurikka of such heating systems' potential dangers. Kurikka turned away immediately and walked away, apparently insulted by my warning."[96] Halminen then wonders, trying to make sense of the past, "Did that test lead to the installation of the heating ducts, which afterwards became so fatal/momentous to that unhappy building and its residents? Let's say so."[97]

ACCIDENTS AND BLAME

The coroner's inquest immediately deemed the fire accidental, though the cause was not noted.[98] Early media reports stated that the fire had been caused by an overturned lamp in a bedroom, but the blame then shifted to the heating system.[99] The wood stove was burning on one end of the building and the outside door was open on the other, creating a strong draught.[100] "Without doubt," Aili Anderson claimed, "the fire was started by the heating pipes that led through the walls from the oven."[101] Halminen likewise concluded that the ductwork "caused the fire – it, and nothing else."[102] However, when faced with tragedy and destitution, simple explanations of the accidental were hard to accept.

As Halminen explained: "In the ensuing turmoil, having lost their ability to judge with discretion and driven to desperation, people's minds began to be haunted, [wondering] if there was something to the cause of the fire, even outright arson."[103] Rumours circulated that Matti Kurikka and the company treasurer, August Oberg, had intentionally set the fire to destroy the financial records. In return, Kurikka published (and presented at a community meeting) a fierce diatribe against the rumours and his opponents. In his long, fiery lecture, he reminded members that they had moved to Sointula "to find friends and to build friendships" and that "enemies do not always have horns on their heads, hooves on their feet, claws on their paws, or sharp fangs in their jaws."[104] Kurikka marked the fire as a turning point in the community's relations: "Then came the fire and all the hellish forces were unleashed because of distress and need. Those who hoped for benefits from the company and had until then patiently controlled their interiors no longer saw it necessary to conceal their wickedness, and now we see the backside of the Finnish national character in all its ugliness."[105] Kurikka's tirade appeared in the 1 December 1903 issue of *Aika*, the first issue published following the fire. In the entire issue, this was the only mention of the fire. Though several months had passed, it is striking that there were no mentions of the deceased or the injured, no empathy expressed for all that had been lost.

The devastating fire challenged Finnish migrant socialist understandings of *vahinko*. Precarity, it seemed, had followed the Sointula residents from their days of "wage slavery." Occurring in the budding utopia, outside of capitalist society, blame could not as easily be placed on an exploitative structure. In the accusations of arson, though, we find fears that cruel, selfish capitalist desires might have infiltrated the community. Such suspicions were difficult to integrate into personal and collective understandings of Sointula and made comprehending the loss even more troubling. Instead, the deaths of community members and destruction of communal housing had to be made sense of through the logic of building flaws or simply by submitting to uncontrollable fate. Perhaps this difficulty in comprehending the accident resulted in the misfortune/*onnettomuus* becoming largely unspeakable and unwritable. As such, the fire has found little space in the cultural memory of Sointula. Between constant financial problems and the irreconcilable rift that emerged in the fire's aftermath, the utopian community envisioned by Kurikka, Mäkelä, and other Kalevan Kansa founders never came to fruition. As the original colonization company and its dream faded, so too did the official memory of the fire and its subsequent role in studies of Sointula's history.

CONCLUSION

Accidental fire was a regular and even expected feature of early twentieth-century life in Canada, as it had been for previous generations. The ordinariness of fire perhaps explains why historians rarely delve directly into its forms, meanings, and consequences. Yet by examining cases of fire, we gain valuable historical understanding of culture, society, and daily life. In twentieth-century Canada, wood and fire were essential components in building settler lives, and the navigation of risk was constant. Despite familiarity, however, when fire did strike, it marked significant and terrible moments in people's lives. As I have shown, fire could serve as a class, ethnic, and settler unifier, as in the case of the Finnish socialist press's reader letters and grassroots mutual-aid efforts, but it was also a divider when it challenged the logic of progress, as in the case of the Sointula fire. In the aftermath of fire, networks of family and community were activated to ease suffering and to redraw the porous boundaries of belonging. Fire was likewise followed by the serious work of trying to make sense of why it had happened and, as the other contributions of this collection also make clear, figuring out who or what could be held accountable. Such work often required a consideration of potential supernatural, environmental, and human factors.[106] By examining these available responses, we begin to historicize fire.

This process of making sense also called into question understandings of the "accidental." For Finnish migrants exploring the potentials of socialist or utopian life, accidental fire was interpreted through the lens of class. In the pages of *Toveritar* and *Vapaus*, fire not only marked a *vahinko* – accident/injury/damage – but was especially a "considerable *vahinko* for the worker."[107] In this worldview, the accidental was understood as a result of the capitalist order, which always and inherently resulted in the further subjugation of the working class. Yet in the case of the Sointula fire, the accident had to be reconciled with the utopian world the community was working to build. At the time of the fire, however, the Kalevan Kansa had not achieved its goal of existing outside of the oppressive confines of capitalist society and was entangled in insurmountable financial troubles. In this light, perhaps the deadly fire at the fledgling utopia can also be understood as a "*vahinko* for the worker," still striving for something greater.

This case study of Finnish migrant-settler socialists shows the intimate ways that fire affected daily lives and shaped worldviews. Accidental fires and the language of the accident provide exciting and promising openings to explore the workings of community and people's negotiations of place and belonging. As I have demonstrated, both the lens of the accidental and the social history of fire can lead us to constructive new ways of approaching and understanding Canada's settler history.

ACKNOWLEDGMENTS

I thank Megan Davies and Geoffrey Hudson for including me in this great project, as well as the rest of the contributors to this book and the anonymous reviewers for inspiring new ideas. I acknowledge the generous support of the Kone Foundation that has allowed me to carry out this work.

NOTES

1 *Toveritar*, 21 February 1922. All translations by the author.
2 I am invested in situating the history of Finnish migrants within the history and ongoing legacies of Canadian settler colonialism and am working through which terminology best suits this work. The term "migrant" usefully captures the mobility, transnationalism, and unsettledness of the early decades of Finnish migration and settlement, while "settler" recognizes the differing processes of settlement underway. In this article, I use the terms "migrant," "settler," and "migrant-settler."
3 See also the dictionary of the Institute for the Languages of Finland, available online, https://www.kielitoimistonsanakirja.fi/#/vahinko; also *Suomen etymologinen sanakirja* (Finnish Etymological Dictionary), https://kaino.kotus.fi/suomenetymologinensanakirja/?p=article&etym_id=ETYM_7b212ebfb328de1ef1bbbdf3b7dd3e11&word=vahinko.
4 Pyne, *Awful Splendour*, xxv.
5 MacEacheran, *Miramichi Fire*.
6 Pyne, *Awful Splendour*, 418.
7 Fahrni, "Glimpsing Working-Class Childhood."
8 Saarinen, "Perspectives on Finnish Canadian Settlement," 22.
9 For the role of Finns in the Canadian socialist and labour movements, see Beaulieu, Harpelle, and Penny, *Labouring Finns*; Beaulieu, Ratz, and Harpelle, *Hard Work Conquers All*.
10 Huhta, "Toward a Red Melting Pot," 32.

11 Pilli, *Finnish-Language Press in Canada*, 9.
12 On the Finnish migrant socialist press, see Huhta, "Toward a Red Melting Pot";
    Saramo, "Capitalism as Death."
13 I have analyzed issues of *Toveritar* from January 1916 to December 1922, available
    through the Library of Congress's Chronicling America portal, https://chroniclin-
    gamerica.loc.gov/lccn/2011260133/.
14 Kaunonen, *Challenge Accepted*, 40; Pilli, *Finnish-Language Press in Canada*, 24n52.
15 As an example of the significance of *Toveritar*, see Lindström, "The Radicalization of
    Finnish Farm Women," 74–6.
16 I have analyzed the January 1921 to December 1929 issues of *Vapaus*, available through
    Simon Fraser University's Digitized Newspaper collection at https://newspapers.lib.
    sfu.ca/Vapaus2500-1/Vapaus.
17 For the organization's history, see Eklund, *Builders of Canada*.
18 Pilli, *Finnish-Language Press in Canada*, 127.
19 Ibid., 195–6.
20 *Vapaus*, 2 May 1929.
21 *Vapaus*, 17 November 1928.
22 For example, *Vapaus*, 9 January 1929 and 5 May 1925.
23 *Vapaus*, 5 May 1925, and, for example, 4 August 1924, 11 September 1923, 5 May 1925;
    Toveritar, 18 January 1921 and 29 November 1918.
24 *Toveritar*, 11 February 1919.
25 *Toveritar*, 19 September 1922.
26 On the dangers of working-class life in this period, see Holdren, *Injury Impoverished*;
    Saramo, "Capitalism as Death"; Rosenow, *Death and Dying in the Working Class*.
27 For more on the Hollinger tragedy in the context of the Finnish North American left,
    see Saramo, "Capitalism as Death," 677–82.
28 The royal commission ultimately agreed with what *Vapaus* had immediately asserted,
    finding "gross negligence" on the part of Hollinger Mine.
29 See Saramo, "Capitalism as Death," 671.
30 *Vapaus*, 16 February 1928.
31 *Vapaus*, 13 February 1928.
32 For example, *Vapaus*, 14 and 20 February 1928.
33 *Toveritar*, 22 April 1919.
34 *Toveritar*, 18 October 1917.
35 *Toveritar*, 14 November 1916.
36 *Vapaus*, 5 May 1925.
37 *Toveritar*, 9 April 1918.
38 For example, *Toveritar*, 28 March 1922.
39 *Toveritar*, 17 July 1917.
40 Note the interesting shift away from "I." *Vapaus*, 5 May 1925.
41 Saramo, "Making Transnational Death Familiar," 12.

42 On the growth of the insurance industry in Canada in this period, see Baskerville, "The Worth of Children and Women; Swiss Re Group, "History of Insurance in Canada" (2017). Available online at https://www.swissre.com/dam/jcr:64b0fdca-f4d8-401c-a5bd-9c51614843c0/150Y_Markt_Broschuere_Canada_web.pdf.

43 *Toveritar*, 26 August 1919.

44 *Vapaus*, 9 January 1929.

45 *Vapaus*, 17 November 1928.

46 *Toveritar*, 9 April 1918.

47 *Toveritar*, 29 November 1918

48 *Toveritar*, 25 October 1921.

49 *Toveritar*, 30 January 1917.

50 *Toveritar*, 19 February 1918.

51 Wilson, "'Little Comrades.'"

52 *Vapaus*, 2 May 1929.

53 *Vapaus*, 18 June 1925.

54 *Vapaus*, 15 September 1925.

55 *Toveritar*, 28 August 1917. For dangers of stovepipe sparks, see Sandwell, "Fear and Anxiety on the Energy Frontier," 39.

56 My thinking on "migrant settlerhood" is influenced by Madokoro, "On Future Directions."

57 MacFayden, "Hewers of Wood."

58 For women's home-safety responsibilities, see Tarr and Tebeau, "Housewives as Home Safety Managers," 196–233; Sandwell, "Pedagogies of the Unimpressed."

59 For example, Mavis Hiltunen Biesanz wrote about her mother's relentless worry and fear about fire, having experienced a house fire earlier in life. In Biesanz, *Helmi Mavis*, 84, 133.

60 *Toveritar*, 14 November 1916.

61 Key academic works on Sointula include Kolehmainen, "Harmony Island"; Wilson, "Matti Kurikka and the Utopian Socialist Settlement"; Lindström, "Utopia for Women?"; Saikku, "Utopians and Utilitarians."

62 The notable exception is Wild's general-audience book *Sointula*, which devotes ten pages to the fire and its aftermath.

63 Wild, *Sointula*, 62. It is hard to know the exact number, as people were continuously arriving and leaving and, additionally, some members of the Kalevan Kansa Colonization Company did not live on the island. The Kalevan Kansa's census lists were lost in the fire.

64 Wild, *Sointula*, 62.

65 Halminen, *Sointula*, 89; Anderson, *History of Sointula*, 8.

66 Anderson, *History of Sointula*, 8.

67 Wild, *Sointula*, 69.

68 *Vancouver Daily Province*, 2 February 1903.

69 I searched newspapers available through the University of British Columbia's BC Historical Newspapers open collection, at https://open.library.ubc.ca/collections/bcnewspapers.

70 *Hawaiian Gazette*, 3 February 1903.

71 *Vancouver Daily Province*, 2 February 1903.

72 *Delta News*, 7 February 1903.

73 *Nelson Daily News*, 3 February 1903.

74 Halminen, *Sointula*, 35–8.

75 *Vancouver Daily Province*, 2 February 1903.

76 *Nelson Daily News*, 3 February 1903.

77 *Vancouver Daily Province*, 2 February 1903.

78 *Delta News*, 7 February 1903. On the colony's gender ideals versus realities, see Lindström, "Utopia for Women?"

79 Wild, *Sointula*, 71.

80 *Nelson Daily News*, 3 February 1903.

81 *Vancouver Daily Province*, 2 February 1903.

82 Wild, *Sointula*, 73.

83 *Vancouver Daily Province*, 5 February 1903.

84 Ibid.

85 Provincial Constable Walter Wollacott to the attorney general of British Columbia, 24 February 1903, GR-0429, British Columbia Archives. Thanks to Colin Coates for sharing this and many other pertinent documents with me.

86 *Victoria Colonist*, 3 February 1903.

87 Even in contrast to the documentary evidence on the 1932 Sointula funeral procession and mourning for A.B. Mäkelä. See, for example, Wild, *Sointula*, 137–8.

88 Wild, *Sointula*, 70, provides photo of a shared gravestone for fire victims but does not comment on it and it is not mentioned in any other sources I have come across.

89 Kaapro Jääskelainen (pseud., A.B. Mäkelä), *Muistoja "Malkosaarelta,"* 85.

90 Halminen, *Sointula*, 90–1. Halminen cleverly repeats the word *viruivat* to get at both senses of the word: crawling/creeping and crying.

91 Ibid., 91.

92 Ibid., 92.

93 Ibid., 93.

94 Saramo, *Building That Bright Future*.

95 Halminen, *Sointula*, 88.

96 Ibid., 89.

97 Ibid., *Sointula*, 89.

98 Coroner's inquest, 30 January 1903, GR-0429, BC Archives.

99 For example, *Nelson Daily News*, 3 February 1903.

100 Halminen, *Sointula*, 91; Wild, *Sointula*, 75–6; Anderson, *History of Sointula*, 9.

101 Anderson, *History of Sointula*, 9.

102 Halminen, *Sointula*, 92.

103 Ibid., 92.
104 *Aika*, 1 December 1903, 54 (available at the Migration Institute of Finland Archive).
105 Ibid.
106 For an example of this collective process, see MacEacheran, *Miramichi Fire*, 87–95.
107 *Toveritar*, 25 January 1921.

BIBLIOGRAPHY

Archival Sources

British Columbia Archives, Victoria, BC
Migration Institute of Finland Archive, Turku, Finland

Newspapers and Periodicals

Aika
Delta News
Hawaiian Gazette
Nelson Daily News
Toveritar
Vancouver Daily Province
Vapaus
Victoria Colonist

Other Sources

Anderson, Aili. *History of Sointula*. Vancouver: Sointula Centennial Committee, 1958.
Baskerville, Peter. "The Worth of Children and Women: Life Insurance in Early Twentieth-Century Canada." In *The Dawn of Canada's Century: Hidden Histories*, edited by Gordon Darroch, 452–80. Montreal and Kingston: McGill-Queen's University Press, 2014.
Beaulieu, Michel S., David K. Ratz, and Ronald N. Harpelle, eds. *Hard Work Conquers All: Building the Finnish Community in Canada*. Vancouver: University of British Columbia Press, 2018.
Beaulieu, Michel S., Ronald N. Harpelle, and Jaimi Penny, eds. *Labouring Finns: Transnational Politics in Finland, Canada, and the United States*. Turku: Migration Institute of Finland, 2011.
Biesanz, Mavis Hiltunen. *Helmi Mavis: A Finnish American Girlhood*. St Cloud: North Star Press, 1989.

Eklund, William. *Builders of Canada: History of the Finnish Organization in Canada, 1911–1971.* Toronto: Finnish Organization of Canada, 1987.

Fahrni, Magda. "Glimpsing Working-Class Childhood through the Laurier Palace Fire of 1927: The Ordinary, the Tragic, and the Historian's Gaze." *Journal of the History of Childhood and Youth* 8, no. 3 (Fall 2015): 426–50.

Halminen, Matti. *Sointula – Kalevan Kansan ja Kanadan suomalaisten historiaa.* Mikkeli: Kustantaja Mikko Ampuja, 1936.

Holdren, Nate. *Injury Impoverished: Workplace Accidents, Capitalism, and Law in the Progressive Era.* Cambridge: Cambridge University Press, 2020.

Huhta, Aleksi. "Toward a Red Melting Pot: The Racial Thinking of Finnish-American Radicals, 1900–1938." PhD diss., University of Turku, 2017.

Jääskelainen, Kaapro [pseud., A.B. Mäkelä]. *Muistoja "Malkosaarelta."* Helsinki: Työmies, 1907.

Kaunonen, Gary. *Challenge Accepted: A Finnish Immigrant Response to Industrial America in Michigan's Copper Country.* East Lansing: Michigan State University Press, 2010.

Kolehmainen, John I. "Harmony Island: A Finnish Utopian Venture in British Columbia." *British Columbia Historical Quarterly* 5, no. 2 (May 1941): 111–25.

Lindström, Varpu. "The Radicalization of Finnish Farm Women in Northwestern Ontario, 1910–1930." In *I Won't Be a Slave: Selected Articles on Finnish Canadian Women's History,* edited by Varpu Lindström, 34–58. Beaverton, ON: Aspasia Books, 2010.

– "Utopia for Women? The Sointula Experiment, 1901–1905." *Journal of Finnish Studies* 4, no. 2 (December 2000): 4–25.

MacEacheran, Alan. *The Miramichi Fire: A History.* Montreal and Kingston: McGill-Queen's University Press, 2020.

MacFayden, Joshua. "Hewers of Wood: A History of Wood Energy in Canada." In *Powering Up: A History of Fuel, Power and Energy in Canada, 1800–2015,* edited by Ruth Sandwell, 129–61. Montreal and Kingston: McGill-Queen's University Press, 2016.

Madokoro, Laura. "On Future Directions: Temporalities and Permanency in the Study of Migration and Settler Colonialism in Canada." *History Compass* 17 (January 2019). https://doi.org/10.1111/hic3.12515.

Pilli, Arja. *The Finnish-Language Press in Canada, 1901–1939: A Study in the History of Ethnic Journalism.* Turku: Migration Institute of Finland, 1982.

Pyne, Steven. *Awful Splendour: A Fire History of Canada.* Vancouver: University of British Columbia Press, 2008.

Rosenow, Michael K. *Death and Dying in the Working Class, 1865–1920.* Champagne: University of Illinois Press, 2015.

Saarinen, Oiva. "Perspectives on Finnish Canadian Settlement." *Siirtolaisuus – Migration* 3 (1995): 19–25.

Saikku, Mikko. "Utopians and Utilitarians: Environment and Economy in the Finnish- Canadian Settlement of Sointula." *British Columbia Studies* 154 (Summer 2007): 3–38.

Sandwell, Ruth. "Fear and Anxiety on the Energy Frontier: Understanding Women's Early Encounters with Fossil Fuels in the Home." RCC *Perspectives: Transformations in Environment and Society* 1 (2020): 37–41.

– "Pedagogies of the Unimpressed: Re-educating Ontario Women for the Modern Energy Regime, 1900–1940." *Ontario History* 107, no. 1 (Spring 2015): 36–59.

Saramo, Samira. *Building That Bright Future: Soviet Karelia in the Life Writing of Finnish North Americans.* Toronto: University of Toronto Press, 2022.

– "Capitalism as Death: Loss of Life and the Finnish Migrant Left in the Early Twentieth Century." *Journal of Social History* 55, no. 3 (Spring 2022): 668–94.

– "Making Transnational Death Familiar." In *Transnational Death*, edited by Samira Saramo, Eerika Koskinen-Koivisto and Hanna Snellman, 8–22. Helsinki: Finnish Literature Society, 2019.

Tarr, Joel A. and Mark Tebeau. "Housewives as Home Safety Managers: The Changing Perception of the Home as a Place of Hazard and Risk, 1870–1940." In *Accidents in History: Injuries, Fatalities and Social Relations*, edited by Roger Cooter and Bill Luckin, 196–233. Amsterdam: Rodopi, 1997.

Wild, Paula. *Sointula: Island Utopia.* Madeira Park, BC: Harbour Publishing, 1995.

Wilson, J. Donald. "'Little Comrades': Socialist Sunday Schools as an Alternative to Public Schools." *Curriculum Inquiry* 21, no. 2 (Summer 1991): 217–22.

– "Matti Kurikka and the Utopian Socialist Settlement of Sointula, British Columbia." In *Pitkät jäljet: Historioita kahdelta mantereelta*, edited by Eero Kuparinen, 367–85. Turku: University of Turku, 1999.

2

The Accidental Underground

Death and Injury in Ontario's Mining Industry

John Sandlos

Few workplaces in Canada have proven more dangerous than mines. Workers in the underground environment faced a startling array of threats to life and limb, whether falling rock, the collapse of tunnels or rooms, noxious gases, moving vehicles, dangerous machinery, a fall down an open shaft, objects falling down a mine shaft (tools, timber, or even other miners), or collisions with the rapidly moving cage. Coal miners dealt with unique dangers as they worked seams of ancient carboniferous material that routinely emitted methane gas (or firedamp), causing massive explosions when sufficiently concentrated and combined with an ignition source such as a spark, dynamite shot, or open-flame lamp. Miners' drilling also produced large amounts of coal dust, a flammable material that could ignite in underground explosions. In the aftermath of these blasts, those who survived faced possible poisoning from afterdamp, a toxic mixture of carbon dioxide, nitrogen, and carbon monoxide. Add in the dangers inherent in the use of the explosives common to almost all mines, including faulty fuses, drilling into holes with unexploded dynamite, and workers remaining at the blast site too long (or returning too soon), and one begins to grasp how omnipresent the possibility of death or injury was.[1]

The number of mining accidents in Canada accelerated in the late nineteenth and early twentieth centuries as coal production increased fivefold between 1890 and 1913 to fuel industrial expansion, and hard-rock mining operations multiplied to exploit new sources of precious and base metals.[2] If the casualty rates in the mines were not quite those resulting from military combat, the number of people killed in large-scale disasters or aggregated over long periods of time is shocking. In Alberta, for instance, 773 fatal mining accidents occurred between 1906 and 1930, many of them in the coal industry.[3] The Nova Scotia Archives has created a database containing the names of 2,584 workers who died in the province's mines between 1838 and 1992, the vast majority of them coal miners.[4] While accident rates have fallen in the industry since Canada's under-regulated early industrial period, 268 people died in mining accidents between 1988 and 1993. At the time, underground mining still held top place as the most dangerous occupation in Canada.[5]

How do we interpret this history of death and injury in Canada's mines? Certainly relevant is the Marxist idea that, as industry became more heavily capitalized in the nineteenth century and workers lost control of the means of production, industrialists squeezed profits out of their operations by skimping on costly safety measures.[6] Ian McKay's doctoral dissertation implicitly challenged this perspective (without denying its importance), arguing that the tendency to romanticize miners as perfect proletarian victims, and underground mines as a particularly acute form of working-class hell, obscures the fact that coal miners maintained a high degree of autonomy and agency in their workplace, able to make judgments (and sometimes misjudgments) about safety.[7] Many coal-mining historians have pointed out, however, that the unique craft culture and the autonomy afforded to coal miners was tempered by the fact they were paid by the ton, forcing them to weigh safety versus income and internalize the employer's desire to make production the first priority.[8] Suggesting that the root of most accidents was workers' carelessness – not more systemic issues such as poor training, lack of supervision, or the failure to mitigate danger in the challenging underground environment – became a common way for management and owners to normalize accidents and thus avoid responsibility for them.[9] As Roger Cooter and Bill Luckin have argued, the general public in the industrial world of the nineteenth century increasingly attributed workplace accidents to human causes rather than divine intervention, opening a door for the owners of capital and their allies in government to blame accidents on workers' negligence or the supposedly unavoidable dangers of the modern work environment.[10]

In his compelling book on coal mining in Colorado, Thomas Andrews contends that the material and environmental dimensions of mining accidents deserve more attention. Mines are an extreme environment, he suggests; work underground is akin to the experience of scuba divers underwater or astronauts in space because elaborate support systems – pumping in fresh air, building roof supports, providing artificial light – are necessary to maintain human life. Risk was inherent in these underground locales as miners constructed "workscapes" that were "shaped by the interplay of human and natural forces."[11] Mine accidents were the most severe consequence of human technological interactions with nature underground. As McKay described it, "the environment of the coal mine was so harsh, it rewarded the slightest miscalculations with disproportionate pain."[12] Even in metal mines (which lack the omnipresent dangers of flammable gas), many accidents, particularly those involving falling rock or collapsing roofs, resulted from the workers' primary task of destabilizing the very rock in which they were enveloped. Mining industry officials and government regulators have used the supposed naturalness of mine hazards as another way to evade responsibility for accidents, dismissing them as the product of the "ordinary danger" associated with working underground.[13] In the case of the 1956 explosion in Springhill, Nova Scotia, a royal commission identified its cause as "an unfortunate combination of circumstances for which no blame can be attached to any one individual," even though it was sparked by an electrical wire known to be faulty coming into contact with methane gas and dust.[14] Of course, mining accidents are not just a product of nature, or happenstance: many, if not most, result from the choices mine owners make about how to organize work, apply technology, and mitigate risk amidst the largely known risks in the underground environment.

One gap in the historical literature on mining accidents is the result of an almost exclusive focus on major disasters in the coal industry rather than the smaller fatal events that occurred more frequently. As a general rule, fatalities from major disasters account for only a small proportion of deaths in the industry. Most mining accidents affect a very small number of miners, often killing only one individual at a time.¹⁵ Add in the much larger number of incidents that are non-fatal, and comprehension of the full range of actions and inactions that cause mining accidents becomes a tremendously difficult task. The sheer volume of accidents, even at a single mine, can be staggering, and company and government records often reveal very little about the likely causes.

Fortunately, while searching for sources amid pandemic lockdowns that made archival research nearly impossible, I stumbled on eighty years' (1891–1971) worth of highly detailed mine accident reports at the GeologyOntario website of the Ministry of Energy, Northern Development, and Mines.¹⁶ As a major producer of base and precious metals, Ontario provides an important sub-national mining jurisdiction in which to study mining accidents without having to focus on the coal industry's large-scale disasters. While one disastrous fire at the Hollinger Mine in Timmins claimed thirty-nine lives in 1928, the vast majority of accidents took the life of only one worker, hardly ever more than three.¹⁷ The reports contain reams of data on the immediate causes of fatal and non-fatal accidents in the province's mines, a lengthy report on each fatality, some record of culpability for each accident in the form of inquest results, and records of prosecutions. Taken together, the data suggest two key lessons. First, a large percentage of Ontario's accidents occurred because of the interaction of nature and technology in the underground environment (though certainly some resulted from accidents with machinery, tools, and vehicles that could have occurred in any industrial workplace). Second, state authorities and the justice system tended in most cases to dismiss accidents, even those types that occurred with startling repetition over the years, as nobody's fault, one of the unavoidable, ordinary dangers that occurred in the mines.

THE "SLOW" DISASTER IN ONTARIO'S MINES

The history of Ontario's hard-rock mining industry has largely failed to capture the public imagination in a manner similar to the gold rushes of the BC Interior and the Klondike, where individual sourdoughs who struck it rich panning for gold suggested that the little guy could actually get ahead in the competitive world of late-nineteenth century capitalism. In

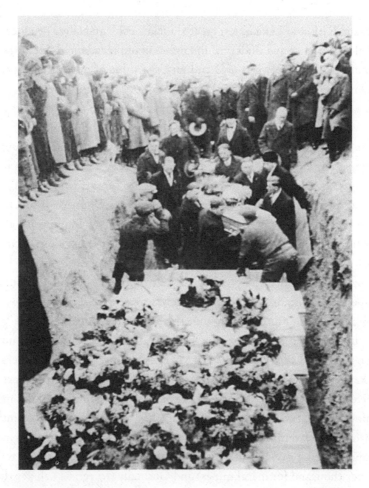

Fig. 2.1 Common grave with coffins of nine of the thirty-nine miners who died in a fire at the Hollinger Mine, Timmins, Ontario, February 1928.

Ontario, the flood of US capital that accompanied the development of the nickel deposits at Sudbury in the 1880s signalled something new: the development of massive and heavily capitalized underground operations to exploit the hard rock of the Canadian Shield.[18] Ontario's mining boom from the very beginning was a product of corporate capitalism, with large-scale investment in heavy equipment a prerequisite to break through the tough shield rock. Subsequent major developments at Cobalt in 1903, Timmins in

1910, and Kirkland Lake in 1911 created nickel, gold, and silver producers of global significance and underground mines of unprecedented size and scale in the province.[19] Between 1898 and 1913, the value of mineral production in Ontario rose from $7,235,877 to $53,232,311. The mining workforce increased from 7,495 to 20,315 over the same period, and more workers than ever were exposed to the dangers of the underground environment.[20]

As mining activity in Ontario grew dramatically, so too did the numbers of injuries and deaths. In 1892, for example, there were five deaths in all the mines, metallurgical works, and quarries in Ontario, but by 1913 that number reached sixty-four fatalities. However, as Ontario's inspector of mines, E.T. Corkill, noted in 1909, there were very few high-profile disasters in the mines: "In metalliferous mining an accident seldom occurs in which a considerable number of men are killed, the fatalities usually being one or two at a time, though in the course of a year they may amount to a large total." Because the accidents were spread over time and dispersed geographically in mines throughout the province, Corkill reported "public opinion is therefore not aroused; the management of the mine is not so much impressed with the importance of careful supervision; the miners are awakened for a few days, and then forget, and the same conditions prevail as before."[21] To drive home his point about dangers of underground metal mining in Ontario, he cited mining mortality rates from several countries showing that coal mining was only marginally more dangerous than metal mining in the United Kingdom (1.46 per thousand in the coal mines versus 1.08 per thousand for metal mines) and Germany (1.7 versus 1.29 per thousand), and equally as dangerous in the United States (3.22 per thousand in the metal mines versus 3.21 for coal).[22] Ontario's accident rate in 1909 seemed to bear out Corkill's argument that crisis conditions prevailed: 4.66 workers per thousand lost their lives that year in the province's mines, metallurgical works, and quarries – a total of forty-nine people. Corkill attributed the high accident rate in part to the "boomtown" conditions that existed at new mining locations in northern Ontario, particularly the silver developments at Cobalt. He argued that a combination of "disorganization, lack of discipline and loss in efficiency of both the men and those in charge" created an unsafe environment, noting that thirty-two of the forty-seven mining accidents in the previous year had occurred at Cobalt.[23]

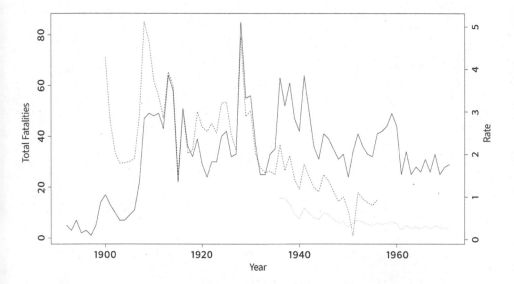

Fig. 2.2 Total deaths and the fatality rate in Ontario's mines, metallurgical works, and quarries, 1892–1971. Solid line represents the number of deaths on an annual basis; dashed line represents the number of workers who died per thousand in province; dotted line represents deaths per million person hours. Figures derived from the Ontario Department of Mines' *Reports on the Mining Accidents in Ontario* and the annual reports of the Ontario Mine Inspection Branch, 1892–1971.

Corkill was likely correct that new mining operations presented unique dangers owing to a sudden influx of inexperienced miners, poorly developed safety training and procedures, and the multitude of new companies. Nonetheless, even as the industry matured, in Ontario the mining accident rate remained stubbornly high – consistently above two out of every thousand workers annually until 1932 (higher than the UK and Germany in 1908) and not dropping consistently below one per thousand until 1948 (see fig. 2.2). Indeed, death remained a constant threat to Ontario's mine workers even as the mortality rate dropped, the relatively slow rate of workplace fatalities adding up to a startling total over time. Between 1892 and 1971, 2,640 workers died through an accident at Ontario's mines, metallurgical works, and quarries, most of these in the mines. (This figure does not account for the hundreds of miners – 1,303 from 1926 to 1972 – who died

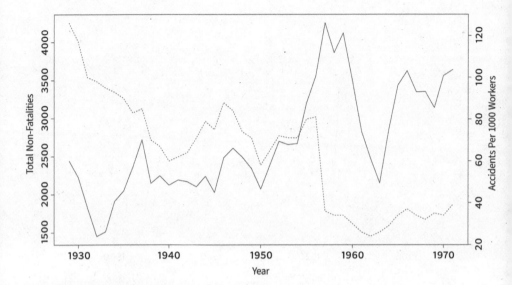

Fig 2.3 Total non-fatal accidents (causing lost-time injury) in Ontario's mines, metallurgical works and quarries, 1929–1971. Solid line represents the total number of accidents, dashed line the number of accidents per thousand workers. Figures derived from the Ontario Department of Mines' *Reports on the Mining Accidents in Ontario* and the annual reports of the Ontario Mine Inspection Branch, 1892–1971.

in Ontario due to silicosis.) While the mining accident reports from the Department of Mines did not always separate out accidents in the mines from those in metallurgical works, complete data exist from 1923 to 1971. Over this span, the total number of deaths that occurred at mines was 1,462, while the total deaths at mines, metallurgical works, and quarries was 1,883. A small proportion of the deaths at mines occurred at the surface, but the vast majority occurred underground.[24]

Many thousands more of Ontario's miners suffered injuries in their workplaces. Between 1927 and 1971, 124,852 workers in mines, metallurgical works, and quarries were injured in 119,982 separate accidents, most of them serious enough to be classified as "lost time" incidents requiring recovery away from work. The annual rate of non-fatal accidents per thousand workers did show a general decline over time, falling from a high of 126 per thousand workers in 1929 (the first year the figure is included in the reports) to a low of twenty-four per thousand in 1962, only to show a rising trend over the next decade back up to thirty-nine per thousand in 1971 (see figure 3.3).[25] While overall improvement in accident rates is significant, this does not change the fact that Ontario's miners faced the very real possibility of death or injury every day that they toiled in the underground environment.

REGULATING DANGER IN ONTARIO'S MINES

In many respects, accident reports adopted a neutral tone when it came to the debate over who was responsible for accidents in Ontario mines, criticizing companies *and* individual workers for unsafe practices. Corkill's 1910 report, for instance, pleaded with the companies to hire more "technical men" to resolve safety issues before deadly accidents occurred. Yet he also criticized those "reckless miners" who put themselves and others at risk by working under loose rock or stealing rides up or down the shaft on the ore bucket or skip.[26] The next year, the chief inspector's report contained two lists – perhaps designed to emphasize his neutrality – cataloguing seven ways that companies frequently breached the Ontario Mining Act but also seven ways that miners did the same.[27]

Such apparent impartiality on the part of inspectors featured more in their rhetoric than in reality, as the legal regime surrounding mine safety in Ontario was heavily weighted in favour of mine owners. Ontario's Mining Act (which consolidated an array of mining legislation as the Mines Act in 1906 and was then revised as the Mining Act in 1908) contained health and safety regulations, but as the chief inspector, T.F. Sutherland, admitted in 1913, enforcement was weak. "The policy so far," he acknowledged, "has been to take action only in flagrant cases where life has been endangered."[28] In practice, the regulatory emphasis within government and industry was on voluntary initiatives, education directed at workers, and self-regulation by the companies. Indeed, Ontario's mining industry played a significant role in drafting the safety regulations in the Mining Act, pressing policies favourable to its bottom line through the Mine Accident and Prevention Association of Ontario, an organization made up of mining company representatives that maintained close ties to the industry key lobby group, the Ontario Mining Association. Although the interests of management and labour converged on some initiatives, such as the funding of mine rescue teams (and the ever-popular rescue competitions) or the creation of joint safety committees (where management invariably controlled the membership and the agenda), unions were relatively powerless.

Organized labour often challenged management's tight control over the health and safety agenda. Mostly they were ignored, especially prior to the period of high public salience on industrial health and safety that began in the 1970s.[29] But by the early twentieth century, safety strikes (some of them wildcat protests) were common in maritime and western coal mines, owing in part to the miners' awareness of the acute dangers associated with mining coal.[30] Such actions were not as common in the less obviously dangerous hard-rock mines of Ontario, with demands for wages and union recognition dominating the agenda in the years before and immediately after World War I. Safety issues were nevertheless important to the miners. Cobalt's miners, for example, successfully pressed the government in 1914 to reduce the workday from ten to eight hours as a means to reduce accidents.[31] The strike at Kirkland Lake's Macassa mine in 1941 has mostly been remembered for inspiring the Ontario government to enshrine union recognition in law, but it also occurred in part because of the International Union of Mine, Mill, and Smelter Workers' concerns over the "ghastly" number of mining accidents in the region.[32] Most famously, a wildcat strike on safety issues at Elliot Lake's Denison Mine in 1974 resulted in the Royal Commission on the Health and Safety of Workers in Mines, and ultimately in the passage of a modernized Occupational Health and Safety Act in the province in 1979.[33]

When workers or labour organizations attempted to take legal actions, the justice system was hardly a champion of health and safety. As Eric Tucker has noted, Ontario's courts largely adopted a doctrine of individual worker responsibility with respect to dangerous factory work from the mid-nineteenth century to 1914, a framework that limited successful legal action against negligence on the part of the mining companies. When the province introduced workmen's compensation in 1915, the standardized system of recompense further removed the threat of liability lawsuits for mining accidents. For this reason, and also because they had to pay the same rate into the workmen's compensation program regardless of how much capital and effort they invested in safety initiatives, many mines disbanded their safety committees.[34] Although fatal workplace accidents were subject to an inquiry by a coroner's jury, these proceedings constituted a non-adversarial attempt to establish the cause of death rather than to assign legal liability to individuals or a corporate entity. So, despite the veneer of technocratic neutrality the mining inspectors infused into their reports, the broader system of mine administration in Ontario worked against the miners' safety.

Nonetheless, coroner's juries and mine inspectors at times employed harsh rhetoric and recommended charges in cases where they believed management had neglected to implement safety measures or when action (or its absence) obviously contravened the safety regulations in the Mining Act. In September 1903, for instance, the inspector described the death of two miners at the Look Lake Mine in the Algoma area as "a most inexcusable calamity" because management had encouraged miners to descend into the shaft while riding on the ore bucket in contravention of regulations. According to the report, two miners, William Pelkonen and Peter Thompson, crashed to their deaths after the bucket became stuck and the brakeman shook the rope, causing it to slacken and the bucket to go into free-fall down the shaft. In cases where mines had reinforced the prohibitions against riding the bucket (or the skip) through training and signage, inspectors blamed the workers, but in this instance the mining company had failed to provide any other safe means of descent other than unstable temporary ladders.[35] In a similar accident in November 1908, two miners, Andrew Osman and John Aha, fell to their deaths from a bucket; local authorities charged and fined Beaver Consolidated Mines under the Mining Act because, once again, the operator had failed to provide a safe ladderway to access the shaft.[36]

Such criticism by mine inspectors rarely resulted in any legal consequences for the companies. In keeping with their weak enforcement of Mining Act regulations, between 1925 and 1971 provincial authorities laid only fifteen charges (twelve resulting in conviction) against mining companies, thirty-five charges against managers or foremen (twenty-six successful), and three successful prosecutions of company presidents. These compare with 224 prosecutions of mine employees in the same span of time, with 216 resulting in a conviction.[37] Most of the charges, whether directed at companies or workers, arose from violations of regulations prior to any kind of accident; the majority resulted only in minor fines, suggesting that the mine inspectors used prosecutions primarily as a preventative means of imposing discipline, mostly on the mine workforce.

Certainly, the authorities were reluctant to lay charges against mining companies for more consequential safety violations that resulted in severe injury or death, and the courts were even more hesitant to find them guilty in the small number of prosecutions that did occur. A case from 1941 suggests the lengths to which local courts went to avoid convicting senior mine officials. On 2 July of the previous year, miner Clifford Carter died from carbon-monoxide poisoning at the Wolfe Lake Mines near Kirkland Lake. The source of the poisoned air was a gasoline motor a mine manager had placed underground to operate a pump, contrary to the regulations of the Mining Act. The crown took the unusual step of charging D.F. Pidgeon (president and manager), E. Wride (manager), and Otto May (manager) with manslaughter under the Criminal Code. May pleaded guilty to lesser charges and paid a fine of $200, and then acted as a witness in the trial of Pidgeon and Wride, claiming he acted on his own initiative when he installed the gasoline-powered pump in the mine. According to the accident report for 1941, Judge A.W. Green dismissed the charges against Wride owing to a lack of evidence. He then instructed the jury in the Pidgeon trial that "it was necessary for the Crown to prove gross negligence and wanton disregard for others and that if they considered there was any care shown by the accused for the safe operation of the gasoline engine, the accused should be found not guilty."[38] In this trial, Judge Green set a very high bar for criminal prosecution, one where the defense could invoke even the smallest shred of evidence pointing to a duty of care on the part of the company (regardless of whether it was flouting the regulations of the Mining Act) as a means to avoid responsibility for fatal accidents.

In another case five years later, miner Edward Jones died at the massive Hollinger gold mine when he was driving a motorized vehicle and hit a door stuck in the open position, a problem that workers had observed for some time. The coroner's jury cited negligence on the part of the company for "a lack of supervision of mechanical devices." But when asked about criminal charges, the crown attorney suggested that the problem was Jones's failure to close the door.[39] Once again the justice system shied away from charging

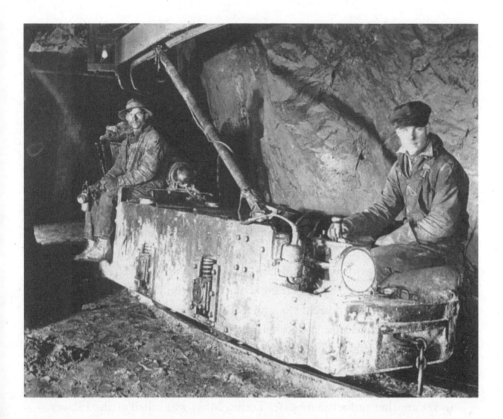

Fig. 2.4 Miners ride an early electric locomotive, Hollinger Mine, Timmins. Such motorized vehicles were one source of the many dangers miners faced in their workplace.

mine officials based on the systemic safety problems that caused accidents, preferring instead to blame workers for death in the mines.

Mine workers certainly did commit acts of carelessness that led to accidents. There were instances where miners died because they did not wear required equipment such as safety belts.[40] Workers also took shortcuts, illegally riding a bucket or a skip from one level of the mine to the next, cutting through unsafe and restricted areas, entering a blast area before the expiration of a mandatory wait period, or drilling into an old hole after a blasting operation to avoid starting anew in hard rock, thus raising the risk of an explosion caused by contact with unexploded powder or dynamite. From a legalistic viewpoint, one could plausibly argue that companies were not at fault when miners wilfully broke safety rules. At the same time, individual accident reports very often downplayed or omitted contextual factors that raised questions about more systemic issues, such as the quality of safety training, pressure from management to increase productivity, or self-imposed compulsion to hurry in response to the lure of pay incentives. In July 1963, for instance, a coroner's jury examining the case of Konstantyn Sabala was one of the few to allude to the pressure to produce when it noted that the miner's failure to take precautions while removing support timbers from the Hollinger Mine could be attributed to "his undue haste to get as much done as possible."[41]

In a relatively small number of cases, the cause of mine fatalities could be attributed to circumstances beyond anybody's control. In August 1913, a bizarre explosion killed Louis del Favero at the Magpie Mine in Michipicoten, caused by a lightning strike on the compressor house, which then sent an electric current along an air line where miners had hung wires connected to dynamite.[42] Another seemingly random incident occurred when a miner, Edward Fleming, died in September 1925 at the Hollinger Mine while having an epileptic seizure (a condition he did not know he had) after he lit the fuse for a blast, preventing him from leaving the blast area.[43] In yet another unfortunate case, Teemu Maki was killed at the Howey Gold Mine in January 1929 when an air hose inexplicably blew off its header and struck the miner in the forehead.[44] In other cases, the mining accident was only a proximate cause of death. When, for example, Ernest Littlejohn had his right index finger crushed while trying to steady a swinging bucket, an injury that required an amputation, he died on the operating table because of a reaction to the anesthetic.[45] Amid the hundreds of fatality reports, there were sixteen deaths from infections that led to fatal conditions such as gangrene, septicemia, or pneumonia, most of these concentrated in the decades before the 1940s antibiotics revolution. In some cases, these infections originated from relatively minor injuries such as lacerations and fractures, but as the introduction to this volume notes, the long distances between remote extractive sites and hospitals in Canada could delay medical treatment and potentially compound the threat from infection. Even if one supports the notion that mining accidents are generally not accidental, but result from systemic safety issues within a mine, some accidents did result from circumstances that would have been difficult for workers or a company to foresee or control.

The question of who was responsible for mine accidents came to a head in Ontario in 1958 with the revelation of very high accident rates in the uranium mines of Elliot Lake. From January to August, the compensable accident rate at Elliot Lake's mines was 53.9 per million man hours compared to 37.1 across the province's mining industry. Over the entire year, twenty-one of thirty-four fatal underground mining accidents in Ontario occurred in the Elliot Lake uranium mines.[46] In a brief to a special committee established in 1958 to inquire into the situation, the Ontario Mining Association summed up the industry's position, stating that "96 percent of all accidents are due to human error and only 4 percent due to mechanical failure or the like."[47] The giant mining company Rio Tinto similarly claimed that "every accident has an element of carelessness and most are completely the result of carelessness. An organization must be built up that protects the workers in spite of themselves." The company also quoted an article from the *Globe and Mail* suggesting that "undesirable persons" had moved into Elliot Lake, confirmed by high numbers of auto accidents, routine violence, and a general atmosphere of lawlessness permeating the area.[48] With such an unruly mob working in the uranium mines, Rio Tinto argued, how could anyone but the workers be responsible for the workplace accidents that led to injury and death?

As one might expect, labour unions took an opposite view from management. The International Union of Mine, Mill and Smelter Workers (Mine Mill) highlighted the systemic issues that inevitably led to death and injury in the mine rather than ineptitude of individual miners. The union pointedly argued that management's harping on carelessness was "specious ... really an attempt by management to evade responsibility by pointing in other directions." According to Mine Mill, "the primary concern of management has been with the meeting of contract requirements, or more properly production schedules, and ... the safety and well-being of the men has come a poor second."[49] The United Steelworkers of America (USWA) adopted much the same tone (despite its reputation as being the less radical of the two rival unions), claiming, "The emphasis has been on getting the properties into production and insufficient consideration has

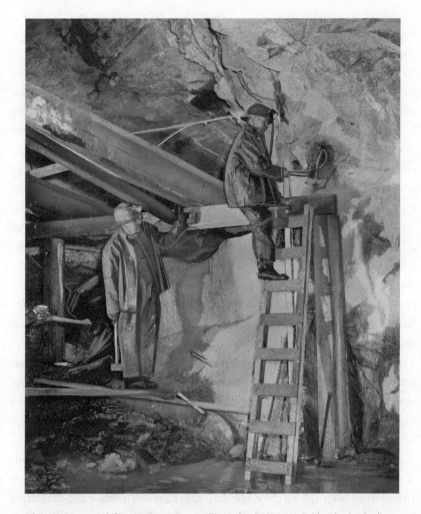

Fig. 2.5 More work for uranium miners, Elliot Lake. Controversies beginning in the 1950s over high rates of accidents and industrial disease contributed to improved occupational health and safety legislation in Ontario.

been given to the safety problems in this type of mining."[50] As evidence, both unions pointed to similar lists of challenges: poor handling and storage procedures with explosive powder; demands from management to proceed with mucking and drilling before the holes and muck were checked properly for residual explosives; problems with falls of loose rock due to inadequate rock bolting methods and overly wide tunnels; poor traffic controls for underground vehicles; a bonus system that incentivized haste over safe practices; inadequate training programs for new workers; variable standards for hoisting equipment; and poor supports for high powered drills and slushing machines. Add to this poor ventilation and the consequent threat of industrial disease from silica dust and radiation, and it is easy to see why the miners would not accept facile admonishments about individual workers' responsibility for health and safety in the mines.[51]

As much as Ontario's mine accident reports attempted to straddle the stark division between labour and capital on many issues, the mine inspectors and coroner's juries weakly nudged mine owners to address safety problems. Surprisingly, the reports only compiled aggregate data on culpability for fatal accidents during a brief period from 1908 to 1913. While the reports' authors did not divulge their method of assigning blame for individual fatalities, they did highlight worker carelessness as the leading cause of fatal accidents (45.3 percent), while apportioning blame in 22.5 percent of cases to the neglect of management, and 30.3 percent to the danger of inherent to the work.[52] To build a larger dataset reflecting the official apportionment of blame for Ontario's mining accidents, I tracked who was held responsible in each of the individual fatal accident reports from 1925 to 1971 (years for which there is consistent format for the reports, including excerpts from the specific rulings of inquest juries). In Ontario, these inquests were public hearings conducted by a coroner before a five-member jury.[53] Out of 1,277 fatalities during this period, the jury blamed the company in only seven cases, and a manager or shift captain in seven others. In contrast, juries blamed employees for negligence in their own deaths or the deaths of others in 135 cases.

While this stark difference in assigning responsibility suggests a clear bias toward mine owners, the more startling revelation is that in 972 (72 percent) of the cases, juries ruled that nobody was to blame for the fatal accident. When combined with the 123 additional cases where neither the coroner's jury or the accident report discussed who was responsible for a miner's death, it is evident most accidents were interpreted as the product of random misfortune.

But even this point is tempered by the fact that, in 282 cases, the inquest juries tried to address some systemic safety issues in the mines, including pointed (albeit unenforced) advice to companies on safety improvements. Most suggestions pointed to serious safety issues in the mines: failure to notify miners of dangerous areas, improper ventilation after blasting (to prevent carbon-monoxide poisoning), a dearth of carbon-monoxide detectors, the absence of safety covers on exposed cable systems or machinery, uncovered vats containing dangerous material, and loose rock on the roof of the mine that was improperly scaled (i.e., removed) or secured.[54] The fact the inquest juries and mine inspectors tried to address such serious safety issues with friendly recommendations rather than enforcement certainly underscores the toothless nature of the mine safety regulatory system in Ontario. On the other hand, the frequency of these suggestions roughly doubled each year beginning in 1958, coincident with the heightened concern over safety issues in Elliot Lake and a broader push from labour unions on occupational health and safety in the 1960s and 1970s. In many ways, inquest juries and mine inspectors tried to find a middle ground between labour and capital, playing a more assertive advisory role without rocking the boat on mine safety issues.

At the same time, the most common assertion on the part of the inquest juries – that nobody was to blame – stems in large part from the fact that accidental deaths and injuries had been naturalized as inherent to the nature of work in the underground environment. By taking on such work, miners accepted these inevitable dangers, at least in the eyes of those who managed and regulated the industry. In particular, inquest juries and mine inspectors typically labelled accidents involving falling rock, or rocks that burst due to geological pressure, as accidents where nobody was responsible. Certainly, this type of accident was one of the hardest to get under control in Ontario's mines, as the proportion of accidents attributed to falls of ground (i.e., rock falling from the roof of the mine) increased from 21 percent of total fatal accidents between 1908 and 1940 to 33 percent of the total between 1955 and 1971. The proportional increase reflected major improvements in other areas (particularly a decline in accidents with explosives from 20 percent to 6 percent of the total over the same two time periods). Yet fatality rates from falling rock did not also improve in

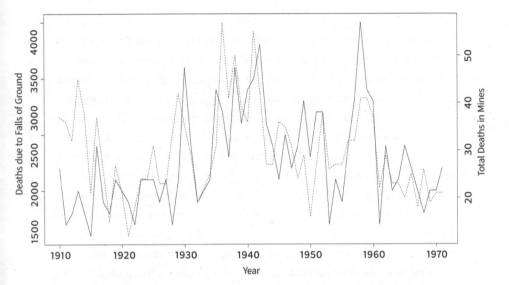

Fig. 2.6 Total deaths due to falls of ground (solid line) in Ontario's mines, 1910–71. Dotted line shows total fatalities in the mines (underground and surface) over the same period. Deaths from falls of ground fluctuated roughly in lockstep with total deaths. Several peaks between the 1930s and 1960s suggest the mining industry had no effective way to address the problem for several decades. Figures derived from the Ontario Department of Mines' *Reports on the Mining Accidents in Ontario* and the annual reports of the Ontario Mine Inspection Branch, 1892–1971.

any dramatic way over time, accounting for 41 percent of total fatalities in the mines in 1971. Falling rock was also the leading cause of non-fatal injuries in Ontario's mines between 1925 and 1971, accounting for 21 percent of incidents in underground mines, nearly double the amount of the second-place cause, falls of persons (see figure 2.6). Mine owners and regulators also conveniently interpreted other types of accidents through the lens of inevitability. No matter how many safeguards were in place, some miners were bound to fall prey to vertical drops in the mines, with others crushed by equipment or rock in the narrow mine workings and still others suffocating from noxious gasses. Even if mine inspectors and coroner's juries recognized some of the systemic safety problems in the mines, in most cases they accepted that a certain amount of death and injury was intrinsic to this tough, masculine line of work.

CONCLUSION

Historian Ted Steinberg has argued that natural disasters are never truly natural but a consequence of the way human-built environments interact with the natural world. Moreover, the damage wrought by disasters usually reflects the political priorities of those in power. So, for example, trailer-park communities in the hurricane zones of the southern United States get levelled not only because of the storm but because of weak building codes that allow developers to maximize profits by selling cheap housing for low-income people. Or, in the case of storm surges, it is often low-income and racialized neighbourhoods that have been pushed onto poorly protected low ground, as was the case with New Orleans' Lower 9th Ward during Hurricane Katrina in 2005.[55] The political dynamics that governed mine accidents and disasters have operated in much the same way. Blaming mine accidents on nature, or careless workers, was a means to deflect blame away from the failure of mine owners to invest the necessary capital to reduce or eliminate certain types of mine accidents. While mining companies did improve some practices, particularly ventilation and the safety of underground blasting, the notorious case of corporate negligence that led to Canada's last major explosion at Nova Scotia's Westray Mine in 1992 suggests that the industry took a long time (more than a century, in the case of coal-mine explosions) to learn from its mistakes.[56]

Except for the occasional critical comments of mine inspectors, or the scattered but friendly advice of the coroner's juries, Ontario's accident reports rarely abandoned their dispassionate tone. In large part, the reports affirmed the core beliefs of an industry that accepted death and injury as inevitable. The reports confirm that some types of accidents, notably those involving falling rock, falling people, and shaft accidents (usually involving a fatal encounter with the cage) occurred year after year in Ontario with no concerted attempt on the part of industry or government to address the issue.

At times, the reports did step beyond the idea that mine accidents were the result of natural causes or workers' negligence, pointing to the fatal choices mine owners made about how and where to unearth minerals. Inspector Corkill noted in 1909 that accidents involving falling rock often occurred because scaling operations to remove loose rock were "so lax as to be absolutely useless." He also suggested that the pursuit of low grade ore at ever-increasing depths had left "men working under a hanging [i.e., the upper wall of a vein] of probably two, three or four hundred feet, which has not been scaled in years, and is, in fact, impossible to scale properly" – a situation that was tantamount to "sacrificing human life to commercialism."[57] The mine accident reports sporadically recommended improvements to rock bolting or timber framing as a means to better support tunnels and hanging walls. They also occasionally addressed the root causes of other underground threats, pleading for operators to install guard rails at shaft openings, post human guards at entranceways to blast areas, or improve signal systems (or even install closed-circuit television) so cage operators could avoid hitting their fellow workers. Human intrusion into the underground environment had created conditions ripe for injury and death among workers. The mine accident reports acknowledged, to some extent, the failure of mining companies to invest in further interventions to lessen the danger of working underground.

Of course, the inspectors who wrote the accident reports were the same officials who had only weakly enforced the regulations of the Mining Act. Their scattered calls for systemic change rang somewhat hollow when juxtaposed with a weak enforcement regime that allowed fatal threats to linger at the mines. Because the number of fatalities in Ontario's mines remained a slow trickle, however, mine owners and provincial regulators never had to face the public scrutiny that accompanied the coal-mining accidents, and companies made only slow and halting attempts to address the dangerous conditions in the mines that killed and injured workers year after year.[58] The complacency of government and the mining industry persisted at least until the late 1950s, when the occupational health disasters that accompanied the uranium rush at Elliot Lake forced at least some reckoning with the accident issue (and also industrial diseases such as silicosis and lung cancer). Unfortunately, Ontario's mine workers bore the consequences of the sluggish response to the threat of mining accidents. Their safety too often mattered less than squeezing more production and profit out of the mines before the boom turned to bust.

ACKNOWLEDGMENTS

Many thanks to Yolanda Wiersma for teaching me the coding skills necessary to produce the three graphs using the statistical software R. Thanks
also to the three attentive peer reviewers and especially to Megan Davies
and Geoffrey Hudson for shepherding this project to publication.

NOTES

1 For general overviews of coal mining and accidents in Canada, see Belshaw, *Colonization and Community*; DeMont, *Coal Black Heart*; Newsome, *Coal Coast*. Miners also died from dust and fibre in underground and (in some cases) open-pit mines. While not often interpreted as accidents, miners' exposure to substances such as silica dust, coal dust, and asbestos produced an array of lung diseases (silicosis, black lung disease, asbestosis, etc.) that could be considered a form of slow-motion accident, or "slow violence," in the words of Rob Nixon. See Nixon, *Slow Violence and the Environmentalism of the Poor*.
2 G. David Quirin, "Historical Statistics of Canada, Section Q: Energy and Electric Power," accessed 27 July 2023, http://www.statcan.gc.ca/pub/11-516-x/pdf/5220018-eng.pdf.
3 Buckley, "Death, Dying and Mourning in the Crowsnest Pass," 201.
4 "Men in the Mines: A History of Mining Activity in Nova Scotia, 1720–1992," Nova Scotia Archives, https://archives.novascotia.ca/meninmines/.
5 Katherine Marshall, "A Job to Die For," *Perspectives (Statistics Canada)*, catalogue no. 75-001-XPE (1996): 26–31.
6 Tucker, *Administering Danger in the Workplace*; Tucker, "Making the Workplace 'Safe' in Capitalism."
7 McKay, "Industry, Work and Community in the Cumberland Coalfields"; McKay, "Realm of Uncertainty."
8 Buckley, *Danger, Death and Disaster in the Crowsnest Pass Mines*; Whiteside, *Regulating Danger*.
9 Dodd, "Blame and Causation in the Aftermath of Industrial Disasters." For the same phenomenon in a global context, see Cooter and Luckin, *Accidents in History*.
10 Cooter and Luckin, "Accidents in History: An Introduction," in Cooter and Luckin, *Accidents in History*, 1–16.
11 Andrews, *Killing for Coal*, 125. For a discussion of the ecological context for occupational health and safety in industry more broadly, see McEvoy, "Working Environments."
12 McKay, "Industry, Work and Community in the Cumberland Coalfields," 649.
13 Buckley, *Danger, Death and Disaster in the Crowsnest Pass Mines*.
14 Quoted in Dodd, "Blame and Causation in the Aftermath of Industrial Disasters," 253.
15 Benson, "Mining Saftety and Miners' Compensation in Great Britain; Farrenkopf, "Accidents and Mining," 193–211.

16 See https://www.geologyontario.mndm.gov.on.ca.

17 An account of the fire can be found in Sutherland, *Report on the Mining Accidents in Ontario*. For further discussion, see Saramo's chapter in this volume.

18 Clement, *Hard-Rock Mining*; Swift, *Big Nickel*.

19 Barnes, *Fortunes in the Ground*; Sandlos and Keeling, *Mining Country*.

20 Archibald Blue, director, Bureau of Mines, *Eight Report of the Bureau of Mines, 1899* (Toronto: King's Printer, 1899), 6; Thomas Gibson, Deputy Minister of Mines, Ontario, *Twenty-Third Annual Report of the Bureau of Mines, 1914* (Toronto: King's Printer, 1914), 3.

21 Thomas Gibson, Deputy Minister, Department of Lands, Forests and Mines, Ontario, *Eighteenth Annual Report of the Bureau of Mines, 1909* (Toronto: King's Printer, 1909), 73.

22 Ibid.

23 Ibid., 73, 78. For an overview, see Baldwin, "Study in Social Control"; Baldwin and Duke, "'Grey Wee Town,'" 71–87.

24 The data were taken from Ontario Department of Mines, Reports on the Mining Accidents in Ontario, published annually between 1923 and 1957 (Toronto: King's Printer), and Ontario Mine Inspection Branch, Annual Reports for the years 1958 to 1971 (Toronto: King's Printer).

25 Data taken from Ontario Department of Mines, Reports on the Mining Accidents in Ontario, 1927–1957, and Ontario Mine Inspection Branch, Annual Reports, 1958–1971. The Department of Mines did not keep consistent data on injuries prior to 1927. Most reports after 1927 include figures for mine injuries alone, but for some years the numbers are missing. To give an idea of the proportion of non-fatal accidents in mines, 61,734 incidents were reported in the mines between 1934 and 1964, but 81,474 incidents in mines, metallurgical works, and quarries during the same period. In most years, the non-fatal accident statistics concentrated on "lost time" injuries that would require payments under the workmen's compensation program.

26 Department of Lands, Forests and Mines, Ontario, *The Bureau of Mines Twentieth Annual Report* (Toronto: King's Printer, 1911), 78.

27 E.T. Corkill, Chief Inspector of Mines, Ontario, *Report on the Mining Accidents in Ontario in 1911* (Toronto: King's Printer, 1912), 6.

28 T.F. Sutherland, Chief Inspector of Mines, Ontario, *Report on the Mining Accidents in Ontario in 1913*. Bureau of Mines (Toronto: King's Printer, 1913).

29 Corbeil, "Mining Ontario." The idea that the state was in effect a client of the mineral industry is not limited to the realm of health and safety regulation. Throughout Canada, provincial governments adopted a supportive role towards the mining industry through subsidies, infrastructure development, and limited regulatory oversight (especially in the early period of growth prior to World War II); see McAllister and Alexander, *Stake in the Future*; McAllister, "Shifting Foundations in a Mature Staples Industry; Nelles, *Politics of Development*; Yudelman, *Canadian Mineral Policy Formulation*. For a broad analysis of the state's industry-friendly approach to regulating occupational health and safety issues in Ontario, see Tucker, *Administering Danger in the Workplace*.

30 McKay, "Strikes in the Maritimes"; McCormack, *Western Canadian Radical Movement*.

31 Baldwin, "Study in Social Control," 86.

32 MacDowell, *Remember Kirkland Lake*, 103. The quoted reference to the "ghastly" accident rate came originally from a union brief on working conditions in Kirkland Lake.

33 MacDowell, "Elliot Lake Uranium Miners' Battle." See also further discussion on Elliot Lake below in the chapter.

34 Tucker, *Administering Danger in the Workplace*.

35 Thomas Gibson, Director, Bureau of Mines, Ontario, *Report of the Bureau of Mines, 1904* (Toronto: King's Printer, 1904), 40.

36 Thomas Gibson, Deputy Minister, Department of Lands, Forests and Mines, Ontario, *Eighteenth Annual Report of the Bureau of Mines, 1909* (Toronto: King's Printer, 1909), 59.

37 Data taken from Ontario Department of Mines, Reports on the Mining Accidents in Ontario, 1925–1957, and Ontario Mine Inspection Branch, Annual Reports, 1958–1971.

38 W.O. Tower, Chief Inspector of Mines, Department of Mines, Ontario, *Report on the Mining Accidents in Ontario in 1940* (Toronto: King's Printer, 1941), 19–20; W.O. Tower, Chief Inspector of Mines, Department of Mines, Ontario, *Report on the Mining Accidents in Ontario in 1941* (King's Printer, 1942), 15.

39 W.O. Tower, Chief Inspector of Mines, Department of Mines, Ontario, *Report on the Mining Accidents in Ontario in 1946* (Toronto: King's Printer, 1947), 35.

40 Mine Inspection Branch Staff, *Ontario Department of Mines Bulletin 151, Report for 1955* (Toronto: Queen's Printer, 1956), 23–5.

41 Mine Inspection Branch Staff, *Mines Inspection Branch Annual Report, 1963; Ontario Department of Mines Bulletin 163* (Toronto: Queen's Printer, 1964), 20.

42 T.F. Sutherland, Chief Inspector of Mines, Ontario, *Report on the Mining Accidents in Ontario for July, August and September, 1913* (Toronto: King's Printer, 1913), 8.

43 T.F. Sutherland, Chief Inspector of Mines, Ontario, *Report on the Mining Accidents in Ontario in 1925* (Toronto: King's Printer, 1926), 24.

44 D.G. Sinclair, Chief Inspector of Mines, Ontario, *Report on the Mining Accidents in Ontario in 1929* (Toronto: King's Printer, 1930), 22.

45 T.F. Sutherland, *Report on the Mining Accidents in Ontario in 1925* (Toronto: King's Printer, 1926), 35.

46 The accident rates are from R.G.K. Morrision, A.V. Cortlett, and H.R. Rice, *Report on the Special Committee on Mining Practices at Elliot Lake*, bulletin 155, Department of Mines (Toronto: Queen's Printer, 1959), 7. The deaths from the Elliot Lake Mines were reported in Mines Inspection Branch, *Ontario Department of Mines Bulletin 157, Report for 1958 on Accidents* (King's Printer, 1959).

47 Morrision, Cortlett, and Rice, *Report on the Special Committee on Mining Practices at Elliot Lake*, 125.

48 Ibid., 108.

49 Ibid., 85.

50 Ibid., 89.

51 For a broad overview of the Elliot Lake controversy, see MacDowell, "Elliot Lake Uranium Miners' Battle."

52 A small number of accidents (3.5 per cent) could not be classified. See Thomas Gibson, Deputy Minister, Department of Lands, Forests and Mines, Ontario, *Eighteenth Annual Report of the Bureau of Mines, 1909* (Toronto: King's Printer, 1909), 72; Gibson, *Nineteenth Annual Report of the Bureau of Mines, 1910* (Toronto: King's Printer, 1910), 57; Gibson, *Twentieth Annual Report of the Bureau of Mines, 1911*, 60; Gibson, *Twenty-First Annual Report of the Bureau of Mines, 1912*, 56; Gibson, *Twenty-Second Annual Report of the Bureau of Mines, 1913*, 62; Gibson, *Twenty-Third Annual Report of the Bureau of Mines, 1914*, 53.

53 Wood, "Discovering the Ontario Inquest," 243–66. See also R. Blake Brown's chapter, this volume.

54 These incidents were noted in D.G. Sinclair, Chief Inspector of Mines, Ontario, *Mining Accidents in Ontario in 1936* (Toronto: King's Printer, 1937), 50; W.O. Tower, Chief Inspector of Mines, Ontario, *Report on the Mining Accidents in Ontario in 1945* (Toronto: King's Printer, 1946), 37; D.G. Sinclair, Chief Inspector of Mines, Ontario, *Mining Accidents in Ontario in 1938* (Toronto: King's Printer, 1939), 20, 44, 53; Thomas Gibson, Deputy Minister, Department of Lands, Forests and Mines, Ontario, *Eighteenth Annual Report of the Bureau of Mines, 1909* (Toronto: King's Printer, 1909), 68; Mine Inspection Branch Staff, *Mines Inspection Branch Annual Report 1970, Ontario Department of Mines Bulletin 170* (Toronto: Queen's Printer, 1971), 38; Mine Inspection Branch Staff, *Mines Inspection Branch Annual Report 1970, Ontario Department of Mines Bulletin 160* (Toronto: Queen's Printer, 1960), 54.

55 Steinberg, *Acts of God*; Colten, *Unnatural Metropolis*. See also Knowles, "Learning from Disaster?"

56 Richard, *Westray Story*; Tucker, "Road from Westray."

57 Corkill's assessment of mine accidents also included a dose of ethnocentrisim, as he blamed foreigners "lacking in sufficient intelligence" for poor scaling in the mines. His comments are contained in Thomas Gibson, Deputy Minister, Department of Lands, Forests and Mines, Ontario, *Eighteenth Annual Report of the Bureau of Mines, 1909*, 74–8, at 74.

58 Mark Aldrich has similarly argued in *Death Rode the Rails* that the prevalence of small workplace accidents in the American railway system made it easier for companies and regulators to render safety issues invisible or to blame individual workers rather than systemic failures of health and safety regulation.

BIBLIOGRAPHY

Archives

Ontario Department of Mines GeologyOntario website, www.hub.geologyontario.
mines.gov.on.ca/

Other Sources

Aldrich, Mark. *Death Rode the Rails: American Railroad Accidents and Safety,
1828–1965.* Baltimore: Johns Hopkins University Press, 2006.

Andrews, Thomas G. *Killing for Coal: America's Deadliest Labor War.* Cambridge,
MA: Harvard University Press, 2008.

Baldwin, Doug. "A Study in Social Control: The Life of the Silver Miner in
Northern Ontario." *Labour / Le Travail* 2 (1977): 79–106.

Baldwin, Douglas O., and David F. Duke. "'A Grey Wee Town': An Environmental
History of Early Silver Mining at Cobalt, Ontario." *Urban History Review* 34,
no. 1 (2005): 71–87.

Barnes, Michael. *Fortunes in the Ground: Cobalt, Porcupine and Kirkland Lake.*
Erin, ON: Boston Mills Press, 1986.

Belshaw, John Douglas. *Colonization and Community: The Vancouver Island Coalfield
and the Making of the British Columbian Working Class.* Montreal and Kingston:
McGill-Queen's University Press, 2002.

Benson, John "Mining Safety and Miners' Compensation in Great Britain,
1850–1900." In *Toward a Social History of Mining in the 19th and 20th Centuries:
Papers Presented to the International Mining History Congress, Bochum, Germany,
Sept 3–7, 1989,* 1026–38. Munich: C.H. Beck, 1992.

Buckley, Karen Lynne. "Death, Dying and Mourning in the Crowsnest Pass:
An Examination of Individual and Community Response to Danger and
Death in the Mines, 1902–1928." Master's thesis, University of Calgary, 2002.

Buckley, Karen Lynne. *Danger, Death and Disaster in the Crowsnest Pass Mines,
1902–1928.* Calgary: University of Calgary Press, 2004.

Clement, Wallace. *Hard-Rock Mining: Industrial Relations and Technological Changes
at INCO.* Toronto: McClelland & Stewart, 1981.

Colten, Craig E. *An Unnatural Metropolis: Wrestling New Orleans from Nature.*
Baton Rouge: Louisiana State University Press, 2005.

Cooter, Roger, and Bill Luckin, eds. *Accidents in History: Injuries, Fatalities and
Social Relations.* Amsterdam: Rodopi, 1997.

Corbeil, Matthew. "Mining Ontario: Corporate Power, the Mining Industry,
and Public Policy in Ontario." PhD diss., York University, 2020.

DeMont, John. *Coal Black Heart: The Story of Coal and the Lives It Ruled.*
Toronto: Doubleday Canada, 2009.

Dodd, Susan. "Blame and Causation in the Aftermath of Industrial Disasters: Nova Scotia's Coal Mines from 1858 to Westray." In *The Politics of Recognition and Response*, edited by Eric Tucker, 237–76. Amityville, NY: Baywoood Publishing Co., 2006.

Farrenkopf, Michael. "Accidents and Mining: The Problem of the Risk of Explosion in Industrial Coal Mining in Global Perspective." In *Making Sense of Mining History: Themes and Agendas*, edited by Stefan Berger and Peter Alexander, 193–211. London: Routledge, 2019.

Knowles, Scott Gabriel. "Learning from Disaster? The History of Technology and the Future of Disaster." *Technology and Culture* 55, no. 4 (2014): 773–84.

MacDowell, Laurel Sefton. "The Elliot Lake Uranium Miners' Battle to Gain Occupational Health and Safety Improvements, 1950–1980." *Labour/Le Travail* 69, no. 1 (Spring 2012): 91–118.

– *Remember Kirkland Lake: The Gold Miners' Strike of 1941–42*. Rev. ed. Toronto: Canadian Scholars' Press, 2001.

McAllister, Mary Louise. "Shifting Foundations in a Mature Staples Industry: A Political Economic History of Canadian Mineral Policy." *Canadian Political Science Review* 1, no. 1 (June 2007): 73–90

McAllister, Mary Louise, and Cynthia Alexander. *A Stake in the Future: Redefining the Canadian Mineral Industry*. Vancouver: UBC Press, 1997.

McCormack, A. Ross. *The Western Canadian Radical Movement, 1899–1919*. Toronto: University of Toronto Press, 1977.

McEvoy, Arthur F. "Working Environments: An Ecological Approach to Industrial Health and Safety." *Clio Medica* 41, no. 2 (1997): 59–89.

McKay, Ian. "Industry, Work and Community in the Cumberland Coalfields, 1848–1927." PhD diss., Dalhousie University, 1983.

– "The Realm of Uncertainty: The Experience of Work in the Cumberland Coal Mines, 1873–1927." *Acadiensis* 16, no. 1 (1986): 3–57.

– "Strikes in the Maritimes, 1901–1914." *Acadiensis* 13, no. 1 (1983): 3–46.

Nelles, H.V. *The Politics of Development: Forests, Mines and Hydro-Electric Power in Ontario, 1849–1941*. 2nd ed. Montreal: McGill-Queen's University Press, 2005.

Newsome, Eric. *The Coal Coast: The History of Coal Mining in B.C., 1835–1900*. Victoria, BC: Orca, 1989.

Nixon, Rob. *Slow Violence and the Environmentalism of the Poor*. Cambridge, MA: Harvard University Press, 2018.

Sandlos, John, and Arn Keeling. *Mining Country: A History of Canada's Mines and Miners*. Toronto: James Lorimer, 2021.

Steinberg, Ted. *Acts of God: The Unnatural History of Natural Disaster in America*. New York: Oxford University Press, 2000.

Sutherland, T.F. *Report on the Mining Accidents in Ontario in 1928*. Toronto: King's Printer, 1929.

Swift, Jamie. *The Big Nickel: Inco at Home and Abroad*. Kitchener, ON: Between the Lines, 1977.

Tucker, Eric. *Administering Danger in the Workplace: The Law and Politics of Occupational Health and Safety Regulation in Ontario, 1850–1914*. Toronto: University of Toronto Press, 1988.

– "Making the Workplace 'Safe' in Capitalism: The Enforcement of Factory Legislation in Nineteenth-Century Ontario." *Labour / Le Travail* 21, no. 21 (1988): 45–85.

– "The Road from Westray: A Predictable Path to Disaster?" *Acadiensis* 28, no. 1 (1998.): 132–9.

Whiteside, James. *Regulating Danger: The Struggle for Mine Safety in the Rocky Mountain Coal Industry*. Lincoln: University of Nebraska Press, 1990.

Wood, J.C.E. "Discovering the Ontario Inquest." *Osgood Hall Law Journal* 5, no. 2 (1967): 243–66.

Yudelman, David. *Canadian Mineral Policy Formulation: A Case Study of the Adversarial Process*. Kingston: Centre for Resource Studies, Queen's University, 1984.

3

Coroner Morton Shulman versus Dr Edward Shouldice

Medical Malpractice in 1960s Canada

R. Blake Brown

Patient safety has been defined as "the reduction of risk of unnecessary harm associated with healthcare to an acceptable minimum."[1] In the twenty-first century, the patient safety movement in medical practice and education has in Canada and elsewhere included significant study of contemporary accidental injury in medical care.[2] The relevant history of the previous century has been less studied.

In Ontario in the mid-1960s, the muckraking chief coroner of Toronto, Dr Morton Shulman, and the well-known hernia specialist, Dr Edward Earle Shouldice, locked horns over the quality of medical care needed to prevent unnecessary deaths. The battle between the two men started in 1963, when a patient, Horace Burnett, aged seventy-one, died at the Shouldice clinic after undergoing a hernia procedure. Shulman took part in the resulting coroner's inquest, which recommended that Shouldice reform his medical practice to prevent future deaths. Shouldice, however, steadfastly refused to undertake these changes and successfully challenged the legality of the inquest. Shulman nevertheless pressed Shouldice to undertake the inquest recommendations. Shouldice responded by asking the Ontario attorney general and the premier to order Shulman to stand down. This appeal to provincial authorities, though successful, eventually led Shulman to publicly allege political interference. Examining this battle between Shulman and Shouldice highlights how law and legal institutions contributed to Canadians' understanding of what was an accident and what was careful medical care. It also shows how medical professionals, for financial reasons and out of concerns to protect reputations, sometimes fiercely resisted efforts to mitigate risk.

In exploring this subject, this chapter contributes to the history of accidental injury in health care including the historiography on medical malpractice law in Canada. The question of how the law determined where, how, and why medical professionals would be held legally accountable for poor medical outcomes has received relatively little attention.[3] In addition, historians have largely overlooked the operation of the coroner system in investigating suspicious deaths in the twentieth century.[4] The battle between Shulman and Shouldice illustrates several trends in the institutional and legal responses to allegations of medical mistakes. First, the high bar established by the civil courts to successfully sue a doctor for malpractice motivated a desire to use alternative avenues to pursue concerns with poor treatment. The coroner system provided one such avenue, particularly if the coroner took an aggressive stance to investigations. Second, steps that might avert preventable deaths were frequently weighed against the cost and inconvenience of such measures. Third, physicians' and surgeons' ability to defend themselves against claims of their legal responsibility for accidental injuries or deaths highlighted the uneven financial resources, social standing, and knowledge of the parties that allowed medical professionals to avoid many deaths and injuries being defined as requiring compensation or changes in medical practice. These factors contributed to what the editors of this volume identify as the "typically slow and incomplete" efforts of the Canadian state and court system to mitigate risk.[5]

In shedding light on the fight between Shulman and Shouldice, I draw upon sources held at the Archives of Ontario, including the transcript of the coroner's inquest into the death of Burnett and the jury's verdict, as well as correspondence between Shouldice, Shulman, and various government officials. Published materials employed include medical journals, news-paper reports, legal publications, legislation, and the report of a royal commission that examined Shulman's allegations of political interference.

SHOULDICE CLINIC AND HERNIA SURGERY

Horace Leslie Burnett, seventy-one, was not worried. The long-time butcher was to have a hernia operation at Toronto's internationally famous Shouldice Surgery on 10 July 1963. "He thought there'd be nothing to it and wanted to drive himself there," his wife, Annie, later recalled.[6] Burnett walked into the operating room. The procedure, done under local anesthet-ic, lasted two and a half hours, after which he walked back to his recovery room. The surgery was successful in repairing his hernia, but a few hours later he was dead.

Burnett's confidence probably stemmed from the reputation of Edward Earle Shouldice and the other doctors at his hospitals. Born in Ontario in 1890, Shouldice moved with his family in 1901 to Alberta. He completed medical school at the University of Toronto in 1916. After graduating, he went to Europe to join the war effort. Following his return, he served as a demonstrator in anatomy at the University of Toronto medical school. In 1930, he became the head of the Outpatient Department at the Toronto General Hospital and began investigating the disappointing results of hernia surgeries. A hernia is a displacement and protrusion of an internal organ through the lining of a cavity in the body. Although surgeons had completed procedures to address hernias for decades, many patients suf-fered recurrences, infections, and postoperative issues such as pneumonia and blood clots. During World War II, when Shouldice served as a war-time consulting surgeon to the Canadian army, he was concerned about the number of men rejected for service because they suffered from hernias. He began operating on men with hernias wanting to join the military and in doing so pioneered methods that eventually made him famous.

In 1945, Shouldice founded a private hospital at 626 Church Street in Toronto, where he focused on treating hernias. He opened a second hos-pital in 1963 in a large three-storey house on Bayview Avenue in Thornhill. He and his staff substantially reduced the rate of hernia recurrence. He innovated in using local anesthesia during hernia repairs, thus allowing for the procedures in a day-surgery setting, and emphasized the importance of ambulation immediately after surgeries; usually his patients walked back to their recovery rooms. This was a marked departure from traditional practice in which patients were confined to their beds for days, sometimes leading to deaths from pulmonary embolisms. Shouldice also took aggressive measures to prevent infections. He travelled extensively to lecture and demonstrate his techniques.[7] By all accounts, he and his hospitals were successful. Still, Horace Burnett was dead: what happened, and was his death a preventable accident?

MORTON SHULMAN AND THE CORONER SYSTEM

The Ontario Coroners Act required Burnett's death to be reported to a coroner. The act dictated that everyone who knew of a death in certain circumstances notify the coroner, including situations that suggested "negligence" or "malpractice" or occasions when a person died "suddenly or unexpectedly." The coroner took possession of the body of the deceased and conducted "further investigation" to determine whether an inquest was necessary.[8] This preliminary inquiry often ended the investigation, but a coroner who believed further inquiries were necessary could issue a warrant for an inquest, which was conducted by the coroner and five jurors. Coroners did not conduct autopsies (pathologists did autopsies), but coroners and juries determined when, where, and how a person died. The coroner could demand the presence of witnesses to be questioned by the jurors, coroner, or, if present, crown attorney. The regular rules of evidence used in court did not apply in a coroner's inquest. At the end of the inquest, the coroner summed up the evidence to the jury, and the jury then came up with a verdict concerning the cause of death. By the early 1960s, coroners' juries in Ontario often made recommendations meant to improve public safety, although these findings were not binding on individuals, organizations, or the government.[9] The discretionary aspects built into the system (such as when to hold an inquest, what witnesses to call, how to question witnesses, and how to sum up evidence) allowed an aggressive coroner to pursue public-safety reforms.

Morton Shulman was intent on using the coroner system to improve public safety. Born into a Jewish family in Toronto in 1925, Shulman graduated from medical school at the University of Toronto in 1948. He established a busy family practice in Toronto's west end, where he offered services to the area's diverse ethnic communities. In 1952, he became one of Toronto's many coroners. Coroners were paid on a fee-for-service basis and usually completed this work as a supplement to their regular practice. Shulman kept a low profile as a coroner, but that changed after he became Toronto's chief coroner in 1963. He used the coroner system (and the press) in fights with doctors, hospitals, government officials, politicians, and medical regulators. His actions angered many, who accused him of seeking attention and caring little for the reputational harm experienced when he drew attention to questionable medical care. His term as Toronto's chief coroner was short-lived, as the Ontario government dismissed him in 1967. He went on to become a New Democratic Party member of the Ontario legislature, serving from 1967 to 1975, and then hosted a talk show on CityTV, *The Shulman File*. He was also a successful investor and a best-selling author on how to invest in stocks and art. He was appointed to the Order of Canada in 1993 and died in 2000.[10]

As I have explored elsewhere, Shulman used the position of Toronto's chief coroner to urge policy changes to improve public safety, not just to explain the cause of deaths.[11] For example, he encouraged changes in automobile design to protect drivers and passengers and sought to improve safety at construction sites. To publicize his work, he produced an annual report of the coroner system in Toronto, in which he pushed his policy beliefs and criticized people and organizations that impeded his initiatives. He also examined deaths that might have resulted from medical malpractice: cases of children who died during or after tonsillectomies, for example, and patients treated with ineffective cancer serums. He often accused medical professionals of failing to provide careful care and for participating in a "conspiracy of silence" by refusing to give evidence about malpractice by other doctors. This was important because unlike other areas of tort law altered by statute (such as the law of workplace accidents discussed by Auger-Day in this volume), common law rules still shaped medical malpractice litigation. Patients wishing to sue a doctor for negligence had to prove that the doctor had failed to meet the required standard of care, which was defined as the skill and care offered by the ordinary competent doctor. A bad result in and of itself did not establish a failure to meet the standard of care. To prove that a doctor's treatment had fallen short of the standard usually required a patient to get expert testimony from doctors who would define the appropriate standard of care and then testify that the doctor had failed to meet that standard. These hurdles contributed to a very low rate of successful lawsuits; moreover, many physicians belonged to the Canadian Medical Protective Association, an organization that pooled resources to help defend against malpractice claims.[12]

THE CORONER'S INQUEST INTO BURNETT'S DEATH

Coroner Dr Elie Cass investigated Burnett's death and decided that an inquest should be held. Inquests were open to the public, and the investigation of Burnett's care at the Shouldice Hospital attracted media coverage. The inquest took place over two days in September 1963. Dr Cass presided over the inquest, though he was joined by Dr Shulman. Twenty witnesses appeared. As in all coroner's inquests, an important witness – the dead patient – was unavailable, and thus the jury's decision and recommendations would be based largely on the evidence of doctors and nurses who worked at the Shouldice Hospital, as well as on the testimony of expert witnesses brought before the inquest. Crown Attorney William MacVannell conducted much of the questioning of the witnesses, although at various times Dr Cass and Dr Shulman also asked questions, as did some jurors. A pathologist reported on his autopsy of Burnett, and a police detective entered into evidence pictures of the hospital and its equipment.

Witnesses discussed the care given to Burnett. These included Burnett's surgeon, Dr Nicholas Obney, and Dr Byrnes Shouldice (Earl Shouldice's son), who assisted in the operation. Earle Shouldice, who had joined the surgery when it took longer than anticipated, also testified. Further witnesses included Dr Alfred Browne, who conducted the preoperative examination of Burnett, and several nurses employed at Shouldice Surgery. Expert witnesses gave evidence that either supported or criticized the care provided to Burnett. Shouldice was represented by lawyer Nathan Phillips,

who had served as mayor of Toronto from 1955 to 1962. Phillips's participation was unusual, in that parties in such inquests had no legal right to
question witnesses or have counsel. However, Phillips asked permission
to participate because Shouldice and his clinic were "world-famous and his
reputation may be affected by this Inquest."[13] He was permitted to query
witnesses, though Shulman and Cass frequently chided him for attempting to ask "questions" that were actually efforts to give evidence himself.[14]

The inquest provided extensive details of Burnett's treatment. Burnett
had undergone hernia surgery in 1946, but a recurrence sent him to
Shouldice Surgery on 8 July 1963. Dr Byrnes Shouldice examined Burnett,
and a surgery to address the hernia was scheduled in August. However,
Burnett began to suffer more pain in the affected area, and reported vom-
iting on 9 July. As a result, on the morning of 10 July, he returned to the
Shouldice hospital at 626 Church Street. Dr Browne examined Burnett
and determined that the condition of the hernia had become critical. Some
basic tests were conducted, including taking Burnett's temperature, blood
pressure, and pulse and listening to his lungs, as well as a urinalysis.[15]
The doctor who would undertake the surgery, Dr Obney, consulted with
Shouldice, and they decided that an operation should be conducted right
away. Obney was an experienced surgeon, having worked at Shouldice
Surgery since 1946. (He would go on to complete more than 32,000 hernia operations by the time he retired in 1988.)[16] With Dr Byrnes Shouldice
assisting, Obney began Burnett's surgery at 3:00 p.m. Burnett received a
sleeping pill, the painkiller Demerol, and a local anesthetic, Novocaine. A
registered nurse, Kate Brawn, monitored Burnett's condition, while a second nurse, Elizabeth Brown, handled instruments. The procedure proved
complicated, and Earle Shouldice came to assist. The bowel was strangulated as it protruded through the hernia, cutting off blood to the affected area.
The surgeons also had difficulty putting the bowel back in place. While a
normal hernia procedure took forty minutes to complete, the operation on
Burnett dragged on to two and half hours.

As was the usual practice at Shouldice Surgery, Burnett walked back
to his recovery room after the completion of the operation. He initially
seemed fine, but just after 9:00 p.m., the duty nurse, Mary Fowler, discovered that he was bleeding from the nose and mouth, had poor colour, and

was having trouble breathing. She started Burnett on oxygen and gave him an injection of coramine, a respiratory stimulant.[17] She then called another Shouldice Surgery doctor, Aleksander Georgievski, who set out to the Church Street location to help, arriving in twenty or twenty-five minutes. Burnett, however, died soon after Dr Georgievski arrived. A pathologist pointed in his autopsy to three factors in Burnett's death: acute coronary insufficiency (i.e., heart disease); congestion and oedema of the lungs (i.e., excess fluid in the lungs); and pneumococcal pneumonia. The pathologist's identification of these underlying health issues raised the question of whether Shouldice Surgery should have ensured that Burnett was healthy enough to undergo a lengthy hernia operation.

The key issues at the inquest became whether Shouldice Surgery could or should have prevented Burnett's death by providing better preoperative screening and post-operative care. As well, the inquest investigated whether the hospital should alter the equipment available during surgery in case of an emergency, and whether it enlisted the appropriate surgical staff. This emphasis made the investigation more a consideration of possible nonfeasance (a failure to act) by Shouldice Surgery than malfeasance (an act of wrongdoing). The hospital's doctors and nurses testified to their qualifications, skill, and care, sometimes appearing defensive of the hospital and its reputation. The doctors defended themselves by pointing to the thousands of procedures conducted at their hospital and the small number of deaths. Dr Obney, for example, said that he had completed 13,800 hernia procedures; he explained the rationales for the hospital's procedures and asserted that there had been very few patient deaths.[18] Shouldice staff reported having completed 42,000 operations and stated that only eleven patients had died under their care. The invocation of statistics shedding light on the probability of patient death was meant to suggest that Shouldice Surgery's quality of care was acceptable. It did not, however, answer the question of whether Burnett's death could have been prevented.

The inquest questioned whether Shouldice Surgery had completed a sufficient preoperative examination of Burnett. The staff reported that Burnett had shown no evidence of illnesses prior to the surgery other than the hernia. Dr Browne claimed the pre-op examination was acceptable, though he admitted that that he had mostly conducted a chest exam and taken Burnett's blood pressure. Dr Cass asked questions that elicited Browne to confirm that he had not done blood tests nor requested an electrocardiogram or chest x-rays.[19] Dr Cass pressed Dr Browne on the extent of the pre-op exam:

> DR CASS: "How old was this man?"
> DR BROWNE: "He was seventy-one."
> DR CASS: "And you knew this man required surgery?"
> DR BROWNE: "Yes."
> DR CASS: "You didn't think it was necessary to do as complete an examination as possible?"
> DR BROWNE: "I felt I did a complete examination."
> DR CASS: "In other words you think listening to a man's chest and heart and a few other simple tests are all that is necessary preoperatively?"[20]

This questioning took aim at the fact that Burnett was suffering from pneumonia and heart disease and thus at risk of suffering a poor outcome. The Shouldice Surgery doctors responded that further tests would not have exposed his underlying health issues. Moreover, they claimed that even if those health issues had been discovered, the fact that Burnett's bowel was strangulated made it imperative that the surgery take place immediately.

One of the expert witnesses who defended Burnett's treatment provided evidence that undermined the practice and equipment of Shouldice Surgery. Dr Roderick A. Gordon, a professor of anesthesiology at the University of Toronto, stated it was reasonable to use local anesthetics for hernia procedures. However, under questioning from Dr Shulman, Gordon stated that lab work should be done for every patient undergoing the kind of hernia operation done by Shouldice Surgery.[21] The inquest also brought to light that Shouldice Surgery operated without some staff and equipment useful in some emergency situations. For example, the hospital did not employ an anesthetist; rather, regular doctors delivered anesthetics, and a nurse supervised the condition of the patient during the surgery. This information led to questioning to determine whether a two-and-a-half-hour hernia surgery was a "major" surgery that necessitated the presence of a trained anesthetist. Moreover, Shouldice Surgery did not employ a resident doctor, in part because of the small size of the hospital and also because of the belief that doctors on call could quickly get to the hospital if a patient's health suddenly deteriorated. The questioning also highlighted that Shouldice Surgery did not have some equipment such as intubation tubes that might be used in rare circumstances.[22]

An expert witness, general surgeon Donald Cameron, harshly criticized Shouldice Surgery's facilities, staffing, and procedures. For example, Dr Cameron asserted that local anaesthetics were not generally used in Canada for "major surgeries." "In most hospitals – in all hospitals I think an anesthetist is in attendance at major operations," he testified, and in his view hernia surgery was "a major procedure and I think perhaps it was injudicious not to have an anesthetist in attendance."[23] Cameron believed that having a nurse monitor Burnett's condition during the surgery was insufficient. Cameron also stated that laboratory tests should have been done to determine Burnett's condition prior to surgery and that intubation tubes and other equipment should be available during any major surgery.[24] Cameron also noted that Shouldice Surgery had sought accreditation from the Ontario Hospital Services Commission but that it was not granted, thus casting doubt in the jury's mind about the quality of the hospital.[25]

The aggressive questioning of Shouldice and his staff sometimes elicited testy responses. For example, after coroner Cass asked Dr Obney why blood was not available to patients, Obney asserted his expertise: "I have operated on thirteen thousand eight hundred patients and I know that area like the back of my hand. If I ever got into a jackpot like that I would quit operating. Why do you think I have spent so much of my life doing hernias? Because I know every inch of that territory."[26] Earle Shouldice strongly defended the reputation of Shouldice Surgery and the treatment provided to Burnett. Shouldice explained that very serious cases were sometimes sent to the Toronto General Hospital, and thus his hospital should not be criticized for lacking the equipment of larger institutions. Phillips sought to establish Shouldice's expertise, asking him, "I know you are a modest person, Doctor, do you think there is anywhere – any surgeon anywhere who knows more about hernia surgery than you do?"

Shulman intervened before Shouldice could answer, acknowledging "I think we all agree Dr Shouldice knows more about hernia repair than anyone."[27] However, Shulman also showed frustration with Shouldice at times. For example, he said to Shouldice, "Would you just answer the questions, please, and not wander far afield."[28] Dr Shouldice eventually lashed out: "I thought this was an Inquest into the death of a man." He expressed his unhappiness at the focus of the inquest on his hospital: "I think that is out of the field of the Coroner."[29] Despite this criticism, Dr Shouldice also stated, "We are quite prepared to make any changes the jury might recommend" – though he would later backtrack from this commitment.[30]

Dr Cass and Dr Shulman summed up the evidence for the jury, offering harsh criticism of the treatment provided by Shouldice Surgery. Dr Cass noted that Burnett had been given a physical prior to the surgery "in which most attention was directed to the hernia, and little attention was paid to the possibility of co-existent disease of other parts of the body." Dr Cass told the jury, "Now usual tests done before an operation, for example blood tests, were not done."[31] Cass also questioned the wisdom of having a seventy-one-year-old patient walk back to his room after a two-and-a-half-hour surgery. He took aim at the lack of equipment such as breathing tubes, a blood bank, resuscitation tools, and x-ray equipment. He noted that Shouldice Surgery staff said this equipment was not necessary, but he disagreed, for "although most of these operations are routine and last about three-quarters of an hour, occasionally one can run into serious trouble and it is in just these cases that all means and equipment must be on hand to help the patient."[32] Concern with unusual cases also led Dr Cass to tell the jury that it would be preferable to have a resident in the hospital on call twenty-four hours a day. Dr Cass proposed several recommendations to the jury and told them that if they delivered a verdict including these recommendations, they "would be rendering the Shouldice Surgery a great service and they could then reach the high level of service and performance which I am certain they would wish to obtain."[33] Shulman also addressed the jury. Interestingly, he asserted that there was no evidence of any negligence or malpractice in Burnett's death, as the hernia surgery had been performed skilfully. However, he urged the jurors to offer recommendations that could prevent other deaths in the future, such as improvements in operating room equipment.[34]

The jury's verdict concluded that Burnett's cause of death was pneumonia, with pulmonary oedema and coronary heart disease as possible contributing factors. The jury made recommendations related to patient treatment at Shouldice's hospitals. These included that a "more intensive clinical and laboratory examination be undertaken," and that a certified anesthetist be available, particularly in emergency cases. And, the jury urged that a "complete emergency armamentarium" be available.[35] In regard to post-operative treatment, it recommended that a resident doctor be employed, if possible, to handle unforeseen emergencies. The jury's recommendations were meaningful, but for Shouldice they were potentially problematic, expensive to implement, and seemed to suggest that his hospital had provided poor care. The jury's decision risked creating a perception that Burnett's death had been an avoidable accident, even if Shulman had acknowledged that the death was not due to malpractice or negligence. This was a concern given that the coroner's inquest had attracted considerable media attention and Shouldice relied on paying patients for his and his staff's income.[36]

QUASHING OF THE INQUEST
AND SHULMAN'S RESPONSE

Rather than implement the recommendations of the coroner's jury, Shouldice sought to have the inquest quashed by the Ontario Supreme Court (now known as the Ontario Superior Court of Justice) on the ground that only one coroner should have been present at the inquest. The provincial Coroners Act stated that after a coroner issued a warrant to take possession of a body, "no other coroner shall issue a warrant or interfere in the case, except under the instructions of the Attorney General or the Crown attorney."[37] Since Shulman had participated in the inquest called by Dr Cass without the permission of the attorney general or crown attorney, Shouldice believed Shulman's participation should result in the quashing of the inquest. Shulman snapped back, expressing his disappointment that Shouldice was intent on "seeking legal loopholes" rather than "using these energies to improve the situation at his hospital as the jury recommend-ed."[38] Justice E.A. Richardson handed down a decision on 13 December 1963 quashing the coroner's inquest. Richardson found Shulman's participation in the inquest objectionable, saying, "I can't for the life of me see why Dr Shulman was at the inquest. He had no business to be there and he should know it. It was quite irregular." Even more pointedly, Justice Richardson said that Shulman "would be better advised to read the Coroner's Act than to be launching inquests into deaths at hospitals." Finally, he lauded Dr Shouldice's tremendous work and said that he did not believe any med-ical mistake had been made and advised that any issue regarding Burnett's treatment would better be taken up with the Ontario College of Physicians and Surgeons.[39]

Shulman refused to accept the court's decision and immediately con-tacted the provincial attorney general, Fred Cass, to explain that he had attended the Burnett inquest only because Shouldice's lawyer had request-ed his presence. He called Justice Richardson's comments about him a "personal attack" and said that if the government would not appeal the decision, he would like to personally hire a lawyer to do so.[40] Attorney General Cass, however, told Shulman that his office had determined that Justice Richardson's decision was correct. Cass also indicated that he did not approve of Shulman's plan to engage his own counsel for the purposes of launching an appeal. Shulman responded by saying that allowing the judgment to stand would create obstacles in the functioning of his office going forward. He nevertheless did not pursue an appeal himself, though he continued to complain about the attorney general's refusal to challenge the court decision.[41]

Dr Shouldice was not content with the court's judgment and harsh words for Shulman, and he expressed concerns about the dangers that inquests posed for the professional reputation of doctors. In early 1964, he wrote to the chief coroner of Ontario, Dr H. Beatty Cotnam, to draw his attention to the "real and potential dangers that may result from abuse of the functions of the Coroner's Court." While he saw value in coroner's inquests, Shouldice believed that any appearance before a coroner's jury "does carry the suggestion, to the lay mind, that these actions have at least been questionable." This could damage a doctor's reputation and livelihood, particularly since the news coverage was often "slanted toward the dramatic or the sensational rather than being prosaic and factual." He expressed frustration that the Burnett inquest had looked at his procedures and practice even though the cause of death was determined not to have been his fault. He also maintained that evidence that supported the work of his hospital had been ignored. His letter suggested that abuse of the coroner system could "only undermine the confidence of the public in doctors and hospitals, and impair the image of the medical profession as a whole in the eyes of the laity."[42]

Cotnam forwarded Shouldice's letter to Attorney General Cass, noting that it showed that Dr Shouldice was "still very upset about this matter," despite the quashing of the inquest. Cotnam also told the attorney general that in his view the Burnett inquest had been unnecessary and that there "appeared to be unnecessary publicity and persecution by two coroners for personal or other reasons of which I am not aware."[43]

Dr Shouldice also complained about his treatment at the inquest at a meeting of the Ontario Medical Association. The association subsequently undertook a report on the coroner system of Ontario, which offered several recommendations, including the creation of a system to remove coroners, that witnesses be allowed to have counsel, and that steps be taken to help protect the reputations of medical professionals.[44] Shouldice and Shulman both also took to the airwaves to express their divergent views about the staffing and procedures at Shouldice Surgery. In January 1964, both appeared on the CBC program the *Toronto Files*, and Shouldice declared that he would not implement the recommendations.[45] He also claimed that he had not requested that Shulman attend the inquest.

Justice Richardson's pointed judgment contributed to a government plan to abolish the position of chief coroner of Toronto.[46] Shulman publicly defended his participation in the Burnett inquest, saying that Nathan Phillips had requested his presence and that chief coroners of Ontario had in the past sat in on or taken over inquests.[47] The Toronto press came to Shulman's defence, lauding him as a crusading coroner willing to challenge the government, medical professionals, and hospitals to help protect the public. The *Toronto Daily Star* noted that doctors' organizations and hospitals got upset when Shulman ordered inquests into deaths, but concluded,

"We believe Dr Shulman is the kind of coroner the public needs, even if he is not the kind the attorney general's department wants."[48] The plan to abolish the post of position of chief coroner of Toronto was abandoned in the face of such defences.[49]

Shulman, however, refused to leave the Burnett issue alone, and at the end of 1964 attempted to get Shouldice to follow the recommendations contained in the quashed jury verdict. He wrote a letter to Shouldice saying that he believed that once an inquest was quashed, "it legally did not occur," and thus it "would have been quite proper for me to order Dr Cass to hold a new inquest in the case." He had not done this "in order to avoid further unfavourable publicity for your clinic" and because he hoped Shouldice would carry out the recommendations on his own accord. Shulman asked Shouldice which recommendations had been carried out, saying that he was "anxious to prevent future unnecessary mortality."[50] Shouldice did not respond, instead writing to Premier John Robarts, forwarding him a copy of Shulman's letter, which he felt was a "partly concealed threat to my institution." The direct contact with the premier highlighted how well-known physicians could employ social position to defend their interests. Shouldice believed Shulman's letter to be "quite irregular and the demands made are illegal" as the inquest had been quashed. He told the premier about the success of his clinic, for which he believed he "should be honoured and not brow-beaten by your self-appointed 'McCarthyite,' the Chief Coroner of Metropolitan Toronto." Shouldice believed some of his surgeons had become reluctant to take on difficult cases because they feared bad publicity and maintained that some patients had become fearful of surgery and thus suffered or died unnecessarily. Shouldice also contested Shulman's view that his work as coroner had not damaged the reputations of doctors or hospitals and asserted that doctors were "loath to argue with such a psychopathic personality who constantly publicizes himself as the great emancipator of the Medical Profession and Hospitals in Ontario." Dr Shouldice was offended that he had been publicly criticized by two coroners "who appear to be twenty years behind the times." He thus demanded that Shulman be removed "from his position of persecution."[51]

Attorney General Arthur Wishart then instructed Frank Wilson, the assistant deputy attorney general, to call Shulman to inform him that he should not harass Dr Shouldice. This did not deter Shulman. On 22 January 1965, Shulman again wrote to Shouldice, telling him that he was "disappointed that rather than make those simple changes at the clinic which could prevent future deaths, you would attempt to silence me through the Attorney General's Department." He said he would forgo calling another inquest if Shouldice committed to carrying out a portion of the jury's recommendations.[52] Shouldice again did not answer Shulman but wrote once more to the government to complain about Shulman. On 10 February, Attorney General Wishart told Shulman that his letters to Shouldice were inappropriate. Wishart reminded Shulman that the Ontario Supreme Court decision had quashed the recommendations of the coroner's jury and that Shulman's suggestion that he would hold a new inquest unless Shouldice complied with the recommendations "constitutes a threat." Such a "threat by a public servant to a responsible member of our society is, in my opinion, inexcusable, and is inconsistent with your duties as Chief Coroner."[53] Wishart also informed Shulman that he lacked the authority to call another inquest because the statute said that once any coroner issued a warrant for the body, only the attorney general or crown attorney could order another by a different coroner.[54] Shulman responded to Wishart by stating that the hospital accreditation officials had found Shouldice Surgery's facilities wanting and that he had thus "taken every possible effort" to urge Shouldice "to take the simple steps which could prevent future deaths." He further suggested that it should be "equally clear that this is my only interest and that I have tried my best to have these improvements made without any further public criticism of his hospital." Shulman expressed hope that Wishart would decide to cooperate with his efforts to "cut mortality at Shouldice Clinic."[55]

Dr Shouldice died in August 1965, meaning that Shulman would no longer be able to pressure him to change practice at his hospitals. Shouldice was lauded in the *Canadian Medical Association Journal* for his pioneering work in hernia treatment, though obituaries in Toronto's major dailies highlighted the recent inquest into Burnett's death and Shouldice's refusal to adopt the jury's recommendations.[56]

Shulman later claimed that the order not to open a new inquest into Burnett's death constituted improper political interference with his office.

After a series of run-ins with the government and the medical profession, Shulman was finally fired as Toronto's chief coroner in April 1967. He responded with a fusillade of public allegations suggesting coverups of medical errors and political interference. His claims attracted considerable press attention, leading Premier Robarts to appoint a royal commission to investigate. The province appointed Justice William D. Parker as sole commissioner.[57] Shulman prepared a lengthy brief for the commission laying out many allegations, including that Attorney General Wishart and Premier Robarts had tried to suppress the inquest into the death of Burnett. Shulman claimed that the attorney general had prevented him from appealing Justice Richardson's decision to quash the inquest verdict and said that the government had interfered in his efforts to improve safety at Shouldice Surgery. He called the attorney general's efforts to stop him contacting Dr Shouldice "inexplicable" and said that Wishart's actions "completely ignored the moral responsibility to patients using the Shouldice Clinic."[58] Shulman's secretary, Ann Worobec, testified that she had listened in on the call between Shulman and the assistant deputy attorney general, Frank Wilson, in which Wilson had told Shulman that his letters to Dr Shouldice led to the order for Shulman to stop making trouble.[59] Shulman's lawyer alleged that Premier Robarts and the attorney general's office had shown "complete indifference to the objective of protecting the public and reducing mortality" because of a "zealous concern to protect the pride of Dr Shouldice."[60] A lawyer for the Shouldice clinic responded by accusing Shulman of attempting to blackmail Dr Shouldice by threatening to start a new inquest. Burnett's son, Ross, said that the Burnett family believed Shulman had mishandled the inquest (which the family had never wanted) but that his father might have benefited from better post-operative care.[61]

The Parker commission dismissed all of Shulman's allegations and in doing so questioned his truthfulness, methods, and motivations. Parker devoted a chapter to the Shouldice affair in his final report, providing an overview of the correspondence between Shulman and the attorney general's office. He noted that Shulman told *The Toronto Files* that there was no reason to hold another inquest because "we already have all the facts" and said he believed Shouldice was competent.[62] Justice Parker concluded that Shulman's warnings that he would call a new inquest were efforts to "accomplish by threat what he could not accomplish legally," and that the Coroners Act only allowed the province's chief coroner, the attorney general, or a crown attorney to issue a warrant for a second inquest.[63] Parker damned Shulman, saying the threat to use adverse publicity through an inquest "does not conform to the standard of justice." It was "foreign to those basic principles which protect the rights of the individual."[64]

CONCLUSION

By the time the report of the Parker commission was released, Shulman had become a member of the Ontario Provincial Parliament. He lashed out at Justice Parker, calling the report a cover-up.[65] For its part, Shouldice Surgery continued its work. In 1970, the *Globe and Mail* published a celebratory feature on Shouldice's hernia treatment, reporting that none of the 25,000 patients operated on at the Shouldice hospitals since Burnett in 1963 had died.[66] This lack of deaths after 1963 perhaps shows that Shulman's concerns about public safety were unfounded – or, perhaps, the bad publicity received after Burnett's death led Shouldice Surgery to take more precautions with patients. If the latter, Shulman's actions may have helped mitigate risk by drawing public attention to the work of Shouldice's clinic and encouraging more vigilant care.

The controversy surrounding Burnett's death highlights the role of the law in helping to define what was, and was not, an accident in twentieth-century Canada. As the editors of this volume note, an accident is a "contested and evolving public-private category of misfortune where notions of responsibility and meaning play out in an emerging and evolving nation."[67] Malpractice law dictated that a doctor was liable for failing to provide treatment that met a standard of care understood as the skill and care offered by the ordinary competent doctor. In courts across Canada, judges and jurors wrestled with incidents of medical injuries and deaths and asked themselves if the poor outcome was an accident for which no medical professional could be blamed, or whether it resulted from failures to meet the accepted standard of care and thus constituted malpractice. In Burnett's case, Shulman asserted that the surgery had been completed skilfully, but the inquest cast doubt on whether the Shouldice Hospital had the right mix of staff and instruments needed to prevent unnecessary deaths in rare circumstances. The coroner system allowed for activist coroners like doctors Shulman and Cass to call for practice changes to limit such "accidental" deaths, even if hospitals could not be held liable under negligence law. The coroner's inquest system permitted the public and the media to attend and report on allegations of inadequate treatment, meaning that publicity could lead to changes in practice, even though Ontario jury verdicts contained recommendations, not binding orders. Shulman was dogged in pursuing possible instances of malpractice, and further research is needed to show whether coroners in other Canadian jurisdictions made similar efforts to highlight accidental medical deaths. Shouldice contested the portrayal of his clinic's work as inadequate. He leaned on his standing within the medical profession and the public to strongly assert that his experience, professional status, and record meant that he should not have to abide by the views of "lay" jurors untrained in medical practice. His status allowed him to effectively lobby the provincial government to control Shulman. He also used the law of judicial review to quash the findings of the coroner's inquest as a means of erasing the jurors' questioning of his methods. As a result, the official record says that Burnett died of natural causes and his death was thus an "accident" that could not have been prevented.

NOTES

1 World Health Organization, *Conceptual Framework for the International Classification for Patient Safety*, Version 1, January 2009, https://iris.who.int/bitstream/handle/10665/70882/WHO_IER_PSP_2010.2_eng.pdf?sequence=1.

2 Baker et al., "Canadian Adverse Events Study"; Hayward and Hofer, "Estimating Hospital Deaths Due to Medical Errors"; Canadian Patient Safety Institute, *Surgical Safety in Canada*; Canadian Patient Safety Institute, *Measuring Patient Harm in Canadian Hospitals*.

3 For existing studies of medical malpractice, see Mitham, "'Very Truly and Undisturbedly Yours'"; Brown, "Master Mariner's Left Testicle"; Brown, "Canada's First Malpractice Crisis"; Brown and Hudak, "'Have You Any Recollection.'" For examples of American studies of malpractice, see de Ville, *Medical Malpractice in Nineteenth-Century America*;

Burns, "Malpractice Suits in American Medicine before the Civil War"; Mohr, "American Medical Malpractice Litigation"; Hogan, *Unhealed Wounds*.

4 Existing work on coroners focuses on the nineteenth century. See Miron, "Suicide, Coroner's Inquests"; St-Denis, "London District and Middlesex County, Ontario, Coroner's Inquests"; Leslie, "Reforming the Coroner"; Duffin, "In View of the Body of Job Broom."

5 John Douglas Belshaw et al., "Introduction: Framing an Accidental Past," in this volume, 21.

6 "Widow Recalls Painful Memories of Husband's Death," *Toronto Daily Star*, 6 May 1967.

7 Ibid.; Bendavid, "Biography: Edward Earle Shouldice"; "Obituaries," *Canadian Medical Association Journal* 93 (16 October 1965), 888; Rutkow, "Hernia Surgery in the Mid 19th Century."

8 Coroners Act, Revised Statutes of Ontario 1960, c.69, ss.7(1), 10(1); An Act to Amend the Coroners Act, S.O. 1961, c.12, s.3.

9 Wood, "Discovering the Ontario Inquest."

10 Alan Edmonds, "He's Too Rich to Be Cautious, Too Popular to Be Fired," *Maclean's*, 19 June 1965; Shulman, *Anyone Can Make a Million*; Shulman, *Anyone Can Make Big Money Buying Art*; Shulman, *Member of the Legislature*; Dianne Saxe, "Lives Lived: Morton Shulman," *Globe and Mail*, 5 October 2000; Nicolaas van Rijn, "Man of Many Hats Morton Shulman Dies at 75," *Toronto Star*, 19 August 2000.

11 Brown, "'Architects' Mistakes Should Be Covered with Ivy and Doctors' with Sod.'"

12 Meredith, *Malpractice Liability*; Brown, "'Architects' Mistakes.'"

13 Proceedings of an Inquest into the Death of Horace Leslie Burnett, transcript, Sr, 3, September 1963, RG 33, series G-3, box 32, file 32.8, Archives of Ontario (AO).

14 "Ex-Mayor Appears at Inquest as Counsel for Dr Shouldice," *Globe and Mail*, 6 September 1963; "Probe Hernia Death at Hospital," *Toronto Daily Star*, 6 September 1963.

15 Proceedings of an Inquest into the Death of Horace Leslie Burnett, Sr, 20–3.

16 Bill Gladstone, "The Duke of Hernia Surgery," *Globe and Mail*, 17 April 2003.

17 Proceedings of an Inquest into the Death of Horace Leslie Burnett, Sr, 134–6.

18 Ibid., 102.

19 Ibid., 48.

20 Ibid., 49.

21 Ibid., 166–7.

22 Ibid., 66, 116–17.

23 Ibid., 80, 81.

24 Ibid., 81–4.

25 Ibid., 92.

26 Ibid., 126.

27 Ibid., 155.

28 Ibid., 156.

29 Ibid., 159.

30 Ibid., 163.

31 Ibid., 174.

32 Ibid., 175.

33 Ibid., 176.

34 Ibid., 177–8.

35 Ibid., 180.

36 "Overhaul Hospital Practices: Jury," *Globe and Mail*, 11 September 1963; "Jury Urges 5 Changes after Clinic Death," *Toronto Daily Star*, 11 September 1963.

37 Coroners Act, R.S.O. 1960, c.69, s.10(3).

38 "Doctor Seeks to Quash Inquest Urging Change," *Globe and Mail*, 29 November 1963.

39 "Quashes Inquest Rebukes Coroner," *Toronto Daily Star*, 13 December 1963. See also "Chief Coroner Battles Pressure to Cut Hospital Death Inquests," *Globe and Mail*, 14 December 1963; "Court Quashes Hospital Inquest," *Windsor Star*, 14 December 1963.

40 Morton Shulman to Fred Cass, 14 December 1963, RG-33, series G-3, box 30, file 30.2, AO.

41 Fred Cass to Morton Shulman, 19 December 1963, RG-33, series G-3, box 30, file 30.2, AO; Morton Shulman to Fred Cass, 20 December 2963, RG-33, series G-3, box 30, file 30.2, AO.

42 E.E. Shouldice to H.B. Cotnam, 13 January 1964, RG-33, Series G-3, box 32, file 32.6, AO.

43 H.B. Cotnam to Attorney General, 17 January 1964, RG-33, Series G-3, box 32, file 32.6, AO.

44 "Report of the Special Committee on the Coroners Act," *Ontario Medical Review* 33, no. 5 (May 1966): 369–75.

45 "Private Hospital Owner to Ignore Jury's Plea," *Toronto Daily Star*, 22 January 1964; "Will Ignore Jury's View: Shouldice," *Globe and Mail*, 22 January 1964.

46 Geoffrey Stevens, "Will the Outspoken Coroner Lose His Job?," *Globe and Mail*, 16 December 1963.

47 Shulman, *Metropolitan Toronto Coroner's Office Statistical Report*. Frank Wilson took offence to Shulman's effort to vindicate his participation in the Burnett inquest, telling Attorney General Wishart that chief coroners had only been involved in past inquests after the writ of warrant of possession of the body with the approval of the attorney general or crown attorney. Frank L. Wilson to A. Wishart, 10 December 1964, RG 33, series G-3, box 29, file 29.2, AO.

48 "The Embarrassing Coroner," *Toronto Daily Star*, 28 January 1964. Also see "The New Broom," *Globe and Mail*, 29 January 1964.

49 Shulman, *Coroner*, 36–9.

50 Morton Shulman to E.E. Shouldice, 16 December 1964, RG 33, series G-3, box 29, file 29.5, AO.

51 E.E. Shouldice to John P. Robarts, 18 January 1965, RG 33, series G-3, box 29, file 29.5, AO.

52 Morton Shulman to E.E. Shouldice, 22 January 1965, RG 33, series G-3, box 29, file 29.6, AO.

53 A.A. Wishart to Morton Shulman, 10 February 1965, RG 33, series G-3, box 29, file 29.6, AO.

54 Coroners Act, R.S.O. 1960, c.69, s.10(3).

55 Morton Shulman to A.A. Wishart, 16 February 1965, RG 33, series G-3, box 30, file 30.2, AO.
56 "Obituaries," *Canadian Medical Association Journal* 93, no. 16 (16 October 1965), 888; "Obituaries," *Canadian Medical Association Journal* 93, no. 23 (4 December 1965), 1233; "Surgeon Won Renown as Hernia Authority," *Globe and Mail*, 23 August 1965; "Dr E.E. Shouldice, Famed Hernia Specialist," *Toronto Daily Star*, 23 August 1965.
57 "Is Queen's Park Hiding Incompetence?," *Toronto Daily Star*, 10 April 1967; Ontario, Order-in-Council 1456/67 (13 April 1967), file 28.5, box 28, series G-3, RG33, AO; "Robarts Orders Shulman Inquiry," *Toronto Telegram*, 10 April 1967; Ontario, *Report of the Royal Commission to Investigate Allegations Relating to Coroners' Inquests*, v–viii.
58 "Robarts Named in 'Suppression,'" *Toronto Telegram*, 6 May 1967. Also see "Shulman Says Robarts Vetoed New Inquest," *Toronto Daily Star*, 6 May 1967; "Shulman Says He Was Told Robarts Barred One Probe," *Globe and Mail*, 6 May 1967.
59 "Secretary Backs Shulman on Surgery Clinic Warning," *Globe and Mail*, 3 August 1967; "Secretary Says Shulman Told Don't Make Trouble," *Ottawa Journal*, 3 August 1967.
60 "Wishart-Robarts Smear Charged," *Windsor Star*, 22 August 1967. See also "Robarts, Wishart Criticized," *Ottawa Citizen*, 22 August 1967; "Robarts' Role Denounced by Jolliffe," *Globe and Mail*, 22 August 1967.
61 "Surgeon's Letter Labels Shulman as Psychopathic," *Globe and Mail*, 2 August 1967; "Doctor Labels Shulman 'Psychopathic' Person," *Ottawa Citizen*, 2 August 1967; "Dead Doctor Branded Shulman 'a McCarthyite,'" *Toronto Daily Star*, 2 August 1967; "MD's Letter Calls Shulman 'Psychopathic Personality,'" *Ottawa Journal*, 2 August 1967.
62 Ontario, *Report of the Royal Commission to Investigate Allegations Relating to Coroners' Inquests*, 55.
63 Ibid., 56.
64 Ibid., 58.
65 "Shulman Calls Report Slanderous Document," *Globe and Mail*, 23 February 1968; "Charges Parker Probe a 'Whitewash' Job," *Globe and Mail*, 24 February 1968.
66 Joan Hollobon, "After the Operation ... a Nice Walk," *Globe and Mail*, 19 June 1970.
67 Belshaw et al., "Framing an Accidental Past," 11.

BIBLIOGRAPHY

Archives

Archives of Ontario, Toronto

Newspapers and Periodicals

Maclean's
Ottawa Citizen

Ottawa Journal
Toronto Daily Star
Globe and Mail (Toronto)
Toronto Telegram
Windsor Star

Other Sources

Baker, G. Ross, Peter G. Norton, Virginia Flintoft, Régis Blais, Adalsteinn Brown, Jafna Cox, Ed Etchells, et al. "The Canadian Adverse Events Study: The Incidence of Adverse Events among Hospital Patients in Canada." *Canadian Medical Association Journal* 170, no. 11 (25 May 2004): 1678–86.

Bendavid, Robert. "Biography: Edward Earle Shouldice (1890–1965)." *Hernia* 7, no. 4 (December 2003): 172–7.

Brown, R. Blake. "'Architects' Mistakes Should Be Covered with Ivy and Doctors' with Sod': Medical Malpractice, Morton Shulman, and the 'Conspiracy of Silence.'" *Canadian Historical Review* 102, no. 2 (2021): 255–78.

– "Canada's First Malpractice Crisis: Medical Negligence in the Late Nineteenth Century." *Osgoode Hall Law Journal* 54, no. 3 (2017): 777–803.

– "A Master Mariner's Left Testicle and the Law of Surgical Consent in Mid-20th-Century Canada." *Canadian Bulletin of Medical History* 36, no. 2 (2019): 255–80.

Brown, R. Blake, and Magen Hudak. "'Have You Any Recollection of What Occurred at All?': *Davis v. Colchester County Hospital* and the Medical Negligence in Interwar Canada." *Journal of the Canadian Historical Association*, n.s. 26, no. 2 (2015): 131–62.

Burns, Chester R. "Malpractice Suits in American Medicine before the Civil War." *Bulletin of the History of Medicine* 43, no. 1 (1969): 41–56.

Canadian Patient Safety Institute. *Measuring Patient Harm in Canadian Hospitals*. Ottawa: Canadian Institute for Health Information, 2016.

– *Surgical Safety in Canada: A 10-Year Review of cmpa and hiroc Medico-Legal Data*. 2016. https://www.patientsafetyinstitute.ca/en/toolsResources/Surgical-Safety-in-Canada/Documents/Surgical%20Safety%20in%20Canada%20-%20Detailed%20Analysis%20Report.pdf.

De Ville, Kenneth Allen. *Medical Malpractice in Nineteenth-Century America: Origins and Legacy*. New York: New York University Press, 1990.

Duffin, Jacalyn. "In View of the Body of Job Broom: A Glimpse of the Medical Knowledge and Practice of John Rolph." *Canadian Bulletin of Medical History* 7, no. 1 (1990): 9–30.

Hayward, Rodney A., and Timothy P. Hofer. "Estimating Hospital Deaths Due to Medical Errors: Preventability Is in the Eye of the Reviewers." *Journal of the American Medical Association* 286, no. 4 (25 July 2001): 415–20.

Hogan, Neal C. *Unhealed Wounds: Medical Malpractice in the Twentieth Century.* New York: LFB Publishing, 2003.

Leslie, Myles. "Reforming the Coroner: Death Investigation Manuals in Ontario, 1863–1894." *Ontario History* 100, no. 2 (2008): 221–38.

Meredith, William C.J. *Malpractice Liability – of Doctors and Hospitals (Common Law and Quebec Law).* Toronto: Carswell, 1956.

Miron, Janet. "Suicide, Coroner's Inquests, and the Parameters of Compassion in Ontario, 1830–1900." *Histoire Sociale/Social History* 47, no. 95 (2014): 577–99.

Mitham, Peter J. "'Very Truly and Undisturbedly Yours': Joseph Workman and a Verdict of Malpractice against John Galbraith Hyde." *Canadian Bulletin of Medical History* 13, no. 1 (1996): 139–49.

Mohr, James C. "American Medical Malpractice Litigation in Historical Perspective." *Journal of the American Medical Association* 283, no. 13 (2000): 1731–7.

Ontario. *Report of the Royal Commission to Investigate Allegations Relating to Coroners' Inquests.* Toronto: Queen's Printer, 1968.

Rutkow, Ira M. "Hernia Surgery in the Mid 19th Century." *Archives of Surgery* 137, no. 8 (2002): 973–4.

Shulman, Morton. *Anyone Can Make a Million.* Toronto: McGraw-Hill, 1966.

– *Anyone Can Make Big Money Buying Art.* New York: Macmillan, 1977.

– *Coroner.* Toronto: Fitzhenry & Whiteside, 1975.

– *Member of the Legislature.* Toronto: Fitzhenry & Whiteside, 1979.

– *Metropolitan Toronto Coroner's Office Statistical Report, 1963.* Toronto, 1963.

St-Denis, Guy. "The London District and Middlesex County, Ontario, Coroner's Inquests, 1831–1900." *Archivaria* 31 (Winter 1990–91): 142–53.

Wood, J.C.E. "Discovering the Ontario Inquest." *Osgoode Hall Law Journal* 5, no. 2 (1967): 243–66.

4

Pedalling Acceptable Losses

Narratives of Cyclist Accidents in Vancouver, BC

John Douglas Belshaw

Cycling accidents will happen, whether one is competing, commuting, or casually riding about. Historically, however, the character of the bicycle accident – how it happens, how it is understood, how it is treated, and how it is narrated – has changed dramatically. An examination of newspaper accounts of accidents involving bicycles in Vancouver in three periods shows continuity and, also, ruptures set in changing social and technological contexts. Prior to World War I, ca. 1886 to ca. 1914, the emergent city was dominated politically and demographically by adult white male settlers, and its roads saw the golden age of "ordinary" bicycles and their replacement by "safety" bikes that increased accessibility to the sport/activity. The mid-century era (ca. 1940–60) sees the rise of the baby boom population and increased suburbanization, along with a multiplicity of children's and youth's bicycles. The final era – which I have called the "new wave" of the 1970s and '80s – brings the ten-speed bicycle and a more diverse cycling population involving more young adult men and women. These cross-generational comparisons are an advance on existing studies on accidents/collisions involving bicycles, which tend to focus on the ideals and experiences of one generation.[1]

This study complements Cameron Baldassarra's assessment, chapter 8 in this volume, of changing understandings of canoeing accidents over time. While the site and circumstances of cycling accidents in Vancouver

– like incidents along the rivers surveyed in Baldassarra's account – do not change much, the ways in which they are narrativized and interpreted do. In part, this reflects cycling's split personality as both a serious mode of transportation and a thrilling recreational pastime. Baldassarra's recreational canoeists occupy a space vacated by industrial users of the Petawawa River, and they situate their risks in the context of leisure time, not commuting or shifting goods. I argue here that historic forces of change frame accidents and responses to cycling dangers. In each period, accident reports in local newspapers underline distinct qualities. Some of the ascribed causes of mishaps are long-running, while new ones appear as old ones fade away; the solutions proposed to cycling dangers likewise include some hardy perennials and some telling innovations. Technological change is part of the story, but I maintain that these accounts and themes mostly reflect social power and inequalities as well as typologies associated with modernity. A turn-of-the-century cyclist was "thoroughly modern," turned out in bloomers and starched stand-up collars; a mid-century cyclist was a non-citizen casually dressed and playing with a toy; a 1970s cyclist was staring down "the man" and cycling (if not swimming) against the tide.

THE PRE-WAR AGE

A sensational cycling accident captured the front pages of Vancouver newspapers in late September 1900, when Miss Rachel Shannon, a pedestrian in her early fifties, was struck by a cyclist and killed while crossing a downtown street. The post-mortem identified the cause of death as a severe head injury, and an inquest was called the next day to determine whether the cyclist, Edward Blackmore, was guilty of "furious riding." The legal context in this case was city bylaw No. 258, which defined travelling "too fast" on a bicycle as movement in excess of eight miles per hour (about thirteen kilometres per hour). Most of the witnesses believed Blackmore was not moving faster than six miles per hour, although one disagreed. Having said that, moving "very fast, over six miles an hour" was still below the bylaw threshold.[2] In the end, it was determined that Blackmore was not a reckless "scorcher," and a verdict of "accidental death" was rendered. Only a few hours later, he and his father served as two of Miss Shannon's pallbearers.[3]

"Accidents" in this golden age of cycling essentially fell into three types: cyclists and things, cyclists and cyclists, and – the most numerous – cyclists and pedestrians. In 1896, the editor of the *Vancouver Daily World* noted that riders, too, fell into types. The "wabblers" were generally new (and implicitly male) riders of uncertain ability. The notorious "scorcher" was competent but dangerous. The local "wheelwoman" was closely related to the wabbler, though not to the scorcher. "Accidents with wabblers are looked upon as inevitable, and all injuries that occur from them which can be repaired by a blacksmith or a bottle of arnica are regarded as mere casualties incidental to wheeling. When a wheelwoman runs down a wheelman it is an unavoidable mishap. When a wheelman runs down a wheelwoman it is an unpardonable blunder. When two wheelwomen collide it proves to each that neither understands her sport, and is not yet educated for the road."[4] So long as the cyclists hurt only themselves or other cyclists, the accounts (though sometimes comical) were rarely critical. For example, the *Daily World* reported in 1891 that "Fred. Turner was seriously injured by falling off his bicycle this morning. His injuries are about the head and may be dangerous." In October 1903, a "Miss M. Maddock took a spill in Stanley Park, hitting the fence in front of the seal pond. Knocked out cold. Recovered." Gravity, bad luck, and inanimate objects featured in these and other reports.

Collisions with pedestrians, however, were another matter. The killing of Miss Shannon illuminates a few things about cycling in the pre-war era. First, cyclists were more likely predators than prey, more likely the cause of injury than victims. Second, Shannon's death sheds light on the social ecology of turn-of-the-century Vancouver. Several witnesses were called at the inquest, but those whose testimony redeemed Blackmore's reputation were cyclists. The post-mortem that ascribed Shannon's death to her skull cracking on a cobblestone rather than the force of Blackmore's collision was conducted by a cyclist. Some of the witnesses were members of the Terminal City Cycle Club (TCCC), founded by Edward's father and business partner, William Blackmore, a prominent local architect.[5] The gallery at the inquest, moreover, was reportedly populated by many local "wheelmen." The show of solidarity for Edward Blackmore is significant. The Blackmores and their clubmates were drawn from the right side of town. Late nineteenth-century

cycling was dominated by the wealthy and the middle-class, and the organizations that supported cycling were "gentlemanly." Moreover, this elitism
was publicly performed by the TCCC and the Vancouver Bicycle Club (VBC).
"Led by captains, lieutenants, and buglers, they wore expensive outfits of
dark waistcoats, puttees, and little rifleman's caps, finery that cost upwards
of $30."[6] The leadership was drawn from the well-connected. John Moore
Bowell, a champion of organized sports in the glory days of gentlemanly ama-
teurism, had a high-profile appointment as collector of customs in Vancouver
around 1888, secured by his father, the minister of customs (later prime minister) Mackenzie Bowell. J.M. Bowell became VBC president around 1894.[7]
He and Blackmore and their respective clubs participated in parades, organized races, parties, and events, held a fundraiser for victims of the 1895
Fraser River flood, and campaigned for road improvements.[8] Enthusiasm for
cycling spread quickly among those who could afford it, and as early as 1890
there were "large" numbers of middle-class women on bicycles in Vancouver
as well.[9] If Miss Shannon was fated to be killed by a cyclist, it would almost
certainly be a well-to-do one.

The pertinent bylaws were seldom enforced and – at the height of the
bicycle craze in 1897 – the editor of Vancouver's *Daily Province* made the
connection with elitism. Only one in ten of all cyclists obeyed the city's
rules, he hazarded, adding that "the way in which the police close their eyes
to the flagrant transgressions of certain well-known 'bikers' is little short
of scandalous."[10] In 1902, Mayor Thomas Neelands complained to council
that city police were unable to enforce the bylaw meant to keep cyclists off
sidewalks. It was not just boys and young men recklessly careening down
sidewalks, Neelands asserted, "but prominent citizens and merchants." He
cited a case in which "a well known man, who was riding on his bicycle on
the sidewalk, had run over a little child and did not stop to see if the child
was hurt, but had ridden right on."[11] This may well be Vancouver's first "hit-
and-run" story, and its juxtaposition of power and weakness – an ostensibly
respectable male of standing injures a helpless child – manifests a critique
of the young city's emergent social order. It also forms part of a larger tale
of managing mobility.

Regulating cyclist behaviour was one of the first acts of the newly incorporated city council. Bylaw No. 258, "to regulate the use of bicycles"

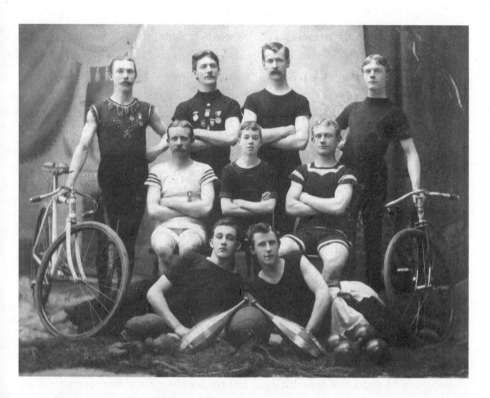

Fig. 4.1 Terminal City Bicycle Club, ca.1896. Witnesses who testified at the Shannon inquest included H. Jones and Richard Tossell (*front row*). Dr McAlpine (*back row, with medals*) performed the post-mortem.

(invoked in the Shannon inquest), was introduced only a month after the 1886 Great Fire.[12] In the 1880s, bicycles were high-wheelers (aka "ordinaries"); difficult to mount, tricky to ride, challenging to (intentionally) stop, they needed to move fast enough to stay upright. The "penny-farthing" thus lent itself to speed and disaster. The first "safety bicycles" – machines with comparably sized wheels and shorter step-over frames – arrived in Vancouver in 1890, broadening cycling's appeal.[13] More riders meant more and different problems. In an 1896 opinion piece rich with playful hyperbole, "Hastings" wrote, "It is no longer a case of risk, but of dead certainty (or certain death)" that pedestrians would encounter a wayward cyclist.[14] A year later, the *Province* complained that the bylaws were not being enforced and that the "sidewalk biker … scorches about Vancouver (with a special partiality for Robson street) and the people fly before him like dust before the gale."[15] In the 1890s, the city responded with a registration requirement and a system of $1 "tags." Cycling organizations would repeatedly claim that the bicycle tax was their idea, intended to fund improved infrastructure. Nevertheless, the *Province* portrayed the licensing scheme as regulatory: "Bicyclists must be prepared to pay a tax on their wheels, and though there will be no big burly with a little wagon and a big net to gather them in, they must pay a license or walk."[16] New rules required "the tintinnabulation of ... bells." Victoria dropped speed limits to five miles per hour, but Vancouver did not follow suit.[17] As well, cyclists were required in 1901 to use headlamps and to keep at least one foot on a pedal at all times so as to be able to brake effectively.[18]

Throughout much of this period – and increasingly in the early twentieth century – fines were held out as the chief means to modify cyclists' behaviour, mainly that of adults, but of children too.[19] Conduct might be reformed, but could infrastructure be as well? Even the largely anticyclist *Province* had to allow that "the pugnacious sidewalk 'biker'" could be a consequence of poor roads.[20] Georgia Street was a morass of "holes, ruts, lumps, mud and a few other things," one reader observed.[21] Improvement of roads was a challenge taken up by local cycling clubs in the 1890s, partly as a response to the "reckless rider" narrative. National organizations such as the Canadian Wheelmen's Association (CWA) and various Good Roads Associations (GRA) influenced local clubs on this score.[22]

While these organizations sought overall improvement of roads, some advocated for separated cycle paths. Cinder tracks were installed on Westminster Avenue (now Main Street) and along a small stretch of Granville Street around 1900. The GRA, armed with $500 from the city, built a path to Greer's (now Kitsilano) Beach.[23] However, cyclists were vocal about their right to a share of the road, improvements on which they believed they had paid for through tags, and cyclist organizations called for efficient collection and expenditure of their tag monies.[24] The GRA stated in 1902 that the city had collected $2,784.50 from cyclists in fees and complained that not enough was going to path upkeep.[25] In 1905, council was considering an end to the bicycle tax, but organized cyclists "were unanimous in wishing the regulations of the present bylaw to continue."[26]

The city engineer, however, claimed that revenues from tags no longer met the cost of cinders for tracks. He felt "it would be well to discontinue the bicycle tax" and, ominously, "not construct any more paths."[27] Improvements in cycling infrastructure as a solution to accidents were at this point largely set aside until the late twentieth century.

When we appreciate the narrow bicycle ownership in this first period and the success of cyclists' early campaigns to improve infrastructure, it is possible to grasp how settler wealth transformed late nineteenth-century cities like Vancouver. As elsewhere in North America, Vancouver's elites supported Good Roads organizations. Elitist cycling clubs joined forces in Canadian Wheelmen branches. They obliged the city to buy road-smoothing equipment. Early and well-placed cyclists pursued their interests while, unknowingly, literally paving the way for automobilism.

The decade from about 1890 to 1903 is widely viewed as pivotal in the history of cycling in Europe and North America.[28] Vancouver may have been at the furthest end of the Canadian supply line, but some of its citizens were quick to take up the new cycling trend.[29] Then the fad slowed and ebbed away. Part of the explanation is likely economic: the middle-class bicycle market had reached saturation point, and early adopters were aging out of scorching and wabbling. However nominal the price of a bicycle tag in the pre-war era might seem, it acted as a financial barrier for some Vancouverites and may have stalled the growth of cycling generally. There was, of course, another trend on its way.

In 1903 the *Province* covered the business tour of G.A. Ferguson of Hyslop Brothers, a Toronto manufacturer of bicycles and automobiles. Ferguson harkened back to the "phenomenal cycling craze of 1896–7" and predicted (wrongly) a return to those glory days. He was also cautiously optimistic for his new line of motorized delivery vans and "probably some private motor carriages." A few months later, the *Province* carried a report of what must be one of the city's first auto accidents: "A new steam motor car, which arrived on Tuesday last, was being given its trial trips. The three owners, one of whom is a former champion cyclist, were in the vehicle at the time of the accident ... in making a sudden turn at the corner of Prior street and Westminster avenue, the steering lever came loose and allowed the front wheels to turn suddenly."[30]

Well-connected cyclists, like the "former champion cyclist" in this early crash, were the bridge between the cycling craze and the new motorized vehicles. Local elites on two wheels were not driven from the streets by automobiles: they were abandoning their bicycles in a rush. Wealthy cyclists like Charles A. Ross led the conversation about cycling hazards in the 1890s and early 1900s and then did the same for automobiles. In that photograph of the Terminal City Bicycle Club, Ross is the giant at the back, muscular and mustachioed. The "genial captain" of the club, Ross was an advocate for better road surfaces, and by 1904 "chief consul" for the province in the national bicyclists' lobby.[31] Eight years later, he was the general manager of the McLaughlin Carriage Company in British Columbia and president of the Vancouver Automobile Club.[32] Historian Robert A.J. McDonald has noted that, by 1912, "In a bigger and wealthier Vancouver, evidence of personal success came to mean fast cars, fashionable recreation and expensive homes. The motor car was a toy for the rich during the early years of the century."[33]

The Bowell family's entrepreneurial story is likewise aligned with the rise of automobility. J.M. Bowell's son, John Mackenzie "Mac" Bowell, co-owned one of the first car dealerships in Vancouver and rose to become the city's most prominent dealer at mid-century as one half of the firm Bowell-Maclean, better known locally as "Bow-Mac." Automobile owners now claimed the high ground or at least the high street. The storyline of cycling accidents as a product of upper-class disregard for the rights of pedestrians fades quickly as the motor vehicle becomes the new barometer of wealth and velocity. This shift sets up a different era of accidents by the late 1930s.

MID-CENTURY

Thanks in part to the car-dealing heirs of the cycling elites, the interwar period saw an increase in automobilism and with it a growing array of dangers. Greater velocity was not matched by greater ability. Motorcars were toppling pedestrians and bicycles and colliding with horses, carriages, and streetcars in an expanded ecosystem of transportation modes. Frank White, a delivery-truck driver in the late 1930s and '40s, recalled, "Most people really didn't know how to drive, they drove around the city like they were on some country road. They hardly obeyed any rules … You just buffaloed your way across most corners."[34] In 1938, 494 motor vehicle collisions with pedestrians, sixteen of them fatal, were recorded in Vancouver; 242 cyclists were hit by motor vehicles, with 183 injured and two killed. Two more Vancouverites died in the 143 crashes involving automobiles and streetcars; by comparison, ten incidents involving horse-drawn vehicles resulted in two injuries.[35] Part of the expansion of automobile use in this period may be explained by the economy and geography. As households relocated to the suburbs beyond the reach of street railways, automobiles became a necessity. Industry was still concentrated along Burrard Inlet and False Creek, and professional, commercial, and retail jobs were still mainly downtown. When the trams were removed in 1950, dominance over the roads tilted even further towards automobiles.

Inevitably, rising numbers of automobiles driven by motorists of varying levels of skill were going to bring trouble. In 1950, the Vancouver Traffic and Safety Council (VTSC) claimed there were 85,000 cars in Greater Vancouver, with about 72,000 in Vancouver City proper.[36] That year 7,000 car crashes were recorded in Vancouver alone. In the decade that followed, an average of 250 children were struck (three to five of them fatally) by cars every year.[37] Reliable statistics are elusive, but there were reckoned to be a hundred bicycle accidents per year in the mid-1940s. Of the nearly sixty bicycle accidents described in local newspapers between 1946 and 1955, probably no more than ten of the cyclists were adults.[38] This was partly a product of demographic and geographic change. The baby boom began in British Columbia around 1938 and peaked in 1957.[39] It fuelled the growth of suburban sprawl and reduced the viability of cycling as a mode of transport for commuting downtown and for waterfront workers. It also had implications for the character of childhood. Getting to school, visiting classmates, and delivering newspapers across lower-density communities had increased the appeal of bicycles for children and youth. The bicycle was no longer a status object of the elite but was now principally an instrument of children's transportation, entertainment, and labour.

Accounts of accidents in this period reinforce the impression that it was children who were mostly on bicycles at mid-century. Described either as "falls" or collisions with automobiles, bike-accident tolls were published daily, and a "Crop of Weekend Mishaps" could be expected in newspapers every Monday. The roll call for 28 November 1950, for example, listed ten separate incidents, including cyclists Fay Bartells (age seventeen) in East Vancouver, Barrie Herrod (ten) of South Main, and Thomas Colvin (forty-three), all of whom collided with cars.[40] Surprisingly minor cycling accidents are included. In 1948, a three-year-old from East Vancouver "received a bump on his nose when his small bike hit a parked car"; a fourteen-year-old "fell from his bicycle when it skidded," resulting in cuts. A seventeen-year-old boy was riding around Windermere Pool when his beach blanket got caught in his front wheel: he wound up with a split eardrum and jaw injuries.[41] These mundane trials set the tone of Vancouverite readers' understandings of bicycle accidents: they happened a lot, they happened to children, and they were due to three main causes: bad bicycles, bad children, and bad drivers.

Back when the local elite had a near monopoly on bicycles, the machines were relatively expensive and generally well-maintained objects associated with status. By mid-century, the state of children's bikes was often said to be poor. For example, in 1949, twelve-year-old Carole Somner was helping a friend deliver newspapers when she fell under the wheels of the Main Street streetcar. The *Sun* held a faulty bicycle pedal responsible.[42] Lorraine Brander's recollection of life in the East End in the 1940s includes an unsafe machine:

> I wanted a bicycle so badly, but they were relatively expensive. Mum finally got me this second-hand bike and a bunch of us would ride down the side streets and along Commissioner, down a path beside the tracks ... one day we were having a little race on – what's the name of the elevator beside Buckerfield's? Union Grain Growers. Well, the brakes weren't working so good on this old bike. There's a low timber curb around the edge of the pier and I hit that and went flying over the handlebars, over the side and down into the water[;] it was about twenty, twenty-five feet down. My bike must have somersaulted because it came down behind me ... The watchman came down the ladder and pulled me out, but the bike is still down there I guess.[43]

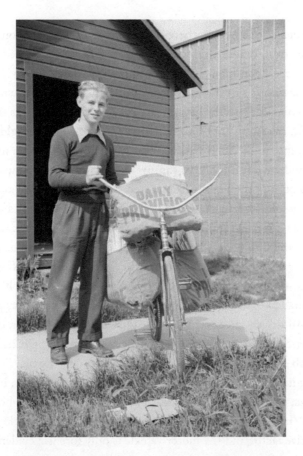

Fig. 4.2 *Vancouver Daily Province* delivery boy with bicycle, ca. 1940–48.

The themes in the Brander account reflect poverty, the absence of safe cycling and play spaces, and a poorly maintained bicycle.

Bad cycling habits, however, got more ink than faulty bikes. In October 1949, the *Province* blamed "dusky autumn evening" collisions on cyclists "who shoot out into traffic from side roads." The reporter reminded readers that regulations required headlamps and rear-wheel reflectors. "There is no excuse for cyclists who persist in ignoring regulations that protect public safety. They are among the worst menaces on the highways and police should remind them of it more forcibly."[44]

The *Province* was wrong: there were much worse menaces on the road. In accounts of automobile-inflicted injuries and deaths at mid-century, hit-and-runs were a common theme. On 19 January 1942, Calvin Wall, aged fourteen, was killed in the 7200 block of Main Street, "thrown from his bicycle in collision with the hit-and-run car, at 11 p.m." This was the second hit-and-run case in twenty-four hours, and Police Chief Donald MacKay was clearly incensed: "Such drivers are just the same as any other murderers. Nothing will be left undone to capture this man who killed with his car and drove off into the night without even stopping."[45] In 1948 alone, there were ten hit-and-runs involving cyclists. Early one morning in February, a sixteen-year-old telegraph messenger boy on his way to work was struck at Robson and Granville. The driver fished out the smashed bicycle from under his car and drove off.[46] In another hit-and-run in November, a fifteen-year-old was "hurled ... 38 feet to his death" on a stretch of the old Trans-Canada Highway near Cloverdale.[47] Newspaper accounts presented hit-and-run drivers as deviant and disgusting. Jack Fletcher, described sympathetically as a "crippled messenger boy," had just parked his bike by the curb on Kingsway when a driver smashed into the bicycle, severely damaging it. The narrative played on Fletcher's vulnerability, his plucky work ethic, and the callous disregard shown by the driver who fled the scene.[48] What stands out in these accounts is that the bicycle ceases to be the active factor and the motor vehicle is only forensic evidence, while the bad driver for once looms large.

Mid-century politicians, officials, and newspapers collectively took the view that automobile and bicycle accidents were a product of moral laxity. As to precautionary measures that might be deployed, fines had been used since the 1880s to rein in reckless cycling, and this strategy was of course extended to automobile drivers. The Vancouver Police Department was the principal arbiter of good and bad road behaviour; it was among several organizations that, at mid-century, called for personal improvement as the preferred method to curtail accidents. Local newspapers paired with the police department in 1938 to promote the goal of "One Hundred Deathless Days," a campaign of shame and willpower. It was an almost immediate failure. Perhaps it had been forgotten by 1955 when the police tried again with "Eighty Deathless Days."[49] The Traffic and Safety Council tried a similar shaming campaign in 1948 that proposed a "blazing neon score-board of death" at the south end of Burrard Bridge.[50] But plans to change the safety environment remained on the margins, although in 1952 a coun-cil candidate, Theresa Galloway, advocated the return of dedicated bike paths.[51] None of these initiatives came to much. Efforts to encourage better motorist habits ended long before eighty days had passed, Mrs Galloway's cycle paths had to wait another half century, and the opportunity to erect a Neon Scoreboard of Death was squandered.[52]

With the failure to reform motorists through gentle suasion or to pro-vide safe cycling spaces, the focus returned to cyclists. In the late 1940s, the police department and some city councillors touted the idea of a cyclist court for young offenders.[53] Police also called for inspections of bicycles, "just as motor vehicles are checked at the testing station."[54] In March 1949, the *Sun* ran a near-full page piece on road safety, ostensibly aimed at all road users but focusing heavily on the need for educating child cyclists. The feature directed children to obey stop signs, ride in single file close to the right-hand curb, and never to "double." It merely urged drivers to "Always 'Give the Kids a Brake.'"[55]

Other scholars have examined aspects of these mid-century devel-opments. Tamara Myers, for example, has observed that "the 'enemy' of children became the accident – not the automobile, not the motorist."[56] David Pomfret concurs and notes that automobilism and the rise in motor vehicle-related deaths changed childhood, claiming, "Children's ur-ban lives more generally were recast in terms of endangerment."[57] Mona Gleason argues that responsibility for the safety of the twentieth-century child shifted from the private to the public domain to figures outside of the family. In Vancouver, those figures included teachers, organizations like the Vancouver Traffic and Safety Council, the police, and newspapers.[58] These authorities sought to "immunize" children against accidents through training and safety-shaming. A careful reading of mid-century safety pre-cautions, however, reveals that their goal was in actuality safer and more efficient motoring.

To recap one theme so far, the pre-war era saw aggressive campaigns for improved roads and cycle paths as a means of reducing bicycle acci-dents and, implicitly, getting cyclists off the sidewalks in the interests of pedestrian safety. By the mid-century, this was certainly no longer the case. Infrastructure was no longer held out as a problem nor as a solution: the problem was the rider, the bicycle itself, or bad people behind the wheel of motor vehicles. Injuries that adult cyclists inflicted on one another or on pedestrians circa 1900 were, fifty years later, supplanted by injuries inflicted on cycling children by adults. In hardly more than a decade, the situation would change again.

THE NEW WAVE

Four incidents involving bicycle accidents in the period between the late 1960s and the mid-1980s highlight some of the ways in which cycling culture in Vancouver had transformed. The first of these involved three adult male cyclists riding single file across the Lions Gate Bridge, heading for work downtown in 1971. Before the bridge sidewalks were widened in the 1990s, cyclists had to travel in the traffic lane. The first cyclist hit a pothole and fell, causing a pile-up, at which point all three were hit by a truck.[59] In August 1981, a provincial small-claims court judge, aged fifty-eight, was struck while commuting in Point Grey.[60] Two cycling fatalities involving twenty-year-olds made the pages of the *Sun* in January 1985: a young man was hit by an impaired driver at Main and Pender in Chinatown, and two weeks later a UBC student was the victim of a hit-and-run on West Broadway.[61] There are, to be sure, stories of children involved in bicycle accidents, but we are seeing here something new: cycling's demographics had changed and become "respectable" once again.

The 1970s ushered in a second North American boom in cycling. The invention and popularization of multi-gear bicycles – known universally at this time as ten-speeds – coincided with maturing baby-boom demographics to produce a nicely matched supply and demand. In some histories, this "new wave" of cycling is tied to counterculture questioning of mainstream assumptions, widespread concern for air pollution, mistrust of big corporations (such as leading automakers), and a growing body of literature about aspects of urban sustainability (including Jane Jacobs's *The Death and Life of Great American Cities* and E.F. Schumacher's *Small Is Beautiful*).[62] This changed intellectual landscape led to the emergence of "biketivists," most

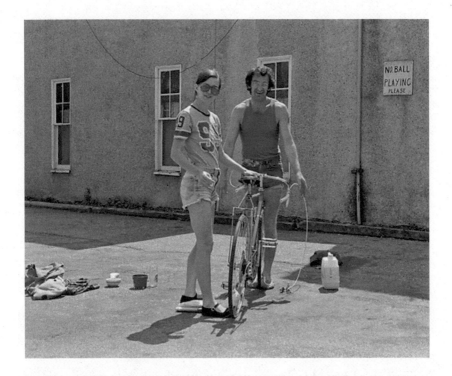

Fig. 4.3 Man and woman doing maintenance on ten-speed bicycle, ca. 1970. Cut-offs and T-shirts were standard cycling wear.

of whom pursued an anti-car agenda animated by the OPEC oil crisis of 1973 and premature forecasts of the end of the "gas-guzzler."[63] This was not entirely a fringe phenomenon: an October 1970 photograph in the *Province* shows Mayor Art Phillips pedalling a foldaway bicycle around City Hall Annex, alongside Alderman Brian Calder, who claimed to commute daily from his home in Marpole on his ten-speed.[64]

Local factors were also at play in Vancouver. Young baby-boom adults were drawn to urban life in Vancouver's Kitsilano and the West End and away from the suburbs and automobile dependency. A mild climate and a homegrown environmental movement were other considerations.[65] In 1983, the Vancouver Police Department reckoned there were 150,000 bikes in the city, more than one for every three residents.[66] A transit strike in 1984 intensified matters as it "forced cyclists on to city streets in record numbers."[67]

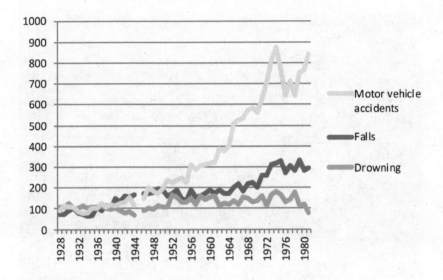

Fig. 4.4 Accidental deaths by external causes, British Columbia, 1928–81.
Source: J.M. Macdonald, "Vital Statistics in British Columbia: An Historical Overview
of 100 Years, 1891–1990," *Vital Statistics Quarterly* 4, no. 1 (June 1994): 19–48, at 40–1.

This third period is distinguished in part by sharply rising accident
numbers. In 1931, there were 111 motor vehicle deaths; for the first time,
this category of accidental and external causes of death passed all the
others. By the 1950s, motor-vehicle deaths as a category were aggressive-
ly in the lead. As figure 4.4 shows, the number of motor vehicle deaths
rises to 1974, growing in real terms but also on a per-capita basis. There's
some respite in the late 1970s, but the pace resumes in the early 1980s.[68]
Among these rising totals were significant numbers of incidents involving
cyclists. Of course, police reports capture only part of the story and need
to be augmented. One study at North Vancouver's Lion's Gate Hospital
in July and August 1970, for example, counted 135 visits arising from cycling accidents, of which fourteen required hospitalization. Nearly 70 per
cent of the accidents involved boys, and of those, 75 per cent were under
ten years of age.[69] The situation only continued to worsen. The head of the
police traffic division reported in 1981 that 11 per cent of traffic fatalities in
the first eight months of the year involved cyclists. The first six months of
1982 saw fifty-nine accidents involving bicycles, twenty-six of them in June

alone. What lay behind this "terrible frequency," as the chair of the Bicycle Advisory Committee observed, was simply "an increase in cycling."[70] By this time, the press too acknowledged a change: "Since the 10-speed boom of the early 1970s, cyclists and motorists have been on a collision course in the Lower Mainland."[71] The two modes were now seen as competing users of a grudgingly shared public space.

In this new-wave era, both cyclists and motorists articulated their relationship in the language of rights and entitlement. In 1970 a *Province* correspondent claimed, "A lot of drivers have been irritated recently by having to lose valuable seconds in transit because of the large number of cyclists on the road." He added, "It behooves [cyclists] to remember that the roads were made for cars, not bicycles."[72] His views were echoed thirteen years later when a North Vancouver man wrote to the *Province*:

The cyclists writing to you seem unaware that the roads were designed and built for motor vehicles and paid for by motor vehicle owners through extortionate taxes on gasoline, car license fees, etc. As the owner of a Buick Electra, I am paying more than my fair share of road maintenance through gasoline taxes, thus subsidizing the cyclist who crawls ahead of me at 10 mph in a 30 mph zone. If I drove my car in such a fashion I could receive a traffic ticket for obstructing traffic – and rightly so.[73]

The writers' complaints invoke ideas like prior claim and paid usership. The second motorist also protests cyclists' slowness in traffic. Gone is the "scorcher." Gone too is the child on a bicycle. The target is the adult cyclist who – at 10 mph – would have been fined for speeding in the pre-war era.

Three overarching trends in reporting accidents stand out in this last era. First, the dynamic of accidents changes. The bicycle no longer "collides with" the automobile; in case after case, the cyclist is "struck by a car." Also, motorists – particularly in fatal circumstances – are accorded agency: they are present in accounts as "the driver."[74]

Second, the list of cycling "bad habits" changes somewhat. Cycling after dark without headlights continues to be a source of comment, but riding on the left-hand side of the road emerges as *the* issue of this era. Newspaper delivery boys and girls who ride the streets early every morning and after school every evening are singled out for "cycling everywhere but the right side of the road."[75] This behaviour is a particular target of the Vancouver Police Department in the early 1980s.[76]

Third, there is a mysterious absence of accident reports overall in newspapers. A cyclist hitting a hay bale in the middle of Pender Street could no longer expect a column inch or two; the weekly "Toll of Mishaps" had also disappeared. Despite an apparent consensus that the streets were increasingly dangerous and real friction was growing between road users, barely a report of a cycling accident appears between 1978 and 1985. That silence did not, however, stand in the way of advice from newspapers and others for new and renewed precautions.

The "expert study" as regards cycling safety makes its appearance in this period. Perhaps nothing is more "modern" than the "expert," and by the 1970s and early 1980s, there were plenty who would claim that title: credentialed and quasi-credentialed safety engineers, club cyclists, and civic officials. These authorities continued to call for better-lit bicycles and better-quality – or at least better-fitting – bicycles. One Ontario study in 1970 identified oversized bikes – hand-me-downs or grow-into models – as a source of cycling peril for children.[77] Remarkably, 1970s reports on accidents largely ignored innovations in bicycle design; reporters, editors, and correspondents instead turned their attention to helmets. When James D. Craig wrote to the *Province* in 1970, he demanded that cyclists be "required to wear helmets for their own protection." Purpose-built bicycle helmets did not, however, exist until 1975, when Bell Auto Parts produced the first of its eponymous helmets. The Canadian Standards Association began reviewing helmet quality in the 1970s but took a decade to approve any products.[78] It was only in 1982 that a significant uptake in helmet use occurred.[79] According to a Norco representative, sales of helmets increased tenfold over that year, largely thanks to the growing popularity of bicycle touring.[80]

Was there something that could be improved at the street level? The role played by cycling advocacy groups in advancing change took a strange turn in the 1970s. The venerable Vancouver Bicycle Club, the Bicycle Association of British Columbia (BABC), and the Veterans' Bicycle Club were all active.[81] Along with some smaller groups, they united in 1979 under the Bicycle

Alliance, an umbrella organization that broke new ground by calling for "space for bicyclists on some forms of public transit, improved bike paths," and other accommodations.[82] Another body that appeared in this period – again with overlapping memberships with the other organizations – was the Bicycle Advisory Committee. According to contemporaries' recollections, the committee "was independent of city hall, but through singular, favourable relationships with sympathetic public officials, they had its ear."[83] There was also a bicycle subcommittee of city council, chaired in 1980 by Alderwoman Helen Boyce who called for a civic "bicycle transportation program" and a "part-time bicycle coordinator to implement it."[84] This all sounded promising.

Material results, however, are difficult to identify. According to one ally, members of the Bicycle Advisory Committee were disregarded by civic authorities: "People just thought they were all nutters. Well, they dressed like they ... were hippies. Big time."[85] Moreover, many of the biketivists in the new-wave era in Vancouver were informed by the writings of British-American engineer John Forester (1929–2020). Forester was hostile to separated bikeways, promoted "vehicular cycling" (which maintained that "cyclists fare best when they act as, and are treated as, operators of vehicles"), and championed "Effective Cycling" education.[86] The BABC and the Veterans' Bicycle Club were drawn to Forester's line of thinking.[87] They focused on fleshing out road infrastructure, connecting networks of accessible highways, and making public transit bicycle-friendly. They mostly spared drivers criticism and instead blamed cyclists.

The president of the BABC in 1983, Gerry Pareja, drew attention to inexpert cyclists: "The average motorist is more skillful than the average cyclist – which isn't surprising. There just isn't much training for cyclists."[88] He reminded *Province* readers that cyclists had rights but also duties equivalent to those of automobilists.[89] An outwardly robust advocacy network thus mainly served to reinforce the view that cyclists were at fault. Going a step further, Pareja, the BABC, and Dan Egan (program coordinator for the Vancouver Safety Council) offered an eleven-week training program to cyclists. Egan was described in 1981 as an advocate for Foresterian approaches: "His office [was] piled high with Effective Cycling manuals." In classic Foresterian language, Egan advised cyclists to "avoid bicycle paths unless they are wide, well-lit and free of debris," which they generally were not. "Paths ... can encourage a false sense of security," Egan warned. In the parlance: "Take the lane" – by which he meant cycle down the middle and do not cower on the side.[90]

This response to accidents was both gendered and ableist. As one 2015 study put it, the "vehicular cycling" approach "bolstered the adult, masculine qualities of cycling, which had been dismissed as childlike behavior for most of the century. Emphasizing confidence, self-control, assertiveness, technical knowledge, and skill, the rhetoric appealed to male cyclists who had ridden in cycling clubs before the boom."[91]

This ethos was evident in Vancouver, where the values of vehicular cycling impeded attention to different abilities. Note, however, that this conversation about cycling safety focused entirely on adult cyclists. If in the pre-war era the focus was on the vulnerabilities of pedestrians, and at mid-century on the powerlessness of children, in the new-wave era, the discourse on accidents attempted to shroud hazardous conditions by treating cyclists simultaneously as newcomers on the streets and as adults capable of making better choices. Individual cyclists called for better infrastructure for riders to make cycling safer, but their requests fell on deaf ears at City Hall and in the Bicycle Alliance.[92] Reports of accidents might emphasize the vehicle as the dynamic factor, and the agency of motorists was regularly underlined, but the response of civic officials and advocates was to treat cyclists as non-conformists who needed to grow up.

CONCLUSIONS

After Jessie McQueen arrived in Rossland, BC, in 1896, she wrote in one letter home to the Maritimes, "Don't be afraid about me & my wheel, mother. I'll never be a reckless rider – have only had it out once as yet, but I see dozens of them about town now – the streets are improved so much." She subsequently travelled by train to Vancouver, bicycle in tow, and did a loop of Stanley Park. McQueen documents improved roads, "dozens" of cyclists in a remote community that did not have a large local elite, awareness that Vancouver was a bicycle-friendly city, and concerns about accidents.[93] She acknowledged the cyclist's responsibility for reducing risk, as the *Vancouver*

Daily World had just months earlier, and both feared the same thing: "reckless riding." Indeed, the *World* squarely addressed cyclists' culpability in collisions and the possibility of a comeuppance in the form of pedestrian retribution: "Fast riding is liable to bring about the imposition of inconvenient restrictions on wheelmen for the safety of pedestrians."[94]

When urban cycling was the preserve of the middle class, a pedestrian uprising looked a lot like a serious challenge to the privileges of the rich. In the post–World War II period, automobilists were regularly reminded to drive safely, but the threat of "inconvenient restrictions" on automobile traffic was absent from the discourse, nor was there any suggestion that children on bikes would rebel against adults in cars. If we explore this theme further, the final era of this study shows us two populations and technologies "on a collision course," as the *Sun* put it in 1983, suggesting two relatively equal forces at odds. New-wave era narratives "level up" the cyclist – as an adult, a judge, a university student, a train of three commuters – while simultaneously denying them the authority of their predecessors in the Edwardian era. Moreover, storylines from the 1970s and '80s could no longer identify a weak, ill-fated character type like 1952's twelve-year-old David Lawrence, whose gym shoes looped over his handlebars got caught in his front spokes, with fatal results.[95] Cycling advocates played to this discourse of a battle of peers by embracing "vehicular cycling" as a claim to pavement equivalence and by taking steps to improve cyclist ability, rather than depicting cyclists as victims or motorists as the source of risk. No surprise, then, that no single accident story from the new-wave era stands out like the killing of Rachel Shannon or Calvin Wall.

Each of the generations examined here approached cycling from different demographic and socioeconomic contexts but, as Glen Norcliffe argues, all were engaged in mobilities in modernity.[96] Jessie McQueen's place in that process is that of an early adopter when the rules and risks were uncertain in ways that they would never again be for future generations. By contrast, the new-wave adult cyclist likely experienced the mid-century's infantilized cycling, and so brought that history forward. Setting one era alongside the other reveals how the act of cycling was contextual. The scorcher, the paper girl, the ten-speed commuter do not make sense otherwise. When we look at victims, casualties, and fatalities in cycling accidents, the same is true: context and demography frame the inequity, the precautions, and the storytelling.

In 1980, *Sun* editorialist David Wright described regular encounters with a Foresterian cyclist. Dressed for the weather and heedless of rain and sleet, he could be found each day plowing his way down East 12th, a fast four-lane car sewer through a residential neighbourhood. Why there? Wright asked. Why not go over a block or two to a nice tree-lined street? "To take it a step further, maybe cycling clubs and associations could put the heat on city hall to designate recommended bike routes and signpost them. I don't mean scenic ones, I mean common-sense routes for bicycles, roughly parallel to the major streets. They could encourage their members to use them. The risk of accidents would be greatly reduced."[97]

Wright is virtually alone in a century of Vancouver journalists reporting on cycling accidents in that he eschewed moral, technological, or didactic solutions to cycling accidents in favour of something structural. In this regard, he added a further wrinkle: spatial contexts matter. The wabbler careening down a cobblestone downtown street in a city of 26,000 people wouldn't recognize the suburbanized mid-century city of a quarter-million, let alone the more densely packed and motorized metropolis of twice that number in 1981. Throughout the periods under study here, however, elite voices – including those in the press – remain prominent. Early wealthy advocates for cycling became early advocates for automobilism; grown-ups dictated the practice and environment of cycling at mid-century; articulate authorities citing expert reports reoriented the conversation in the 1970s and '80s. In these accounts of accidents and risks and the stories they produce, we see the persistence of power dynamics more than the ineffability of physics.

ACKNOWLEDGMENTS

I thank the following individuals: Lani Russwurm introduced me to Eighty Deathless Days and remains a go-to person for details on Vancouver history; Greg Leach admonished me to take a more serious historical view of cycling, and this is a start; Diane Purvey, Amy Walker, Colin Stein, and Norm Fennema all provided feedback on drafts, as did the collection editors. The weaknesses and errors are all my own.

NOTES

1 See Davies, "'Reckless Walking Must Be Discouraged,'" 123–38.
2 "Recognized by Her Picture," *Vancouver Province* (hereafter *Province*), 26 September 1900.
3 "Accidental Death," *Province*, 27 September 1900.
4 "Cycling Accidents," *Vancouver Daily World* (hereafter *Daily World*), 3 June 1896.
5 "William Evans Blackmore," *Biographical Dictionary of Architects in Canada, 1800–1950*, http://dictionaryofarchitectsincanada.org/node/1136.
6 Bouchier, *For the Love of the Game*, 44.
7 *Who's Who in Western Canada: A Biographical Dictionary of Notable Living Men and Women in Western Canada*, vol. 1, edited by C.W. Parker (Vancouver: Canadian Press Association 1911), 120; "$1,350,000 Spent," *Daily World*, 31 December 1888.
8 "Bicyclists Organize," *Daily World*, 31 July 1890. Possibly the earliest bicycle club in Canada was established in Montreal in 1878. This was roughly contemporary with the establishment of the Montreal Amateur Athletic Association (1881) and other organizations associated with elite – and "amateur" – sports and activities. See Lamonde, "Social Relations in Nineteenth-Century Montreal," 765.
9 Barman, *West beyond the West*, 140. On the numbers of women cycling in Vancouver, see *Daily World*, 8 July 1890, 2. What constitutes "large" in this context is unknown.
10 *Province*, 17 July 1897, 3.
11 "Aldermanic Authority," *Province*, 19 August 1902. The mayor added that cyclists "did more damage to the sidewalks than the cows."
12 Davis, *Chuck Davis History of Metropolitan Vancouver*, 20.
13 "For Sale," *Daily World*, 24 July 1890.
14 "Miscellaneous from Vancouver," *Province*, 9 May 1896, also 14 March 1896.
15 *Province*, 27 February 1897, 3.
16 "Taxing the Cycles," *Province*, 5 February 1901.
17 See "A By-Law," *Province*, 5 June 1897, 9, for the full Victoria bylaw.
18 "Bicycle By-Law Goes," *Province*, 12 February 1901.
19 "'Take Off Your Hats,'" *Province*, 3 May 1905, 16.
20 "Miscellaneous from Vancouver," *Province*, 4 May 1903, 14 March 1896.
21 Letter from Reginald Rivers, *Province*, 18 March 1899.
22 "Cycle Path Hobby," *Province*, 5 August 1898. By 1900, the BC branch of the CWA had 372 members.
23 "Cyclists Make Strong Protest," *Province*, 13 June 1902.
24 "Cyclists Plan Reform Campaign," *Daily Province*, 14 July 1905.
25 "Annual Meeting of Bicycle Clubs," *Province*, 13 March 1901; *Province*, 28 May 1901.
26 "Constitutional Question," *Vancouver World*, 17 February 1908; "Why Not Spend Money," *Province*, 15 July 1905.
27 "More Cycle Paths Are Recommended," *Province*, 28 July 1905.
28 Friss, *Cycling City*; Dauncey, *French Cycling*, 5–8.

29 Hobsbawm, *Age of Capital*, 317.

30 *Province*, 10 March 1903; "Motor Car Upset," *Province*, 30 July 1903.

31 "Athletics," *Daily News*, 25 May 1904. Incidentally, it was Ross whom Edward Blackmore was rushing to see when he crossed paths with Rachel Shannon. "Her Death Was Accidental," *Daily World*, 27 September 1900.

32 "Several Reasons for Good Business State," *Vancouver Sun* (hereafter *Sun*), 28 October 1912; "Plan Big Motor Trip to Seattle," *Sun*, 25 March 1912.

33 McDonald, *Making Vancouver, 1863–1913*, 153.

34 Frank White, "Hauling around Town," in Knight, *Along the No. 20 Line*, 104.

35 I believe the number refers to passengers or drivers of buggies, as opposed to the horses themselves. Vancouver Police Archives, Traffic Division Reports, 1938.

36 "Car Accidents Cost Vancouver $3 Million," *Sun*, 25 May 1951.

37 Myers, "Didactic Sudden Death," 470; Read et al., "Epidemiology and Prevention of Traffic Accidents," 689.

38 "Traffic Injures Thirty," *Province*, 20 June 1949. Reporting of fatalities was probably accurate enough, but injuries, particularly those not requiring hospitalization, were no doubt underreported.

39 Belshaw, *Becoming British Columbia*, 133–9.

40 "Accidents on City Streets Injure 10," *Sun*, 28 November 1950.

41 "Blanket Throws Boy Cyclist," *Sun*, 30 July 1952.

42 "Girl Dies in Fall under Streetcar," *Sun*, 14 November 1949.

43 Lorraine Brander, "Dolls, Rollerskates and Dockyards," in Knight, *Along the No. 20 Line*, 187.

44 "Don't Let Them Get Away with It," *Province*, 20 October 1949.

45 "Police Open Drive to 'Crack Down' on Hit-Run Drivers," *Sun*, 19 January 1942.

46 "Man Injured, Car-Driver Faces Charge," *Sun*, 21 February 1948.

47 "Hit-Run Killer Hunted," *Province*, 19 November 1948.

48 "Crippled Boy Assisted in Bike Problem," *Sun*, 14 August 1948.

49 "Eighty Deathless Days," *Vancouver News-Herald* (hereafter *News-Herald*), 15 October 1955.

50 "City May Get Blazing 'Scoreboard of Death,'" *Sun*, 29 April 1948.

51 "May Save Lives," *Province*, 31 December 1952.

52 Christopher Dummitt categorizes these campaigns as "Three Es": engineering, education, and enforcement. In point of fact, there was very little engineering (Dummitt does not go far beyond parking meters), education was not systematic, and enforcement was an old device. Shaming played a greater role. Dummitt, *Manly Modern*, 135–8.

53 "Bike Clubs Can Curb Rising Toll of Mishaps," *Sun*, 30 December 1947; "Schoolboy Courts May Try Cyclists," *Province*, 9 June 1948.

54 "Safety Tests for Bicycles Proposed by Traffic Chief," *Sun*, 29 April 1954. This program was piloted in North Vancouver but not, to my knowledge, in Vancouver.

55 "Bicycles Aren't Built for Two," *Sun*, 12 March 1949.

56 Myers, "Didactic Sudden Death," 458.

57 Pomfret, "'Closer to God,'" 366.

58 Gleason, "From 'Disgraceful Carelessness' to 'Intelligent Precaution,'" 231.

59 "Instruction for Cyclists?," *Province*, 5 July 1971.

60 "Bicycle Accident Fatal for Judge," *Sun*, 13 August 1981.

61 "Police Seeking Hit-Run Driver," *Sun*, 19 January 1985.

62 Reid, *Bike Boom*, 114.

63 For a scholarly study of another Canadian city, see Ross, "'Vive La Vélorution!'"

64 "Pedal Power," *Province*, 8 October 1970.

65 There were roughly 350,000 Vancouverites and another 220,000 in the metro region in 1951. Numbers rose to 426,000 and 600,000 respectively in 1971. The city's population stagnated through the 1970s and actually took a bit of a dip, but the Greater Vancouver numbers continued to advance, from 1,028,334 in 1971 to 1,169,831 in 1973.

66 "Cycling Safety a 2-Way Street," *Sun*, 30 August 1983.

67 "Bikes Face Curbs," *Province*, 3 August 1984. The UBC student who was killed in January 1985 had evidently taken up cycling because of the transit strike. "Police Seeking Hit-Run Driver," *Sun*, 19 January 1985.

68 Macdonald, "Vital Statistics in British Columbia," 40–1.

69 "Instruction for Cyclists?," *Province*, 5 July 1971. The "fancy-style" bikes – mainly Mustangs, with an awkward centre of gravity – were regarded as especially hazardous

70 "Increasing Bicycle Deaths Worry Police Inspector," *Sun*, 11 September 1981; "Cyclists Draw Police Crackdown," *Province*, 28 July 1982.

71 "Cycling Safety a 2-Way Street," *Sun*, 30 August 1983.

72 "Bicycles," *Province*, 11 June 1970.

73 "Roads Rightfully Belong to Drivers," *Province*, 13 May 1983. Responses from cyclists were equally adamant: "Cyclists, Beware! Those Cars Are a Constant Threat," *Province*, 24 May 1983. (A Buick Electra was, even by the standards of the day, an almost comically thirsty vehicle.)

74 "Crash Kills Boy Cyclist," *Sun*, 25 June 1971; "Cyclist Dies in Car Crash," *Sun*, 2 July 1971.

75 "Light Up," *Sun*, 5 January 1970.

76 "Cyclists Draw Police Crackdown," *Province*, 28 July 1982.

77 "Not Funny Says Bike Expert," *Sun*, 22 October, 1970; "Odds Up," *Sun*, 19 November 1970.

78 "It's Time We Used Our Heads and Made Cycling Helmets a Must for Children," *Sun*, 17 January 1987.

79 "Importance of Safe Bike Riding," *Sun*, 14 September 1981; Lapner and Ivan, "Bicycle Injuries among Children," 132.

80 "Survival Instincts Encourage Cyclists to Wear Helmets," *Province*, 12 July 1983. As late as the mid-1990s, helmet wear was held out by "experts" as virtually the only change that would yield results. For an egregious example – one that ignores several other glaring possibilities – see Francis and Justason, *Deaths of Cyclists in British Columbia*, https://helmets.org/bcstudy.htm.

81 The Veterans' Bicycle Club takes several forms over the years. At first it was a largely informal collection of aging but able retired competitive cyclists. The "Velo Veterans"

included Lorne "Ace" Atkinson, whose scrapbooks show it evolving into what is now the VeloVets bicycle club, a less elite organization for riders over the age of fifty-five. Lorne Atkinson Scrapbooks, British Columbia Sports Hall of Fame, Vancouver, vols. 3 and 4.

82 *Province*, 23 September 1979.

83 "Early Voices of Advocacy: The Clubs, the Association & the BAC," Van Bikes: A History Cycling Advocacy, accessed 30 July 202,1 https://www.vanbikes.ca/van-blog/1986-95-early-voices-clubs-association-bac.

84 "Cyclists Get Pledge of Aid on Bridges," *Sun*, 29 August 1980.

85 Nelson McLachlan, quoted in "Early Voices of Advocacy."

86 Quoted in Furth, "Bicycling Infrastructure for Mass Cycling," 114.

87 Stein, *Vanbikes*, 32.

88 "Cycling Safety a 2-Way Street," *Sun*, 30 August 1983.

89 "Cyclists, Beware! Those Cars Are a Constant Threat," *Province*, 24 May 1983.

90 "Bikes: Don't Break the Rules," *Sun*, 28 September 1981.

91 Longhurst, *Bike Battles*, 223.

92 "Bikes: Don't Break the Rules," *Sun*, 28 September 1981.

93 Barman, *West beyond the West*, 140.

94 "Bicycle Accidents," *Daily World*, 17 May 1895.

95 "Bike Fall Fatal to City Boy, 12," *News-Herald*, 27 October 1952. Two weeks later, newspapers were warning local children not to ride with shoes on their handlebars (e.g., "Shoes are better slung around the neck"). "Some Safety Council Dont's' [*sic*] for Young Vancouver Cyclists," *Sun*, 6 November 1952.

96 Norcliffe, *Ride to Modernity*. On mobilities, see Bradley et al., *Moving Natures*, 9–13.

97 David Wright, "Risking His Life to Save Fuel?," *Sun*, 9 July 1980. Some bicycling advocates would take up this challenge and produce the first map of recommended routes for cyclists in 1982.

BIBLIOGRAPHY

Archives

British Columbia Sports Hall of Fame, Vancouver
City of Vancouver Archives
Vancouver Police Archives

Newspapers

Vancouver Daily World (aka *Vancouver World*)
Vancouver News-Herald
Vancouver Province (aka *Vancouver Daily Province*)
Vancouver Sun

Other Sources

Barman, Jean. *The West beyond the West: A History of British Columbia*. 3rd ed. Toronto: University of Toronto Press, 2007.

Belshaw, John Douglas. *Becoming British Columbia: A Population History*. Vancouver: University of British Columbia Press, 2009.

Bouchier, Nancy B. *For the Love of the Game: Amateur Sport in Small-Town Ontario, 1838–1895*. Montreal and Kingston: McGill-Queen's University Press, 2003.

Bradley, Ben, Jay Young, and Colin M. Coates, eds. *Moving Natures: Mobility and the Environment in Canadian History*. Calgary: University of Calgary Press, 2016.

Dauncey, Hugh. *French Cycling: A Social and Cultural History*. Liverpool: Liverpool University Press, 2012.

Davies, Stephen. "'Reckless Walking Must Be Discouraged': The Automobile Revolution and the Shaping of Modern Canada to 1930." *Urban History Review/ Revue d'Histoire Urbaine* 18, no. 2 (October 1989): 123–38.

Davis, Chuck. *The Chuck Davis History of Metropolitan Vancouver*. Madeira Park: Harbour, 2011.

Dummitt, Christopher. *The Manly Modern Masculinity in Postwar Canada*. Vancouver: University of British Columbia Press, 2007.

Francis, Robert P., and Peggy Justason. *Deaths of Cyclists in British Columbia: A Composite View of Cyclist Death Commonalities, Prevention Strategies and Collective Recommendations*. Victoria: Office of the Chief Coroner, 1996. https://helmets.org/bcstudy.htm.

Friss, Evan. *The Cycling City: Bicycles and Urban American in the 1890s*. Chicago: University of Chicago Press, 2015.

Furth, Peter G. "Bicycling Infrastructure for Mass Cycling: A Transatlantic Comparison." In *City Cycling: Urban and Industrial Environments*, edited by John Pucher and Ralph Buehler, 105–39. Cambridge: MIT Press, 2012.

Gleason, Mona. "From 'Disgraceful Carelessness' to 'Intelligent Precaution': Accidents and the Public Child in English Canada, 1900–1950." *Journal of Family History* 30, no. 2 (April 2005): 230–41.

Knight, Rolf. *Along the No. 20 Line: Reminiscences of the Vancouver Waterfront*. Vancouver: New Star Books, 2011.

Lamonde, Yvan. "Social Relations in Nineteenth-Century Montreal: Two Cultural Streams." In *Montreal: The History of a North American City*, edited by Dany Fougères and Roderick MacLeod, 750–75. Montreal and Kingston: McGill-Queen's University Press, 2018.

Longhurst, James. *Bike Battles: A History of Sharing the American Road*. Seattle: University of Washington Press, 2015.

Macdonald, J.M. "Vital Statistics in British Columbia: An Historical Overview of 100 Years, 1891 to 1990." *Vital Statistics Quarterly Digest* 4, no. 1 (June 1994): 19–45.

McDonald, Robert A.J. *Making Vancouver, 1863–1913*. Vancouver: University of British Columbia Press, 1996.

Myers, Tamara. "Didactic Sudden Death: Children, Police, and Teaching Citizenship in the Age of Automobility." *Journal of the History of Childhood and Youth* 8, no. 3 (Fall 2015): 451–75.

Norcliffe, Glen. *The Ride to Modernity: The Bicycle in Canada, 1869–1900*. Toronto: University of Toronto Press, 2001.

Pomfret, David M. "'Closer to God': Child Death in Historical Perspective." *Journal of the History of Childhood and Youth* 8, no. 3 (Fall 2015): 353–77.

Read, John H., E.J. Bradley, J.D. Morison, D. Lewall, and D.A. Clarke. "The Epidemiology and Prevention of Traffic Accidents Involving Child Pedestrians." *Canadian Medical Association Journal* 89, no. 14 (October 1963): 687–701.

Reid, Carlton. *Bike Boom: The Unexpected Resurgence of Cycling*. Washington, DC: Island Press, 2017.

Ross, Daniel. "'Vive La Vélorution!' Le Monde à bicyclette et les origines du mouvement cycliste à Montréal, 1975–1980." *Bulletin d'histoire politique* 23, no. 2 (2015): 92–112.

Stein, Colin. *Vanbikes: Vancouver's Bicycle People and the Fight for Transportation Change, 1986–2011 – An Oral History*. Vancouver: Colin Stein, 2022.

PART TWO | PRECAUTION

5

Life and Death in the Building of Montreal's Victoria Bridge, 1854–1860

Anh-Dao Bui Tran

By all accounts, Englishman James Hodges was an extraordinarily inventive engineer, most famous for Montreal's mid-nineteenth-century Victoria Bridge. But according to assistant engineer Charles Legge, Hodges was also a compassionate employer, deeply regretting the workers injured or killed in accidents accompanying the bridge construction: "There beat not a heart more tender and sympathising than his on the occurrence of any of those fatal or serious accidents to life or limb, which always accompany the prosecution of so great a work," wrote Legge. Fortunately, such occurrences were kept to "a minimum by the effective and careful provision provided in every department."[1]

Regarded as the largest architectural work of its time, the three-kilometre-long structure, built between 1854 and 1860, was the first bridge to cross the St Lawrence River.[2] The tubular bridge, made of wrought-iron plates riveted together, was a crucially important link in the Grand Trunk Railway system, connecting Canada West and Canada East and running to Atlantic seaports and their European destinations. The renowned British contracting firm of Peto, Brassey, Jackson, and Betts built the important Montreal-Toronto section of the railway and the Victoria Bridge, the latter structure designed by Robert Stephenson, with his assistant Alexander Ross, the Grand Trunk's engineer-in-chief in Canada.[3] Construction of

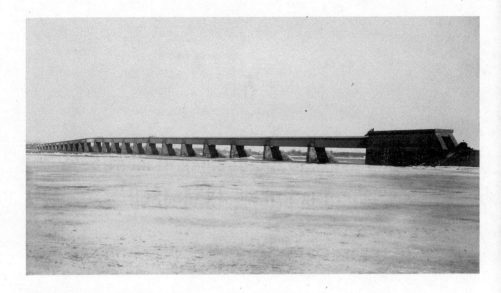

Fig. 5.1 *Victoria Bridge, Montreal.*

this massive bridge at times required the employment of three thousand or more workers.⁴ Legge's remark implies that, while injuries were common on this type of worksite, careful management strategies minimized accidents at the bridge.

Major studies on the Grand Trunk and the Victoria Bridge have emphasized the history of the company, such as Archibald W. Currie's *The Grand Trunk Railway of Canada* (1957), or the construction process, such as Robert Passfield's "Construction of the Victoria Tubular Bridge" (2001), or have examined the living conditions of the workers, such as the 1992 history of the bridge by Stanley Triggs, Brian Young, Conrad Graham, and Gilles Lauzon.⁵ This chapter takes up accidents connected to the construction of this famed railway bridge, a topic that has been overlooked in this literature but sheds new light on the history of large, complex construction sites of the period. Evaluating how risk was defined on this worksite, and the meaning of the term "accident" for Hodges, his colleagues, and the thousands of men who laboured to build the bridge, I argue that risk and risk management formed part of the workers' and employers' working lives and masculine identities. Indeed, the Victoria Bridge project may signal the onset of the transitional moment in the history of risk that Roger Cooter locates in the 1870s and '80s.[6]

My understanding of risk relates to the idea of precaution; that is, as the etymology of the term reflects, to the notion of anticipating – and therefore identifying – risk and danger. Careful provision at the bridge worksite on the part of management was intended to stop accidents from happening, yet the evidence suggests that workers also practised precaution. This notion of precaution – what it meant, whose responsibility it was – is central to this chapter. This case study investigates the "connection between 'risk,' 'accidents,' and modern industrial capitalism" mentioned in the introduction of this volume and discusses the notions of the "tolerance of risk," demonstrating that we can employ the analysis of risk and precaution as a tool to interrogate employers' sources about working conditions, masculinity, and power relations on the nineteenth-century worksite.

The historian aiming to assess the motives and understandings of workers must contend with a scarcity of worker testimonies and a lack of reliable information from companies about injury or risk. Nevertheless, as with John Sandlos's chapter in this volume and in histories of immigrant workers, psychiatric patients, and criminalized women, historians can acknowledge the agency of disempowered people by carefully rereading – "decoding," as historian Roy Porter calls it – the available evidence.[7] The first section of this chapter addresses the silence of the sources on risk and accidents, arguing that the documents detailing the construction of the Victoria Bridge in fact reverberate with stories of danger, skill, and bravery. I then consider the notion of risk and its role on the worksite. After identifying these risks, I analyze the precautions taken on the site and focus more particularly on a care agreement made by the construction firm with a Montreal hospital.

NO ACCIDENTS IN THE SOURCES, NO ACCIDENTS ON THE WORKSITE?

James Hodges's book *Construction of the Great Victoria Bridge in Canada* (1860) is an invaluable source on the project. Step by step, he describes the construction process and details each working season, from the preparation work (1853) to the inauguration of the bridge (1860). Significantly, the word "accident" appears only six times in the book. Three accident references relate to incidents that threatened to delay the completion of the works, a matter of great concern in the short Canadian working season. In an 1859 "accident" that slowed construction by two weeks, thirteen rafts, manned by more than 150 men, were driven against the wooden stagings set up for the project, and a total of 500,000 cubic feet of timber was scattered on the river.[8] There was so much debris that "men were seen walking at the water level."[9] This is the only incidence in which Hodges explicitly acknowledged that no lives were lost, although he makes no mention of injuries.

Conversely, Hodges did not use "accident" in describing how fires nearly burned several stagings, one of which narrowly escaped destruction.[10] He attributed this incident to the carelessness of the "rivet boys" and explained that a water tank and a twenty-four-hour watchman were meant to prevent such fires. They happened, and yet they were not called "accidents" precisely because they were expected – hence the water tank and the watchman – and in the end were kept under control.

A limited conception of accidents also pervades the company's archives. Between 1854 and 1858, engineer-in-chief Alexander Ross's accounts mentioned accidents only three times, referring to train accidents, fire, and delayed completion of the works.[11] Here, "accidents" tended to refer to adverse events that happened at the works rather than damage to labouring bodies. We could interpret this sparse archival record as meaning that few worksite accidents occurred. After all, the death toll was relatively low: twenty-six workers died during the six-year construction, mostly by drowning.[12] These were fatal accidents, at least according to our modern understanding, and yet they were not labelled as such in the texts and documents I reviewed for this chapter.

Examining "the moment of the accident" in late Victorian Britain, Cooter found that accidental injuries were mostly ignored before the 1870s and '80s, when accidents became a matter of public interest and cases of burns or fractures were reclassified as "accident cases."[13] As a consequence, Cooter tells us, accident statistics and hospital records from the 1850s should be treated cautiously, as at this historical moment "the meaning of an 'accident' itself has no stability."[14] The Victoria Bridge employers' sources made no mention of accidents – or, rather, accidental injuries – because the mid-nineteenth-century definition of "accident" did not encompass what would be regarded two decades later as typical industrial injuries. Even Legge, who appeared to reference accidental injuries, used the phrase "accidents to life or limb," implying that "accidents" were perceived as negative events that unexpectedly happened *to* something, in the same way that Hodges regretted that accidents could happen *to* the stagings.

Yet the instability of the definition of "accident" at the Victoria Bridge construction site did not mean that the employers did not acknowledge their obligations to the men who risked their safety in the work.[15] Publications and archival documents about the bridge show how employer benevolence connected to the workers' social, spiritual, and even physical well-being. Hodges provided them with dwellings and a chapel, schoolroom, and library.[16] The biographies of Samuel Peto and Thomas Brassey celebrate the two men's care for workers, providing them with religious education and barracks.[17] Such provisions were not always made. In Britain, railway workers often suffered harsh living and working conditions through employer negligence; the dangerous work and poor living quarters of the Chinese workers who built North American railways are a matter of historical record.[18] However, in the case of the Victoria Bridge site, Hodges's "attention paid to the welfare of the workmen" acknowledged risk and employer responsibility, including medical attendance, an important topic in this chapter's third section.[19]

Such employer benevolence may have been motivated by an awareness that healthy workers' bodies were necessary to the smooth completion of the works. Speaking in Parliament in 1851, three years before the construction of the bridge, Peto defended the Irish labourer: "I know from personal experience that if you pay him well, and show him you care for him, he is the most faithful and hardworking creature in existence ... give him legitimate occupation, and remuneration for his services, show him you appreciate those services, and you may be sure you put an end to all agitation. He will be your faithful servant and the loyal subject of his Sovereign."[20] Peto made a clear connection in his speech between the care provided for workers and the creation of a hardworking, faithful workforce. As Hodges indicated, supporting the welfare of the workers on the Victoria Bridge, including securing shelter and providing medical attention,

guaranteed a peaceful worksite, and a job well done.[21] The sources indicate
an interest in the "many" workmen who suffered sunstroke in summer and
frost-bitten noses, ears, or feet and snow blindness in the winter.[22] Hodges
attributed these injuries to the workers' inexperience with the Canadian
climate, likely referring to the British workers recruited for the project.[23]

Hodges's book may also have offered an opportunity to respond to
public criticism about workmen's welfare raised at the beginning of the
construction.[24] Although the details are few, a report in the *Montreal
Transcript* newspaper, commenting on the Grand Trunk workers' local
strike in May 1855, accused contractors Peto, Brassey, Jackson, and Betts
of imposing long hours and low wages and denounced the impact of a long
workday on the workers' health.[25] Hodges's rebuttal maintained that his
"integrity" had been testified to by the Anglican bishop of Montreal.[26] In
fact, the bishop probably had an interest in protecting the employers: a
letter from the Grand Trunk Company to the Catholic bishop of Montreal
implied that "all religions and other bodies" received benefits from the
Grand Trunk Company until 1860.[27] What is important here is not the
truth of the accusations but that Hodges was concerned with presenting
a positive public image of the bridge project and of himself. The public expected a good Victorian employer to take care of workers' spiritual and
physical well-being. Such benevolence contributed to Hodges's reputation
and therefore had to be advertised.

Notwithstanding Peto's and Hodges's public pronouncements about
the care they took for their employees, it is likely that the risks and
dangers the workers faced were not necessarily perceived as constituting
poor working conditions or ill treatment. In fact, the capacity of workers
to manage risk was regarded as a demonstration of their skills and
masculinity – and here we also find evidence of the spatial dimensions
of dangerous work conditions and a belief that the skill and strength of
male workers would mitigate the risk of accidents. In April 1858, the
spring ice breakup destroyed the dams necessary for the construction of
the bridge and delayed the project.[28] The men worked a series of
exhausting eighteen-hour-days to make up lost time, positioning an average
of ten tons of masonry per hour, or more than two cubic feet per minute.

Engineer-in-chief Ross underlined that it was "an achievement … without a parallel," but he was also describing a calculated capitalist risk: exhausted workers can make dangerous and costly mistakes.[29]

Ross might have wanted to reassure the company's directors that the bridge would be completed on time. But even if he exaggerated the workers' achievements, he appeared genuinely proud of them. Ultimately, the bridge was finished two years ahead of schedule, despite all the challenges.[30] This achievement underlined the exceptional abilities of the workers, but Legge's description of some gangs of riveters who "have been known to make 4 days in about 16 hours, working time, putting in 700 rivets, when 180 constituted the number required,"[31] is also a window into the role of competition and masculinity in the workers' performances. In his essay on logging in Northern Ontario, Ian Radforth shows how cutters and haulers competed among themselves for the highest work output of the day and how their pride, their status among their peers, and their manliness and sense of self depended on it. This "distinctly masculine outlook … increased productivity – and ultimately employers' profits – at the same time as it expressed a commonality of experience."[32]

The Victoria Bridge workers' exploits were rooted in a similar culture that combined workplace skill and masculinity. It is likely that they considered risk part of their work and managed the tasks assigned to them accordingly. The employers' accounts only hint at danger, because managing risk and avoiding accidents was the business of the workers themselves. Legge described "the tube" – the vast interior construction site where iron plates were riveted together to form the tubular beam that became Victoria Bridge – from the point of view of "a person visiting it for the first time," with eight to ten sets of riveters labouring in the dark, hurling rivets to each other and putting them in place.[33] Visitors stumbled over tools and material and trembled in fear of receiving a red-hot rivet in the face. The noise, Legge wrote, was painful and deafening.

In a few lines, Legge described at least three possible worksite accidents. And yet, by detailing accidents that could befall an inexperienced visitor, Legge implied that they did not befall experienced workers. In fact, his description reads like a homage to the abilities of the workers, extraordinary men with superior strength and endurance who could work efficiently and safely in dark, dangerous environments. The Victoria Bridge employers' rhetoric lauded the workers' physical aptitudes as if these were the natural characteristics of these heroic members of the working class. As Michel Pigenet's work on French dockers demonstrates, such stereotypes of masculinity also dehumanized the working class.[34]

Legge's description emphasized space in the construction project, comparing the tube, where the workers belonged, to "Pluto's dark dominion" and establishing a spatial frontier between workers and the "visitor." We see here a physical and social distribution of risk. Accidents could happen to an unaware visitor but, according to Legge, were less likely to befall the workers. Cooter shows that industrial injuries were the lot of the working class, kept out of public view in railway yards or mines or quarries.[35] On the Victoria Bridge worksite, a similar spatial separation likely contributed to the idea that managing industrial risks was mainly part of the workers' job.

The apparent absence of workplace accidents in the textual sources about the bridge worksite, the vast unseen interiors of the construction spaces involved in this massive building project, and the stereotypes attached to the category of "worker" suggest that workers were regarded as existing outside the world inhabited by their employers, Legge's imagined readers, and society's moneyed and professional elites. Historian Georges Vigarello shows how workers' bodies defined their identities: labouring bodies symbolized strength and physical power, but they also bore the scars of labour and fatigue.[36] Consequently, workers' bodies were also at the heart of the issue of accidents. How well their bodies performed, and how much responsibility the employers took for their well-being, characterized the relationship between workers and employers and determined employers' strategies for managing the worksite. In fact, the language employers used to describe the bodies of working men, and the way in which different accidents were perceived, reveal a social framing and understanding of risk. This framing suggests we need to examine the notion of risk on the worksite more precisely.

RISK ON THE WORKSITE

The multiplicity of tasks involved in railway and bridge construction help us establish a taxonomy of risks present at the Victoria Bridge workplace. Hodges described how the quarrying, shaping, and shipping of the stones were important and painstaking steps of the construction process. This was dangerous work. Quarrying was known for its high accident rates and associated chronic illnesses.[37] A 1908 British memoir of an anonymous stonemason includes accounts of falls, burns, and lung disease.[38] The 1853 tramway built to ship stones to the Victoria Bridge site from thirty kilometres up the St Lawrence River would have involved the work of excavators, who were also prone to mishaps. On 29 July 1853, an excavator working on the Quebec-Richmond section of the Grand Trunk had a load of soil dropped on his leg; the limb was eventually amputated.[39] The same newspaper mentioned a worker from another railway worksite whose toes were severed by a wagon wheel.

These examples are but a few instances of what I call typical worksite accidents, and with thousands of workers on the bridge worksite undertaking such dangerous activities over six years, we must assume that these accidents took place with some frequency. Cooter and Luckin demonstrate that businesses and the state "accentuated the normalization of the accident" as part of the "natural order" of industrial society.[40] Clearly, there was a difference between risks that seemed extraordinary to British employers – or "God's will," such as those caused by the extremes of the Canadian climate – and acceptable industrial risks that were simply part of life on the worksite. Typical accidents were normal, or rather normalized, as part of economic development – as Cameron Baldassarra describes accidents that befell loggers on the Petawawa River in the early twentieth century as "a daily part of life" and "mundane hazards of the job."[41]

But how did the Victoria Bridge workers understand risk on the job? I have mentioned the possible consequences of the fatigue due to the necessity to work hard and fast, a strain made worse when contractors were struggling to finish a project. The Grand Trunk directors offered Peto, Brassey, Jackson, and Betts a $300,000 bonus if the bridge could be open by the end of the 1859 work season.[42] It was common for workers to be paid incentives: instead of a daily rate, the riveting gangs were paid the equivalent of a day's wage for driving 180 rivets, an inducement that increased the work pace. The men's work pace and their remarkable achievements, made possible by risk-taking and fatigue, reflect the role of masculinity in the conception and management of risk on the worksite.

Labour historians sketch out these themes across time and geographical locations. Jamie Bronstein shows how masculinity and expectations about manliness underpinned a fatalistic attitude towards workplace accidents among the British working class in the nineteenth century.[43] Workers accepted the risks of drowning or injury due to exhaustion because they considered them part of their job. Here again, accidents were normalized on the worksite. Yet workers paid a high price for their risk-taking. Historians like Bronstein demonstrate the terrible financial and social consequences of debilitating accidents, as disabled male workers were both impoverished and objects of scorn.[44] Reviewing the same period, Bettina Bradbury notes that accidents undermined the masculinity of the Canadian workers whose legal responsibility was to support their families.[45] Craig Heron and Robert Storey also analyze how the gendered division of Canadian labour in the twentieth century distinguished the domestic, unpaid, "feminine" sphere from the public, waged, "masculine" sphere, and how being able to work was constitutive of workers' masculine identity.[46] Risk was a threat not only to workers' physical integrity but also to their social identity and function.

"Fortunately no lives were lost," Hodges wrote about the thirteen rafts carrying timber that crashed into the stagings in 1859.[47] The centre span had been cleared for navigation, suggesting anticipation of an accident with the rafts. However, the outcome of the incident, when it happened, was regarded as a matter of fortune or misfortune. Hodges added that they were "thankful … to escape so lightly."[48] The word "thankful" is not random and echoes the term "fortunately" used to describe the outcome of the same accident. Both words imply that this accident could have had an unhappy outcome, and if everything went well in the end, it was not anybody's responsibility. Hodges understood that the fact that nobody died when the accident occurred was due to something beyond human control, possibly fate or God.

Sociologist Judith Green analyzes how certain misfortunes came to be classified as accidents in the late twentieth century and shows that even with the advent of nosology in 1839, British accidents were still understood as medical misfortunes.[49] Green would thus regard the accidents that happened at the Victoria Bridge worksite as a problem that concerned the employers, and the outcome of accidents that happened to the workers as a matter of individual fate. This does not mean that the bridge workers or employers did not care about what happened when the thirteen rafts went out of control, but rather that they understood that they wielded no control over the course of such an event.

The employers' accounts from the bridge site contain hints of workers adopting precautions against many potential accidents. The risk of drowning was regarded as particularly significant. To build the foundations of the bridge, workers constructed dams and pumped out the water so that the men could work on the riverbed. A number of times during this process, workers narrowly escaped death. In this passage from Hodges, what he describes as curiosity about the colour of the water might well have reflected the workers assessing risk and reacting to danger:

On the 26^{t}h July [1858] the dam was pumped out, and found to be very staunch. The boulders covering the bed of the river were removed, and the excavation commenced, when a blow of the *pick*, within a few feet of the centre of the dam, tapped a spring of thick black water, which at first produced a fountain about as large as a man's finger. This attracted the notice of the workmen, who crowded round to see "a spring of ink" (as they called it) issuing from the bed of the river, but they found it increase in volume so rapidly, that in a few minutes they had to run for their lives, and in a quarter of an hour the dam was full.[50]

Hodges emphasized the dam's soundness and claimed that a worker digging in the wrong place caused the flood. No workers died because they managed to escape. Green demonstrates that the word "accident" is used to "denote certain kinds of outcome."[51] Here, although Hodges gives a glimpse of the risks the workers faced daily, the potentially tragic consequences of the incident, had they not run fast enough, are implied and yet also absent, because the accident did not happen.

The flooded dam was no isolated incident. The risk of drowning inhered in the construction of these temporary structures. As Legge described it, "If the foundation was bad, a break would fill the entire cavity in a few moments, the men forsaking their tools, and, squirrel-like, running up the ladders provided for their escape."[52] The ladders were a protection to save the workers because the risk of a flooded dam was anticipated. But what really saved the workers was their ability to identify the danger and move quickly.

Although landscape architect Heather Braiden shows how a lithograph in *Construction of the Great Victoria Bridge in Canada* "normalizes the ice," Hodges's text explains how river conditions during the spring season could be dangerously unpredictable.[53] When the break-up of river ice happened earlier than expected in March 1859, workers labouring on the river began to run for the shore but eventually thought it wiser to remain on the tube.[54] Three days later, some temporary piers collapsed because of the thaw. According to Hodges, this caused "great alarm to the workmen ... some of whom narrowly escaped from falling off."[55] Hodges remarked that, despite the bad weather, "every man seemed to imagine that success [in completing the works] depended upon his own individual exertion, and all worked with this feeling as if for very life, irrespective of remuneration."[56] Considering the danger of the moving ice, the men probably did believe that their lives depended on how fast they worked. Fear, a recurrent theme regarding the workers in Hodges's book, determined what constituted a risk and a potential accident. The workers' perception and analysis of risk preserved them. Taken from this perspective, the low death toll noted by Hodges is a testament to the workers' ability to keep themselves safe.

Risk management on the bridge site was therefore related to the "good worker." The company discourse presented the Victoria Bridge workers as the best in the world.[57] Hodges was apparently so anxious to keep his top workers on the job that he employed them over the winter.[58] Beyond the obvious propaganda this discourse represented, the ability to avoid injury and death would have been characteristic of a "good worker." The low death toll at the bridge worksite, if accurate, perhaps depended more on the workers' experience (and ability to run fast) than on the safety provisions Legge mentioned. Historian Arwen Mohun extends the concept of vernacular risk culture to study the ways that workers have negotiated the uncertainties of their labour since the eighteenth century, tracing sets of rules, customs, and beliefs passed informally from person to person and noting that, for bridge painters, "skill, carefulness, and attention to duty were the only means to avoid accidents."[59] Similarly, in chapter 6 of this volume, John Matchim observes, "While the Grenfell mission believed that more modern fishing methods and better regulation would improve the safety" of fishers in Labrador, they actually learned about risk and safety from personal experience.[60] People might not have the power to prevent accidents, but they learned to avoid them, and this learning provided an important part of the knowledge base of a nineteenth-century construction worker.

The discrepancy between how the sources present risks and injuries due to weather and typical industrial risks indicates that the latter were normalized by both employers and workers. Accidental injuries and the outcome of accidents seemed to have been a matter of individual fortune or misfortune. The workers were therefore left to deal with risk and danger themselves or among themselves: they had to identify potential accidents and react accordingly. Their ability to avoid accidents was partly what made them good workers. This individualistic and fatalistic conception of risks and accidents influenced their understanding of the notion of precaution.

ANTICIPATING RISKS AND ACCIDENTS
ON THE WORKSITE

The normalization of risk as well as the understanding of accident as a misfortune did not rule out the necessity of taking precautions. Significantly, both Hodges's and Legge's accounts mentioned such safety measures. These texts were intended to be published, and the insistence on the precautions or provisions taken would have been part of the employers' strategy to bolster their reputation. But we need to analyze these measures to understand the notion of precaution on the worksite.

Some precautions were a response to the injuries caused by the cold weather that so impressed the employers at the beginning of the construction. In 1859, workers wore fur caps covering their ears and handkerchiefs on their faces, and they also covered most of their bodies, allowing them to work even at night at temperatures down to at −20 degrees Fahrenheit.[61] A newspaper article describing the body of a deceased Victoria Bridge worker gives an idea of how workers layered their clothing in winter: long boots, stockings, woollen trousers, two shirts, a top coat, a sash plus a necktie, and leather mitts.[62] Close analysis of weather data from the period shows that temperatures followed a similar seasonal pattern from one year to another; however, there could be extreme variations of temperatures in single days or from one day to the next, which probably favoured injuries. This explains why precautions against the cold worked to some extent but not always, despite the workers' acquired experience during construction.[63] Hodges proudly wrote in 1859 that, despite the cold, no terrible accidents had taken place:

> During the erection of this tube, scores of men were frozen in their hands, noses, ears, and face. Some had to go to the hospital in consequence; yet not a man lost either finger or toe; neither was any man seriously injured during the time the tube was in progress. There were, indeed, fewer casualties than usually occurred in the summer season upon similar work. And this is to be accounted for by the excessive precautions that were taken, in consequence of the certain knowledge that the slightest carelessness would produce fearful mutilation, and very probably loss of life itself.[64]

Again, this passage shows that employers evaluated accidents according to the gravity of their outcomes: scores of men needed medical assistance, but because there was no fearful mutilation, the precautions taken were deemed successful. Similarly, some were injured, but not seriously, so accidents were avoided. We see that serious accidents were defined according to the fear and the horror they could inspire, as implied by the "fearful mutilation" and death that, in the end, did not happen. But these precautions did not prevent accidents altogether and indeed a zero-accident score at the Victoria Bridge worksite would have been an impossible achievement. What is striking, though, is that the injuries listed by Hodges in 1859 at the end of construction were the same that he had described in 1854, when explaining that the workers did not have the experience of working in the Canadian climate. Hodges's characterizing the precautions on the worksite as "excessive" is therefore inaccurate.

We know from Hodges and Legge that, although drowning was the greatest threat to life on the bridge site, most workers could swim and there were lifebuoys and boats at hand.[65] Triggs et al. provide the example of the boatman Joseph Vincent, who saved at least ten men who fell from the bridge, and note that the precautions of having boats at the ready probably lowered the death toll.[66] Hodges admitted that when men ended up in the water – which seldom occurred, he added – they were drawn into the eddy by the current and rarely rescued.[67] When he described an accident that involved the thirteen Indigenous workers manning a raft that crashed into the temporary work, he explained that it had seemed impossible to save so many men.[68] Like the ladders in the dams, these limited provisions establish the anticipation of the risk of drowning. But a number of men drowned, and more almost did when they fell from the bridge. It seems that no precautions were taken to prevent falls from the bridge.[69]

Hodges commissioned the noted Montreal photographer William Notman (1826–1891) to document the bridge construction. Braiden tells us that photography became a critical form of communication in mid-nineteenth-century engineering, a medium that facilitated long-distance professional exchanges and information sharing on international construction sites. Notman's photographs were "a communication tool" among engineers based in Britain and in Montreal.[70] Braiden borrows from scholar Susan Leigh Star's application of the concept of boundary objects to discuss Hodges's account, explaining that forms of visual representation of the bridge construction like the lithographs "convey a broader cultural narrative to lay audiences."[71]

Notman shot film at the Victoria Bridge site from 1858 until the end of the construction, official images that represent what the employers thought was appropriate to show as part of that cultural narrative. *Interior of Staging with Tube in Progress* (fig. 5.2) shows workmen sitting and standing on top of the structure. No barrier is evident to prevent them from falling into the river if dislodged from their positions. Although the men undoubtedly posed for this picture, other images, too, suggest that no precautions were taken. Fig. 5.3, for instance, clearly shows that no safety measures were present to keep men from plummeting from the bridge. That does not mean that the employers did not connect the risk of drowning with the risk

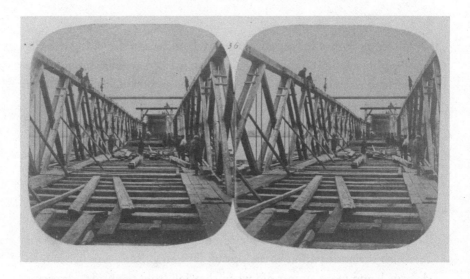

Fig. 5.2 *Interior of Staging with Tube in Progress.*

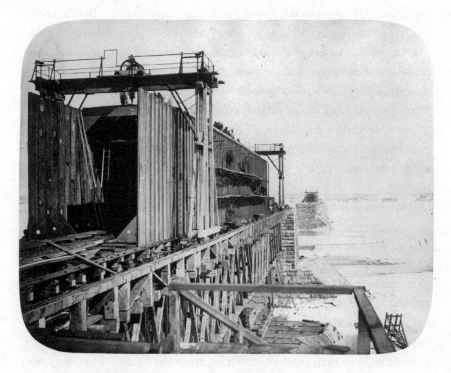

Fig. 5.3 *Centre Tube, March 1859.*

of falling. When a worker, however good a swimmer, fell into the river, it was necessary to save him. However, if a worker fell from the scaffolding or placed himself at risk by standing on the top of the tube, this might have been deemed the responsibility of the employee, not the employer. The precautions taken to protect workers from the cold or the river had a common feature: they did not stop accidents from happening altogether but tried to prevent workers' death or mutilation. In other words, these precautions prevented workers from being unable to work.

A more comprehensive move to mitigate the damage caused by accidents at the site was the contract the employers made with St Patrick's Hospital. Founded in 1852 by Bishop Ignace Bourget of Montreal and managed by the Religious Hospitallers of St Joseph,[72] the hospital was created to provide medical care for Montreal's working-class Irish Catholic community. It was this institution where the injured workers from the bridge and the Grand Trunk Railway were taken to be treated. Newspapers of the period mention the work of the hospital in caring for bridge workers, and Hodges does likewise throughout his account, which concludes with an expression of gratitude to the medical staff.[73] The hospital agreement was a typically paternalistic employer initiative like worker libraries and religious education, but it was also an acknowledgment of the dangerous work involved in bridge building and an institutional innovation to safeguard a skilled workforce in a growing colony.

Employers sending their workers to the hospital and providing them with medical attendance was not new or extraordinary. There was no workers' compensation legislation in Britain until 1880, but employers often compensated injured employees, notably by covering part of their medical costs.[74] Some British and American railway companies of the period provided free medical care or artificial limbs. These provisions were partly meant to discourage the workers from taking political or group action, but paternalism also played a significant role in this process, although much more in Britain than in the United States.[75] Labour historians have shown that companies undertaking large-scale construction projects often financed hospitals. Looking at the construction of canals in North America between 1780 and 1860, Peter Way notes that canal boards hired doctors or established hospitals in cases of epidemics or "to preserve an evaporating labour force."[76] The scheme elaborated by the Chesapeake & Delaware Canal in 1824 consisted of having both contractors and workers pay for the hospital building and its health-care services; this model "became popular on many public works."[77] In Britain, David Brooke shows through detailed examples that railway companies and contractors financed hospitals, although the number of casualties was so significant that their subscriptions "by no means equalled [the hospital] expenses."[78]

The Victoria Bridge contractors were known for their paternalism and even philanthropy. Biographer Arthur Helps emphasizes that when British railway contractor Brassey was dying, navvies came to bid him farewell.[79] Contemporaries testified that Peto took great care of his workers, while some described Hodges as philanthropic and concerned with workers' welfare.[80] Despite obvious hagiographic aspects of their biographies, the paternalism of these employers who provided chapels, Bibles, education, and shelter to their workers was probably genuine, even if somewhat calculated. Providing hospital care for workers injured on the job was another facet of this deliberate paternalism and suggests that employers regarded it as their responsibility to repair damaged bodies rather than to prevent workers from being injured. However, the agreement with St Patrick's Hospital was not just care: it was a precaution, an anticipation of accidental injuries.

The correspondence between the employers, the sisters, and the bishop spells out Hodges's agreement on behalf of the contractors and the hospital. The first available letter, dated October 1853,[81] a response to Hodges who had applied for accommodation in St Patrick's Hospital, shows that the employers moved to make arrangements with the hospital very early in the construction process. They were given "a room or rooms" with twenty-five beds for the exclusive use of Victoria Bridge patients and were required to pay £100 to furnish and set up the rooms. Hodges agreed.

Negotiations continued until February 1854 when Peto, Brassey, Jackson, and Betts accepted the following terms: they would pay £100 to outfit the new twenty-five-bed ward, to be available at all times for workmen who might "require medical attendance"; they would pay two dollars a week for each Grand Trunk railway patient for the duration of their illness; and they would also pay the doctors when the hospital provided medicine.[82] This agreement appears to have been made between the contractors and the bishop rather than between the company and the Committee of St Patrick's Hospital, and records indicate that it continued throughout the construction period.[83]

Booking an entire twenty-five-bed hospital ward for injured workers so early in the history of the construction demonstrated a clear anticipation of accidents.[84] It is distinct from the employers' compensation payments detailed by Bronstein because disbursements were made to the hospital both before and after accidents occurred.[85] It also differs from the company hospitals described by Brooke, where employers chose not to cover the full costs of the workers' medical care: Victoria Bridge contractors invested money in medical care before and throughout the construction period.[86] Hodges often complained about the scarcity of labour in Canada East, and skilled workers were recruited in Britain.[87] The agreement with the hospital was a way to preserve valued skilled workers. Like the lifebuoys, providing hospital rooms aimed at preventing their mutilation or death. It was a significant and rather unusual precaution that did not prevent accidents from happening but ensured that every effort would be dedicated to making broken bodies productive once more.

CONCLUSION

The story of risk and accidents on construction sites like the Victoria Bridge and the Grand Trunk remains largely undocumented, although such worksites have been studied by historians of labour. This chapter demonstrates that workplace injuries, risk, and management of risk were an inherent part of these large, multifaceted work settings. It suggests the beginnings of a move towards the late Victorian reclassification of workplace injuries as accidents and the eventual emergence of twentieth-century state responses like those detailed by Ceilidh Auger-Day in this collection. Investigating these topics thus provides new insights into management strategies and power relations between workers and employers. More significantly, perhaps, it also illuminates precautionary features of working-class masculinity, giving the nineteenth-century bridge worker a role as an active agent in securing an element of workplace safety.

We must take the social distribution of risk into account to understand the notion of precaution. Indeed, the instability of the definition of "accident" does not rule out provision or prevention altogether. On the contrary, the Victoria Bridge employers acknowledged the need to protect workers' bodies to ensure that construction would continue as planned. Risks that could threaten the workers' bodies lay therefore at the heart of the employers' strategy to manage the workers and the worksite. The agreement with St Patrick's Hospital exemplified how the notion of precaution operated in an era when the definition of the accident appeared to be in flux. As anticipatory steps, precautions did not prevent accidents from happening. Yet with precautions in place, drowning men could be saved and broken bodies repaired, and there would be workers to complete the Victoria Bridge.

My research makes clear that historians of the accident need to be adept and painstaking in their research. Sources on the Victoria Bridge, and especially employers' sources, lack mentions of accidental injuries, mainly because there was no stable definition of "accident." But I argue that the silence of the sources in itself constitutes a source of information. Indeed, risks and potential injuries pervade the sources. For example, the historical evidence about the construction of the bridge mentions unusual injuries due to the weather but remains silent about typical risks, demonstrating both a normalization of industrial risks and a dichotomy between extraordinary and ordinary risks. The sources allude to accidents, but at the same time these went unrecorded because the writers reported only positive outcomes.

The ambiguity of the sources examined for this chapter meant that I needed to historicize the perception of risk in order to interrogate the notion of risk itself. Clearly, at the Victoria Bridge worksite, the perception of risk was involved in the complex power relations prevailing on the worksite. The workers should not be regarded as passive victims of terrible industrial risks their employers imposed on them. A culture of masculinity, shared by both workers and employers and encouraged by the gendered division of labour and a patriarchal society, contributed to the normalization of risk.

ACKNOWLEDGMENTS

I am grateful for the help and efforts of Gilbert Langlois and archivist Nicole Bussières (Musée des Soeurs Hospitalières, Montreal, Archives des Religieuses Hospitalières de St Joseph de Montréal), the extraordinary generosity of Gilles Lauzon and Julie Stone, and the support of Fabrice Bensimon and Ian Kerr.

NOTES

1 Legge, *Glance at the Victoria Bridge*, 85.
2 See, for example, "Le Pont Victoria à Montreal," *Le Courrier de Saint-Hyacinthe*, 7 January 1858.
3 I use the word "firm" for the partnership between Peto, Brassey, Jackson, and Betts. In the 1850s, however, revolving partnerships of the big contractors had not yet evolved into the continuing, formal firms of later years. I thank Ian Kerr for this remark. As to why a British rather than a Canadian firm was called on to build and finance this railway, see Currie, *Grand Trunk Railway of Canada*, 11–13; Boxer, *Hunter's Hand Book of the Victoria Bridge*, 28. On the dispute between A. Ross and R. Stephenson over the merit of the design of the bridge, see Boxer, *Hunter's Hand Book*, 20–7.
4 Number of workers in October 1858 taken from "Le Pont Victoria," *Gazette de Sorel*, 28 December 1858,
5 Currie, *Grand Trunk Railway*; Triggs et al., *Le Pont Victoria*.
6 Cooter, "Moment of the Accident," 108.
7 In his seminal 1985 article "The Patient's View," Roy Porter argues that the history of medicine, as well as radical anti-history of medicine, centres on doctors. He defends a "sufferers' history," which a lack of sources (described as a lack of "a historical atlas of sickness experience and response") renders difficult. He proposes to use literate sufferers' diaries, letters, and visual arts but also to read against doctors' testimonies, which he claims should be "decoded to reveal what the sufferers dreaded or demanded" (183). Similarly, in her study of prostitution in early nineteenth-century Montreal, *Beyond Brutal Passions*, Mary Anne Poutanen proposes to "approach criminal justice documents by reading against the grain to locate women's voices and their experiences" (23). See also Dearinger, "Chinese Immigrants, the Landscape of Progress," 67; Reaume, *Remembrance of Patients Past*.
8 Hodges, *Construction of the Great Victoria Bridge*, 69.
9 Ibid.
10 Ibid., 70.
11 Minutes of meetings of stockholders and proprietors, Alexander Ross's account, 24 July 1854, RG30-1026, Library and Archives Canada (hereafter LAC); Ross's

account, September 1855, RG30-1026, LAC; Ross's account, 6 December 1858, RG30-1026, LAC.

12   Hodges, *Construction of the Great Victoria Bridge*, 77.

13   Cooter, "Moment of the Accident," 108.

14   Ibid., 111.

15   Brooke, *Railway Navvy*, 39, shows that it was the contractors' duty to provide housing to the workers, although they were often reluctant to do so.

16   Hodges, *Construction of the Great Victoria Bridge*, 77–8.

17   Peto, *Sir Morton Peto*, 77–80.

18   See, for instance, Fayers, *Labour among the Navvies*, 28–9; Kennedy et al., "Health and Well-Being of Chinese Railroad Workers," 139–41.

19   Hodges, *Construction of the Great Victoria Bridge*, 77.

20   Peto, *Sir Morton Peto*, 57.

21   Hodges, *Construction of the Great Victoria Bridge*, 77.

22   Ibid., 17–18.

23   Brassey, *Work and Wages Practically Illustrated*, 35; Hodges, *Construction of the Great Victoria Bridge*, 26.

24   Hodges, *Construction of the Great Victoria Bridge*, 77.

25   From "The Montreal Strikes," *Montreal Transcript*, 4 May 1855:

> We believe the blame rests not on one side alone; but masters and labourers are alike in fault. For the latter to work twelve hours during the summer, appears to us, so afar as their physical health is concerned, most dangerous and prejudicial. It is stated, and by those who have much experience in such matters, that the twelve hours system is a good one, – injurious neither to master nor men. We are told, in the United States, on the great public works, it is the rule; and that here, unfortunately, the Grand Trunk people made it an exception. At the present time, and with provisions of all kinds at the rate they are, it is a serious thing, and would, doubtless, be felt keenly, even the very thought of oppression. The labourer who is well fed and well paid, rarely grudges working hard; and where his employers are respected, will toil as would a faithful horse, until compelled by exhaustion to cease. But it is said that the Contractors on the two great public works, that have mainly produced the strikes, have not thus behaved towards their workmen; that long hours, low wages, or no pay at all, are the cause of the differences.

26   Hodges, *Construction of the Great Victoria Bridge*, 77. The bishop reportedly pronounced those words in December 1859 during the entertainment provided by Hodges to celebrate the opening of the bridge. "Ouverture du Pont Victoria," *La Minerve*, 20 December 1859, mentions the presence of the Anglican bishop among Hodges's important guests. There is no mention of the Catholic bishop.

27   Joseph Elliott, Secretary and Treasurer of the Grand Trunk Railway Company of Canada to the Bishop of Montreal, 24 July 1860, T75.002, 860–1, Archives de la Chancellerie de l'Archevêché de Montréal (hereafter ACAM).

28 Ross's account, 6 December 1858, RG30-1026, LAC.

29 Ibid.

30 Passfield, "Construction of the Victoria Tubular Bridge," 33.

31 Legge, *Glance at the Victoria Bridge*, 122.

32 Radforth, "Logging Pulpwood in Northern Ontario," 252.

33 Legge, *Glance at the Victoria Bridge*, 121.

34 Michel Pigenet's work on French dockers shows how stereotypes of masculinity associated with these workers were used to both celebrate and idealize the dockers' physical strength and also to portray them as powerful beasts, thus implying that they were less human than members of the middle and upper classes. Pigenet, "A propos des représentations et des rapports sociaux sexués," 56–7, 66.

35 Cooter, "Moment of the Accident," 114.

36 Vigarello, *Histoire de la Fatigue*, 188, 198.

37 Samuel, "Mineral Workers," 42.

38 *Reminiscences of a Stonemason*, 235, 133–4, 87–8.

39 "Accidents de Chemins de fer," *Le Pays*, 3 August 1853.

40 Cooter and Luckin, "Accidents in History: An Introduction," 5.

41 Baldassarra, "'Don't Shoot Crooked Chute,'" in this volume, 228, 236.

42 Passfield, "Construction of the Victoria Tubular Bridge," 33.

43 Bronstein, *Caught in the Machinery*, 88.

44 Ibid., 87.

45 Bradbury, *Working Families*, 80.

46 Heron and Storey, "On the Job in Canada," 9–10.

47 Hodges, *Construction of the Great Victoria Bridge*, 69.

48 Ibid.

49 Green, *Risk and Misfortune*, 71. Nosology is the classification of diseases.

50 Hodges, *Construction of the Great Victoria Bridge*, 49; emphasis in original.

51 Green, *Risk and Misfortune*, 1.

52 Legge, *Glance at the Victoria Bridge*, 100.

53 In a recent article, landscape architect Heather Braiden contrasts the real danger that the "shoving of the ice" represented to Montreal residents to a lithograph in Hodge's book depicting the shove that "normalizes the ice." Braiden, "'Far from Uninteresting,'" 194–216, at 202.

54 Hodges, *Construction of the Great Victoria Bridge*, 60.

55 Ibid., 61.

56 Ibid., 61–2.

57 Ibid., 75. Hodges paid homage to his workers who "worked as British workmen alone can work." The skills and know-how of the Victoria Bridge workers were part of an imperial rhetoric.

58 Triggs, "Le Pont," 48.

59 Mohun, *Risk. Negotiating Safety in American Society*, 1.

60 Matchim, "'Lack of System in Their Work,'" in this volume, 181.

61 Hodges, *Construction of the Great Victoria Bridge*, 57–8.

62 *Pilot*, 13 January 1859, quoted in Triggs, "Le Pont," 49.

63 John Samuel McCord (1801–1865), Activités professionnelles et récréatives, Fonds McCord Family, P001-B3.4_Part17, McCord Museum. Montrealer John Bethune (1791–1872) recorded daily temperature, wind, and precipitation readings from 1838 to 1869. His data are considered accurate and suitable for studying temperature variations on the Victoria Bridge worksite. See Slonosky, "Historical Climate Observations in Canada," 1–18.

64 Hodges, *Construction of the Great Victoria Bridge*, 58.

65 Ibid., 77. Hodges's statement about the swimming abilities of the workforce is surprising. In *Shifting Currents*, Karen Eva Carr states that most Europeans and White Americans in the nineteenth century did not know how to swim, and when they did, they used the breaststroke and backstroke, keeping their faces out of the water even in competition, and therefore did not swim well (388, 390, 397). Carr's point suggests that the workers Hodges mentioned were considered good swimmers because they could swim, which was uncommon enough to be seen as a talent. However, that talent might not have been sufficient for them to survive in the current of the St Lawrence, and it is highly doubtful that the majority of the workforce were strong swimmers.

66 Triggs, "Le Pont," 48.

67 Hodges, *Construction of the Great Victoria Bridge*, 77.

68 Ibid., 63–5. The accident involving thirteen Indigenous workers occurred around 5 May 1859. According to Hodges, none were killed, although some were picked up half a mile further down the river.

69 In an 11 July 2018 email to the author, Julie Stone, who conducts research on the Britannia Bridge (1846–50) at the Menai Heritage (Wales), notes that the weather could be extreme on the Britannia Bridge worksite and that there were wind shields on scaffoldings, which does not seem to be the case for the Victoria Bridge worksite. This fact suggests that Stephenson, who was involved in the construction of both tubular bridges, would have been aware that falls were a common risk on construction sites.

70 Braiden, "'Far from Uninteresting,'" 199–200.

71 A boundary object "allows members of different social groups – engineers, their patrons, and the public – to gain insight into the complex construction project even though the book and their understanding may be quite different." Braiden, "'Far from Uninteresting,'" 200.

72 Lahaise, "L'Hôtel-Dieu du Vieux-Montréal," 51.

73 *Le Pays*, 3 August 1853; Hodges, *Construction of the Great Victoria Bridge*, 77.

74 Bronstein, *Caught in the Machinery*, 3.

75 Ibid., 35, 37.

76 Way, *Common Labour*, 158–9.

77 Ibid., 159.

78 Brooke, *Railway Navvy*, 150.

79 Helps, *Life and Labours of Thomas Brassey*, 172–3.

80 Peto, *Sir Morton Peto*, 78–80; Legge, *Glance at the Victoria Bridge*, 85.
81 Unnamed to Hodges, and Hodges's response, October 1853, Fonds de l'Hôpital St Patrick, Musée des Soeurs Hospitalières, Montreal, Archives des Religieuses Hospitalières de St Joseph de Montréal (hereafter ARHSJM).
82 Jackson, Peto, Brassey, Betts, and Hodges to Rev. T. Plamondon, 17 February 1854, Fonds de l'Hôpital St Patrick, ARHSJM. The Grand Trunk workers included the Victoria Bridge workers, since Hodges thanked St Patrick's medical staff at the end of his book.
83 Religieuses, Hospitalières de St Joseph, 15 April 1854, 525.102, ACAM. A few letters from the sisters to the bishop allude to the Grand Trunk workers throughout the construction period. Until 1857, the sisters regularly complained that the doctors tried to make poor patients pay, arguing that only the Grand Trunk workers and patients in the private rooms were supposed to pay.
84 Out of a total of seventy-five beds. Lahaise, "L'Hôtel-Dieu," 54.
85 Bronstein, *Caught in the Machinery*, 3, 32–9.
86 The examples analyzed by Brooke show that the money spent on medical care by railway companies in Britain did not cover workers' real needs and was much lower than the Victoria Bridge provisions. For instance, the London & Birmingham gave £115 10s. to Northampton General Infirmary to cover costs of £600; the Chester & Holyhead gave ten guineas to Chester Infirmary (but donated £300 for religious and moral instruction), while the Victoria Bridge contractors paid £100 for the room annually, $2 a week for each patient, and £1,000 annually for the medical staff. Brooke, *Railway Navvy*, 150; Hodges, *Construction of the Great Victoria Bridge*, 77.
87 Brassey, *Work and Wages*, 35.

BIBLIOGRAPHY

Archives

Archives de la Chancellerie de l'Archevêché de Montréal (ACAM)
Library and Archives Canada (LAC), RG30-1026, Minutes of meetings of stockholders and proprietors
McCord Museum, Fonds McCord Family, P001-B3.4_Part17
Musée des Soeurs Hospitalières, Montreal, Archives des Religieuses Hospitalières de St Joseph de Montréal (ARHSJM)

Newspapers

Gazette de Sorel
La Minerve (Montreal)
Le Courrier de Saint-Hyacinthe

Le Pays (Montreal)
Montreal Transcript
Pilot (Montreal)

Other Sources

Boxer, F.N. *Hunter's Hand Book of the Victoria Bridge.* Montreal: Hunter & Pickup, 1860.

Bradbury, Bettina. *Working Families: Age, Gender, and Daily Survival in Industrializing Montreal.* Toronto: McClelland & Stewart, 1993.

Braiden, Heather. "'Far from Uninteresting': Getting to Know the St. Lawrence River at Montreal during the Construction of the Victoria Bridge." *Urban History Review* 49, no. 2 (Spring 2022): 194–216.

Brassey, Thomas. *Work and Wages Practically Illustrated.* London: Bell & Daldy, 1872.

Bronstein, Jamie L. *Caught in the Machinery: Workplace Accidents and Injured Workers in Nineteenth-Century Britain.* Stanford, CA: Stanford University Press, 2008.

Brooke, David. *The Railway Navvy: "That Despicable Race of Men."* Newton Abbot, UK: David & Charles, 1983.

Campbell, Robert. "Philosophy and the Accident." In *Accidents in History: Injuries, Fatalities and Social Relations*, edited by Roger Cooter and Bill Luckin, 17–34. Atlanta: Rodopi, 1997.

Carr, Karen Eva. *Shifting Currents: A World History of Swimming.* London: Reaktion Books (ebook), 2022.

Cooter, Roger. "The Moment of the Accident: Culture, Militarism and Modernity in Late-Victorian Britain." In Cooter and Luckin, *Accidents in History*, 107–57.

Cooter, Roger, and Bill Luckin. "Accidents in History: An Introduction." In Cooter and Luckin, *Accidents in History*, 1–16.

Currie, Archibald W. *The Grand Trunk Railway of Canada.* Toronto: University of Toronto Press, 1957.

Dearinger, Ryan. "Chinese Immigrants, the Landscape of Progress, and the Work of Building and Celebrating the Transcontinental Railroad." *California History* 96, no. 2 (May 2019): 66–98.

Fayers, Thomas. *Labour among the Navvies.* London: Wertheim, Macintosh, & Hunt, 1862.

Green, Judith. *Risk and Misfortune. The Social Construction of Accidents.* London: UCL Press, 1997.

Helps, Arthur. *Life and Labours of Thomas Brassey, 1805–1870.* 1872; reprint, London: George Bell & Sons, 1888.

Heron, Craig, and Robert Storey. "On the Job in Canada." In *On the Job: Confronting the Labour Process in Canada*, edited by Craig Heron and Robert Storey, 3–46. Kingston and Montreal: McGill-Queen's University Press, 1986.

Hodges, James. *Construction of the Great Victoria Bridge in Canada.* London: John Wheale, 1860.

Kennedy, J. Ryan, Sarah Heffner, Virginia Popper, Ryan P. Harrod, and John J. Crandall. "The Health and Well-Being of Chinese Railroad Workers." In *The Chinese and the Iron Road: Building the Transcontinental Railroad*, edited by Gordon H. Chang, Shelley Fisher Fishkin, Hilton Obenzinger, and Roland Hsu, 213–41. Stanford, CA: Stanford University Press, 2020.

Lahaise, Robert. "L'Hôtel-Dieu du Vieux-Montréal (1642–1861)." In *L'Hôtel-Dieu de Montréal, 1642–1973*, edited by Michel Allard, 11–56. Montreal: Editions Hurtubise HMH, 1973.

Legge, Charles. *A Glance at the Victoria Bridge, and the Men Who Built It.* Montreal: John Lovell 1860.

Mohun, Arwen P. *Risk. Negotiating Safety in American Society.* Baltimore: Johns Hopkins University Press, 2013.

Passfield, Robert W. "Construction of the Victoria Tubular Bridge." *Canal History and Technology Proceedings* 20 (2001): 5–52

Peto, Henry. *Sir Morton Peto: A Memorial Sketch.* London: Elliott Stock, 1893.

Pigenet, Michel. "A propos des représentations et des rapports sociaux sexués: Identité professionnelle et masculinité chez les dockers français (XIXe–XXe siècles)." *Le Mouvement Social* 198 (2002): 55–74.

Porter, Roy. "The Patient's View: Doing Medical History from Below." *Theory and Society* 14, no. 2 (March 1985): 175–98.

Poutanen, Mary Anne. *Beyond Brutal Passions: Prostitution in Early Nineteenth-Century Montreal.* Montreal and Kingston: McGill-Queen's University Press, 2015.

Radforth, Ian. "Logging Pulpwood in Northern Ontario." In Heron and Storey, *On the Job*, 245–80.

Reaume, Geoffrey. *Remembrance of Patients Past: Patient Life at the Toronto Hospital for the Insane, 1870–1940.* Toronto: University of Toronto Press, 2009.

Reminiscences of a Stonemason; By a Working Man. London: John Murray, 1908.

Samuel, Raphael. "Mineral Workers." In *Miners, Quarrymen and Saltworkers*, edited by Raphael Samuel, 3–97. London: Routledge, 1977.

Slonosky, Victoria "Historical Climate Observations in Canada: 18th and 19th Century Daily Temperature from the St. Lawrence Valley, Quebec." *Geoscience Data Journal* 1 (2014): 1–18.

Triggs, Stanley. "Le Pont." In *Le Pont Victoria: Un lien vital/Victoria Bridge; The Vital Link*, by Brian Young, Conrad Graham, and Gilles Lauzon, 36–73. Montreal: McCord Museum, 1992.

Triggs, Stanley, Brian Young, Conrad Graham, and Gilles Lauzon. *Le Pont Victoria: Un lien vital/Victoria Bridge; the Vital Link.* Montreal: McCord Museum, 1992.

Vigarello, Georges. *Histoire de la Fatigue: Du Moyen Âge à nos jours.* Paris: Éditions du Seuil, 2020.

Way, Peter. *Common Labour. Workers and the Digging of North American Canals, 1780–1860.* Cambridge: Cambridge University Press, 1993.

6

A "Lack of System in Their Work"

Risk, Injury, and Labour in the Grenfell Medical Mission
of Northern Newfoundland and Labrador, 1893–1914

John R.H. Matchim

In 1903, an anonymous author wrote of Labrador, "There is not a spot on the globe where life is harder, or serious accidents of all kinds more frequent than along that stormy stretch of coast."[1] This article in the first issue of *Among the Deep Sea Fishers* (ADSF), the official organ of the Grenfell medical mission of northern Newfoundland and Labrador, recognized that some injuries, such as broken bones and gunshot wounds, "are necessarily frequent" parts of life in Labrador.[2] But the author also believed that the risk of accident and death was accentuated by the domestic and working arrangements of Labrador people. Fishers, for example, used "poor craft" – presumably unsafe or unsuitable for the work required – to conduct the cod and seal fisheries, while primitive first-aid methods did more harm than good.[3] Another writer, Rev. Selby Jefferson, cited a "lack of system in their work and the laziness and mismanagement of their women" to explain the region's poverty and high risk of accident.[4] For both observers, the arrival of Dr Wilfred Grenfell from Britain in 1892 "was the most fortunate thing that happened to Labrador."[5]

The Grenfell mission was established to provide medical support to the thousands of men and women who worked in the vast Labrador cod fishery each summer, finding a livelihood during the rest of the year hunting and sealing. A major part of its work was the treatment of injuries and illnesses at the point of labour near and sometimes on the fishing grounds. Mission physicians and volunteer workers, many of them from urban middle-class backgrounds in the United States and Britain, believed that injuries and accidents were unavoidable realities of fishing and put into place supports and services to mitigate the inevitable outcomes of dangerous working conditions. As the observations of the above writers suggest, the Grenfell mission's approach to work in northern Newfoundland and Labrador extended beyond front-line care. The authors were also certain that the dangers confronted by fishers and their families were accentuated by ignorance and mismanagement, an unfortunate but inevitable result of Labrador's distance from urban "civilization." And they waged professional battles to reshape the health attitudes and practices of local people.

The treatment and prevention of injury and accident in the northern cod fishery created opportunities for Grenfell and other mission workers to regulate the domestic and labour spaces of the local population and attempt to instil in them the values and practices of modern health consumers. The mission's parent organization, the London-based Royal National Mission to Deep Sea Fishermen (RNMDSF), closely associated its work with the success of the British nation, and a concern for national and imperial well-being shaped the Grenfell mission's work in the colony of Newfoundland, albeit in a modified form. Motivated by early twentieth-century (middle-class) sensibilities regarding labour, productivity and citizenship, the mission was part of a broad project to create healthy, self-reliant citizens and fit (male) bodies for industry and war.[6] Mission personnel were practising what John Pickstone calls "productionist" medicine – health practices located at the intersection of health and industrial labour.[7]

As part of the Grenfell mission's improvement project, injury and accident were used to justify its efforts to stamp out alcohol consumption, establish the primacy of the male breadwinner by regulating the involvement of women in the fishery, and replace belief in "superstitious" home remedies with trust in professional medical authority. The training, assistance, and employment that the mission offered people disabled by workplace accidents had less to do with personal well-being than with mitigating the social and economic harm that their "idle" status posed to other individuals and to the state. These interventions, the mission believed, would produce a more respectable labouring class, one that was sober, obedient to authority, observant of separate and appropriate spaces for men and women, and economically productive even in the face of workplace injury. As Rafico Ruiz succinctly writes, the mission's interventions were about "fashioning the right frontier."[8] Interestingly, in the remote and often dangerous setting of northern Labrador, and in the staid pages of ADSF, Grenfell mission workers also refashioned themselves as adventurers and medical heroes, aiming to model healthy bodies and good citizenship on the frontier and sometimes taking risks that placed themselves and those working or travelling with them in danger. As discussed in this volume's introduction, working-class people had little choice but to expose themselves to risks on a daily basis. For the middle-class workers of the Grenfell mission, however, risk was something "voluntarily" accepted, often as an affirmation of a masculine ideal.

Many of these exploits were recounted in the pages of ADSF, a publication that became increasingly important as the mission reoriented its fundraising and recruitments efforts towards the United States in the years preceding the Great War. While ADSF articles were frequently embellished to demonstrate the courage and resourcefulness of Grenfell mission workers and their status as worthy recipients of the reader's financial aid, a careful reading also reveals middle-class ideals concerning appropriate working-class labour and behaviour. Additionally, in its descriptions of everyday life in northern Newfoundland and southeastern Labrador, ADSF provides a unique view of the injuries and accidents encountered by both working people and mission personnel, as well as the sometimes divergent approaches to their treatment. While ADSF was frequently dismissive of home remedies, the magazine's rhetoric – although representative of official mission opinion – was not always shared by clinicians on the ground in Newfoundland and Labrador.

Roger Cooter and Bill Luckin write in their introduction to *Accidents in History* that the study of accidents "must be with the uncompensated individual victim, in terms of his or her experience of injury."[9] While this is not easily achieved, ADSF's extensive archive provides one valuable opportunity to better understand living and working conditions in the cod fishery and fur trade of early twentieth-century Newfoundland and Labrador, and how its men and women responded to the occurrence of both major and "minor" injuries. More broadly, an examination of injury and accident in the regions serviced by the Grenfell mission can contribute to our understanding of scientific medicine and colonialism in the "remote" North. Alison Bashford argues that there was a "logic to modernizing medicine which dovetailed neatly with the logic of Empire and that of expansionist evangelical mission."[10] On the colonial/resource frontier, "modern practice, research and ideas were to be progressively disseminated, displacing older, traditional, and folk techniques associated with unregulated women's and men's practice."[11] This was true of the Grenfell mission in northern Newfoundland and coastal Labrador as well, with its practitioners deploying the incident or risk of injury to displace or reform older medical, labour, and social practices. An examination of accident and injury as it was experienced by mission personnel also reveals interesting parallels with rural-remote physicians and nurses elsewhere in Canada and across the circumpolar North. Motivations for joining the mission in the early twentieth century – adventure, professional ambition, a paternalistic sense of responsibility for "disadvantaged" communities – were, for example, strikingly similar to those of Finnish nurses working in Lapland in the mid-twentieth century, as seen by Marianne Junila in her 2011 study.[12] Tales of medical heroism abound in the pages of ADSF and illustrate how the mission rationalized its own risk-taking while decrying that of local people.

Despite the mission's high regard for the medical and economic opportunities it supplied, local people were not as helpless as ADSF suggested. As we will see, self-care was practised widely in Labrador and Newfoundland, and rather than viewing danger as providential or something entirely outside of their control, men and women learned how to live and labour as safely as possible in their difficult environment. The clinicians and volunteers of the Grenfell mission sought to reform labour practices and ways of life in what they saw as a forgotten colonial frontier, but their sensibilities and interventions were often unsuitable in a subarctic region where survival and safety hinged on intergenerational knowledge and environmental adaptation.

FISHERIES AND THE GRENFELL MISSION

What became the Grenfell medical mission began in 1893 when Wilfred Grenfell, a young evangelical physician employed by the RNMDSF, opened a small hospital at Battle Harbour in southeastern Labrador, one of the centres of the Labrador cod fishery. Initially an extension of the RNMDSF, the Grenfell mission quickly outgrew its parent mission's resources and was incorporated in 1914 as the International Grenfell Association. By this time, as J.T.H. Connor writes, the mission was effectively a "standalone health-care system" organized around a network of small hospitals, nursing stations, the purpose-built hospital ship *Strathcona*, and a sophisticated headquarters hospital in St Anthony in northern Newfoundland.[13] The Grenfell mission was one part of the "massive Anglo-American mission movement" of the late nineteenth century, and Grenfell's annual speaking tours of Britain, Canada, and the United States secured both financial support and the personal assistance of highly qualified medical personnel, with especially strong backing coming from the northeastern United States.[14] However, Jennifer J. Connor notes that while the mission was "essentially Protestant," Grenfell's organization was "not a religious mission with medical missionaries attached; it was a medical mission with social activists attached."[15]

Although famously merged in the public mind with the history and mythology of Newfoundland and Labrador, the mission had its roots in the nineteenth-century British fishing industry. With the construction of a national railway system in the mid-nineteenth century, fresh fish became an affordable staple of working-class towns and cities across Britain, but meeting the increased demand necessitated drastic changes in the technology and labour practices of fishing.[16] Individual fishing voyages were replaced by a new system called fleeting, which involved a group of smacks directed by a fishing "admiral." Every day, and regardless of the weather, small boats transferred fresh fish to sailing cutters that swiftly delivered them to railheads and the urban markets beyond.[17] When steam-power replaced sail on both cutters and trawlers, the increased capital costs were recuperated by fishing in winter as well as summer. Voyages were also longer, with crews remaining at sea for up to eight weeks "of unremitting drudgery and danger."[18]

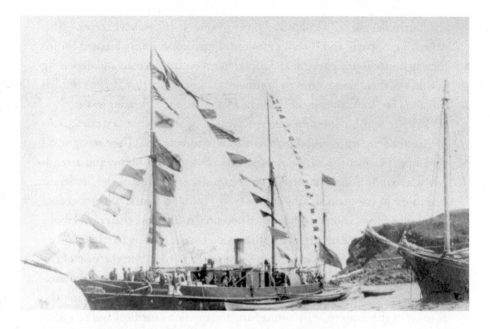

Fig. 6.1 Hospital ship *Strathcona*, flying both British and American flags, early twentieth century. The Grenfell mission continued to employ hospital ships until 1974.

Stephen Friend writes that the late Victorian fishing industry was "acknowledged as the largest and most successful the world had ever known," and it was during this period that "the Church and the public began to take an interest in welfare of the men and women" dependent upon the industry.[19] In 1881, Ebenezer Mather, a member of the Thames Church Mission, was "amazed and appalled" by the miserable conditions he observed while at sea with the Short Blue Fleet.[20] From Mather's brief visit came the RNMDSF, a novel organization that provided spiritual and medical support to trawler crews at sea. By 1900, it had eleven ships under its blue flag, and with one ship always at sea with each of the four main fishing fleets, the mission was able to provide first-aid treatment for broken bones, infected fingers, crushed limbs, and other common injuries. It also provided religious services, reading material, tobacco, and warm clothing as part of a broader effort to stamp out "Dutch copers," vessels from the Netherlands, Germany, and England that travelled to the fishing grounds, often under the Dutch flag, to sell alcohol and pornography to the trawler crews.[21] Also called "bumboats" and "Devil's mission ships," copers were blamed for inflicting unnecessary physical and moral harm on trawlermen and depriving families of their breadwinners, arguments later used to justify the Grenfell mission's attempts to end the trade in alcohol on the Labrador coast.[22]

Mather and his mission were motivated by more than a desire to alleviate the hardships and dangers of trawlermen at sea. They recognized the importance of the national fisheries to Britain's economy, and attendees at RNMDSF annual meetings were proudly reminded of the "constant extension of the great fishing industry."[23] Trawler owners, in turn, recognized that the mission's work had the potential to alleviate their own labour shortage, and the early decades of the RNMDSF were thus partly financed by trawler owners.[24] Imperial security also featured in the rhetoric of the RNMDSF. "The Navy of the Lord," as one mission official called the mission's fleet, provided a "bulwark" of national security by "upholding the seamen of the Empire."[25] By connecting the mission's medical and religious work with the empire, the RNMDSF positioned itself next to prominent military philanthropies like Agnes Weston's Royal Naval Temperance Society, which were rapidly gaining the admiration – and financial support – of the British middle class.

The mission's belief in its imperial and economic value was not merely rhetorical, as its membership included prominent public officials. One such person, Francis Hopwood (later First Baron Southborough), was an assistant solicitor at the British Board of Trade in 1891 when he learned about Newfoundland's precarious dependence on the cod fishery during a meeting with Sir William Whiteway, the prime minister of Newfoundland.[26] After visiting Newfoundland, Hopwood reported on the particularly severe conditions in the Labrador fishery, and the mission agreed to dispatch a hospital ship under the medical supervision of one of its seagoing physicians, Wilfred Grenfell.

The fishery that was observed by Grenfell and the crew of the *Albert* upon their arrival in Labrador in the summer of 1892 was entirely unlike the trawler fishery of the United Kingdom. There were no steam trawlers in Labrador, and the arrival of Arctic sea ice in the autumn meant that there was no winter fishery. Labrador fishers salted their product for later export and so were spared the perils of transferring fresh fish to cutters on small open boats, an especially hazardous task in cold weather. And the Labrador fishery was migratory: in the early 1900s, at the beginning of each season, approximately 14,000 men, women, and children sailed from Newfoundland to the Labrador fishing grounds aboard mail-passenger steamers and small schooners.[27]

Schooner fishers were known as "floaters," and their crews were typically composed of members of the same family and community, including a woman who worked as a cook. Floaters usually lived aboard their vessels and were highly mobile, ranging up and down the Labrador coast in search of the most productive fishing grounds. Fishers who sailed seasonally to Labrador's fishing areas as passengers on steamers and schooners were called "stationers." Unlike schooner crews, who were almost exclusively male, stationers were composed of families who established small shore stations adjacent to their fishing grounds. Finally, there were the permanent residents of Labrador, a small population of approximately four thousand people who included Inuit in the north and Innu in the interior and on the coast at Davis Inlet, along with European settlers and mixed-ancestry families (the result of unions between European men and Inuit women). Fishers in both Labrador and Newfoundland were largely paid in credit, which was extended before the fishing season began and, in principle, paid off when the catch was sold back in the fall. In practice, however, fishers "often found themselves in a state of perpetual indebtedness."[28]

FRONTIER FISHING ACCIDENTS

The risks and hardships particular to fleeting were mercifully absent in the Labrador cod fishery, but life there was nevertheless perilous. Fishing "on the Labrador" was conducted close to the shore using sail and oar-powered craft and the "cod trap," a room-sized box with four walls and floor, constructed of netting and anchored to the shoreline and seabed. Traps varied in size depending on water depth, seabed conditions, and prevailing wind and tide, and fish were trapped after entering the single door. After the cod swam back into deeper waters in the late summer, fishers turned to the jigger, a single or double-barbed hook set in a lead sinker.

After the day's fishing ended, the catch had to be filleted and salted for preservation. On the shore stations, women and children preserved a more lightly salted product by spreading the fish on large wooden platforms called flakes to dry in the sun.

Fishing with schooners, cod traps, and jiggers tested the seamanship of even the most experienced fishers. The risks posed by storms, strong currents, and shoals were heightened by the absence in Labrador of light-houses and other navigational aids, as well as reliable charts. Fishing from schooners and trap boats called for dexterity and constant vigilance as crews worked around numerous moving parts, in confined spaces, and on rigging high above the deck. One fisher, "moaning and groaning in the acutest agony," was left partly paralyzed after falling from the mast of his schooner near Hopedale, while another man was forced to have a leg amputated after it was crushed between two trap skiffs.[29] Conditions below deck on a schooner could be hazardous, too, as one unfortunate skipper experienced when he was scalded in his bunk by a kettle of boiling water tossed by the vessel's motion.[30] His condition, according to the mission nurse who treated him, was made worse by the "cramped, close, unkempt quarters" in the schooner.[31]

More frequent were lacerations inflicted by the common tools of the cod fishery, notably hooks and the long, thin knives used to remove or "split" cod fillets. Painful, deep sores often resulted from the chafing of oilskin clothing against the wrist, a condition colloquially known as "water pups."[32] Far from harmless irritants, the wounds caused by water pups, splitting knives, and fishing tackle resulted in pyogenic infection and blood poisoning, and their treatment constituted the "usual work" of the Grenfell hospital ship during the summer.[33] Grenfell likened the queue of fishers who quickly formed up next to the *Strathcona* to a New York bread line, waiting "not for a cup of coffee, but for the lancet and dressings."[34] Meanwhile, at the St Anthony hospital, overflow tents were frequently constructed to accommodate the summer influx of patients seeking attention "to minor injuries."[35]

Long hours and the intense pace of work no doubt contributed to a high incidence of injury, but experience could reduce the risk of accident. Grenfell recognized this when he wrote that the splitter, "who is a skilled hand, splits the fish and takes out the backbone with a knife like a razor,

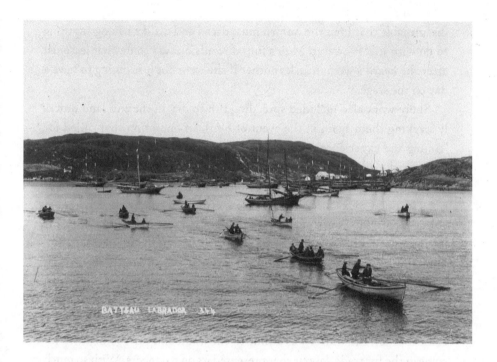

Fig. 6.2 Batteau, Labrador, early twentieth century. Grenfell likened the long lines of boats that gathered next to the hospital ship *Strathcona* to a New York bread line, waiting not "for a cup of coffee, but for the lancet and dressings."

and at an amazing pace" – up to thirteen fish in a minute.[36] But despite the speed and obvious danger of splitting work, Grenfell marvelled that he witnessed only one injury during his first summer in Labrador.[37] Like the praise of visitors for the courage and dexterity of the riveters at the Victoria Bridge building site, described by Anh-Dao Bui Tran in chapter 5 of this volume, Grenfell's account "reads like a homage to the abilities of workers ... who could work efficiently and safely in a dangerous environment."[38]

For women, labouring ashore with the catch and cooking on schooners carried their own hazards. Women, too, participated in splitting fish and shared the risks of the trade. When Ethel Gordon Muir of the Grenfell mission's Needlework Guild of America visited Labrador in the years before the Great War, she was disturbed by the sight of women splitting fish on the bloody, slippery fishing stages: "This work with the fish seemed so disagreeable that I felt the women must dread and dislike having anything to do with it."[39] However, Muir's initial revulsion was somewhat lessened after she heard a woman "ask another if she were not just pining to have a day on the stage."[40]

Shore work also included spreading fish to dry in the sun (and quickly stacking them again in the event of rain), an operation that called for "timing and experience to spread the fish out at the correct time and then build stacks of the right size so that the fish stayed in perfect condition throughout the process."[41] It also demanded stamina, and the repetitive motions strained backs, necks, and bodies.[42] Women employed as schooner cooks spent long hours near stoves and boiling water, often in unstable conditions. Rose Furlong of St Brendan's, Newfoundland, first sailed to Labrador when she was eighteen, and her day began before the fishing started and included baking, cooking, dishwashing, and laundering for ten men. It was, Furlong remembers, "steady go" all day.[43]

Fishing was summer work. For men who lived year-round in southeastern Labrador, the winter was a time to cut wood and earn some extra income in the fur trade, labour that presented its own dangers. With so much wood to cut for building material, heating, and cooking, axe injuries were common. Hunting, either for trade or subsistence, was made more dangerous by the widespread use of old and unstable muzzle-loaders (still common in the early twentieth century) that were liable to explode upon firing, resulting in damaged or destroyed limbs, loss of sight, and death. Trappers also ran the risk of frostbite and accidents sustained on komatiks (winter sleds pulled by teams of huskies), often on remote traplines far from any form of assistance.

In Newfoundland, many fishers supplemented their income by joining the seal fishery in March. By the early twentieth century, this industry had transitioned from schooners to large, purpose-built steamships that could break the Arctic ice and reach the seal-whelping areas.[44] The enormous costs associated with these ships meant that the seal fishery was concentrated in the hands of the same large firms that controlled the cod fishery. To offset their expenses, they pushed crews to their physical limits and stripped ships of any equipment and comforts deemed unnecessary to the hunt, including wireless sets and doctors.[45] While dozens or even hundreds of men were sometimes lost in sealing disasters, notably the *Greenland* disaster of 1898 and the *Newfoundland* disaster of 1914, many more lives were lost to accidents involving a small number of casualties. Enos Squire of Eastport, Bonavista Bay, for example, narrowly escaped injury or death in 1892 on the steamer *Walrus* thanks to a bottle of molasses that leaked in his jacket pocket while a group of men prepared dynamite: "I hastened to the forecastle to unpack and wash my molasses soaked clothes. While I was doing so, a loud explosion shook the ship from stem to stern ... In some manner the dynamite had exploded killing the boatswain and two other men while many others were seriously injured."[46] Such tragedies were commonplace and not enough to delay the *Walrus*, which duly sailed for the sealing "front" a few days later.

Squire would go on to survive the *Greenland* sealing disaster of 1898, but unlike his narrow escape on board the *Walrus*, this time he owed his life to the experience and advice of his father. Squire had been warned by his father, a veteran sealer, to "never leave your ship without taking your oilskins no matter how fine the weather."[47] When a sudden blizzard descended on the ice fields and the *Greenland's* crew, Squire was able to remain warm and protected in his oilskin clothing while many of his fellows became drenched and frozen in their thin woollen sweaters. This example illustrates that local people actively mitigated risk by learning from their "long careers on the water, accumulated experience and skill, and possession of inter-generational expertise."[48] Today we may not immediately associate many of these knowledges with health and safety, but knowing how to tie a knot, identify the right timber for boatbuilding, or read the weather and the behaviour of animals were all essential parts of everyday survival on land and water.[49]

Access to these knowledges and skills mitigated the chances of accident or death, but trapping, fishing, and sealing were inherently dangerous. In many cases, the remoteness of fishing grounds and traplines meant that access to emergency medical care was unlikely, leaving fishers and trappers more exposed than other occupational groups.[50] Under these circumstances, the development of the Grenfell mission with its decentralized network of hospitals, nursing stations, and hospital ships, as well as "some of the best-trained doctors and staff in North America," was undoubtedly welcome.[51] As early twentieth-century schooner fisher Nicholas Smith recalled, if it "were not for these Hospitals and Nursing Stations which have been established along the coast ... many would have been compelled to return hundreds of miles to St John's to receive medical attention, and abandon their summer employment."[52]

Smith's emphasis on the importance of the Grenfell mission to local employment was echoed by the mission itself, which framed its operations as vital to the economic success of fishing families and the colony as a whole. Commenting on life in Labrador before the late nineteenth-century arrival of the mission, one ADSF contributor lamented the "needless physical incapacity which might have been avoided had there been available the services of skilled surgeon and faithful nurse ... to render possible the changing of an almost useless burden into a productive asset."[53] Nor was the potential economic value of a medical mission lost on the colony's merchants, who helped finance the construction of the first hospitals at Battle Harbour and Indian Harbour, nor on its government officials.[54] Superintendent of Newfoundland fisheries Adolf Nielson observed in 1893, "Besides all this loss, suffering, and miseries a sick fisherman has to bear himself, he often causes a great loss to the planter and merchant who supply him, when deprived from prosecuting the fishery, perhaps for the best part of the season."[55]

While Grenfell liked to think of his work as a "productive investment" in the colony, he was strongly opposed to the credit system used by the colony's merchants and was not interested in protecting their narrow economic interests.[56] Rather, the economic value he perceived in his mission's work was mainly focused on fishing families, and on the male breadwinner in particular. Protecting them from injury and sickness was essential to maintaining economic self-sufficiency and – because they did not have to depend on government relief or neighbours for support – their moral integrity. But while the health services made available by the mission were certainly needed, they were not provided unconditionally.

CREATING HEALTHY BODIES AND HEALTHY CITIZENS
ON THE RESOURCE FRONTIER

Prior to the establishment of the Grenfell mission, the people of northern Newfoundland and Labrador had limited experience of professional medicine. Coastal mail steamers carried an overworked medical officer during the summer months, and until 1889 people were sometimes relieved by visiting French physicians supporting France's fishing rights on the western shores of Newfoundland.[57] Schooner crews could also access hospital services in St John's, but as Nicholas Smith notes, such a detour meant sacrificing precious weeks on the Labrador fishing grounds. From its inception in 1893, the mission used hospital ships and small hospitals, and later a network of nursing stations, to make it easier for fishers and remote residents to access outpatient services without compromising their ability to earn a living. This decentralized and mobile system worked reasonably well for the period, but it could not hope to provide complete coverage in a region as large as northern Newfoundland and Labrador.

Uncertain access to medical services meant that ordinary people in the region depended on a variety of self-care practices. In her autobiographical *Woman of Labrador*, Elizabeth Goudie recalls using juniper poultices to successfully treat a serious "carbuncle" (a swelling caused by localized infection) that her husband developed while trapping.[58] When her child fell against the woodstove, Goudie bathed the burns with a juniper-based solution and browned fabric on the stove to provide sterilized dressings. After seeing a physician in Nain, she was told to continue her own treatment: "He told me to carry on with what I was using … He said I had done a marvelous job so my mind was at ease then."[59]

The Grenfell mission, at least officially, had little tolerance for "traditional" treatments, condemning them as ignorant and superstitious: "The folk," one ADSF contributor wrote, "depended for healing upon traditional cures, upon old women who worked charms, upon remedies ingeniously devised to meet the need of the moment, upon deluded persons who prescribed medicines … upon the rough and ready surgery of their own."[60] From this writer's perspective, the continuance of home remedies added another layer of risk, one that was now entirely preventable, to the occurrence of injury.

Mission condemnation of lay treatments was highly gendered, with female elders and young mothers singled out for criticism.[61] A small boy who suffered severe burns after his clothing caught fire was used as an object lesson in ADSF: "What could the unskilled care of a mother, however devoted, have done for injuries such as these?"[62] (Clearly the writer had never met Elizabeth Goudie.) Additionally, mission workers were frustrated by the reluctance of injured fishers to stop their work for medical treatment. "The tragedy of the Labrador fishery," Austin Reeve wrote, "is that during the short season [a man] must fish; even operative cases which should be attended to immediately will wait, getting along the best they can until after the fishing season."[63] One man who refused treatment for an eye injury sustained at the outset of the Great War was condemned as a relic of "the old and dark days" before the Grenfell mission was established in Labrador.[64]

Distrust could operate both ways, as Dr John Mason Little found in 1909 when a local man expressed his belief that doctors kept a separate, more efficacious store of pharmaceuticals for their own use.[65] Nevertheless, Grenfell clinicians and local people often worked closely together, particularly in places that were too small to host permanent medical facilities.[66] Local lay practitioners and clergy frequently performed first aid and even minor surgery before sending their "patients" to a Grenfell mission hospital, and while most of them have been forgotten, fragmentary references to the skilled efforts of "Uncle Cy" and "Parson Woods" survive in the medical records of the Grenfell mission.[67]

The mission briefly attempted to formalize lay treatment of injuries by organizing first-aid classes – "the gospel of splints and bandages" – that would demonstrate the efficacy of mission medicine.[68] In the October 1903 issue of ADSF, Grenfell reported that a Newfoundland man with St John's Ambulance training had saved his injured companion (who had fallen on his axe) by controlling "the hemorrhage in the proper manner ... without either filling the wound with tobacco, flour, or any of the other favorite local hemastatics [sic] and blood poisons."[69] In 1914, "First Aid to the Injured" classes were organized on Pilley's Island, Newfoundland, and Forteau, Labrador.[70] However, the Forteau men's class was later abandoned after local people failed to turn out in sufficient numbers.[71]

ADSF accounts of (mostly male) injured and disabled patients are accompanied by descriptions of their character and their restored ability to work, reflecting the way in which disability was seen as "synonymous with reliance on public dependency, poor citizenship, and the inability to care for oneself or work productively," and echoing centuries-old notions of "deserving" and "undeserving" poor.[72] If persons – particularly men – were unable to fully support themselves and their family due to injury, they nevertheless had no "right to be idle or enjoy the gratuitous support of relatives or of a philanthropic agency."[73] One patient left disabled by a komatik accident is described by Grenfell as "a worthy man" who kept his home clean and orderly and still found a way to support a "small orphan boy."[74] Another man who had his "right hand shot to pieces by an explosion of his gun" recovered sufficiently to "nip a fishing line while he hauled it in with the other hand."[75] ADSF also published letters from grateful former patients such as Newfoundland fisher Patrick Aylward, the "victim of a terrible accident" in the spring of 1902 when his gun misfired.[76] Aylward feared that he would lose his hand and be unable to provide for his family, but after the intervention of Dr Grenfell – who took strips of flesh from his assistant's arm for a skin graft – Aylward said he was "now able to use the injured member at my vocation, which is that of fisherman."[77]

The belief that local people were partly to blame for the occurrence of injury and death was extended to the consumption of alcohol and the direct participation of women in the fishery. Mission interventions sought to protect male breadwinners both from themselves and from the inappropriate presence of women in the dirty and dangerous work of cod fishing. Additionally, the efforts reflected the mission's origins as an extension service of the RNMDSF, which both supported an exclusively male labour force and paternalistically regarded working-class men as childlike in their manners and susceptibilities.

In what may well be an apocryphal accident story, Grenfell wrote that he once "had to tell a woman that she was a widow, and that her children were fatherless, because her husband, gentle and clean living, had been tempted to take 'a drop of alcohol at sea, and had fallen over the side.'"[78] Grenfell added, somewhat defensively, that he had "every right to say that it is inadvisable to have alcoholic drinks among sailors and fishermen," as this group was uniquely prone to its abuse and the injurious consequences of its consumption.[79] In Grenfell's account, the good character and work ethic of the fisher was not in doubt; rather, it was his vulnerability as a "simple" person, exploited by traders, dying from a preventable accident and leaving his family in poverty.[80]

As a justice of the peace in Labrador, Grenfell had the authority to suppress the unauthorized trade in alcohol on the colony's northern coasts, and he did so with enthusiasm. One fisher on the *Strathcona* complained that, if the mission kept this up, "We won't be able to kape an oulde bottle in the house to put a drop of ile [oil] in."[81] But the most powerful symbol of the mission's commitment to protect fishers from alcohol was the King George V Seamen's Institute in St John's, opened in 1912. Like sailors' hostels in the United Kingdom, the institute provided safe lodgings, cheap meals, and recreational opportunities to fishers, sailors, and the thousands of sealers who gathered in St John's each spring to join their vessels. And like British establishments, the Seamen's Institute hoped that, by providing these comforts, it would keep fishers and sealers from their only other source of shelter and food – the public house.[82] By regulating seafaring labour moving through the port of St John's – the "emporium of the trade and fisheries of the colony" – the mission presented its institution as an economic as well as moral asset to the colony and its people.[83]

The risk of accident and injury was also invoked to regulate the transportation and indeed the presence of women engaged in the fisheries. Grenfell wrote that women "very wrongly" joined schooners as cooks and noted approving that the larger and apparently better-built Canadian vessels "carry only 18 men, and no women."[84] However, he was more concerned about women involved in the stationer fishery and their dependence on coastal steamers to reach the Labrador coast.[85] Government officials and Grenfell mission doctors, as well as vessel masters, warned that excessively tight quarters on Labrador steamers could result in suffocation when hatchways were closed in stormy weather.[86] Legislation was passed in 1882 to prevent overcrowding and to provide accommodation for women, and, following a major storm in 1885, the act was revisited by a select committee that called for more stringent vessel inspections and "suitable separate apartments" for women.[87] The changes – if actually implemented – did not

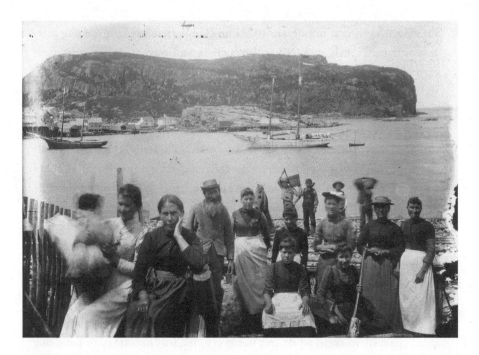

Fig. 6.3 Women drying cod on fish flakes, ca. 1900.

impress RNMDSF physician Eliot Curwen, who wrote ten years later that "women certainly ought not to be allowed to travel in this way."[88] Official concern about the passage of women aboard Labrador steamers reflected contemporary middle-class notions of appropriate gender roles and spaces, but neither the mission nor the colonial government could change the reality that in Labrador all members of the family were needed to successfully carry out fishing work. A neat division of domestic and productive spaces did not and could not exist under the circumstances.

RISKY MISSION WORK AND MEDICAL HEROISM

I have established the Grenfell mission's belief that the risk of accident, injury, and death could be mitigated through health and social reforms. But mission workers themselves undertook unnecessary or questionable risks, sometimes against the advice of local people. Before examining these, however, it is important to acknowledge that working for the mission was inherently dangerous. Physicians and nurses were required to travel long distances by land and sea, often during snowstorms. The physician at Forteau and his dog-team driver, for example, were both frostbitten after enduring "several storms" while conducting visits to remote households.[89] Journeys by water were also hazardous. Besides the constant threat of storms, uncharted shoals and strong currents, the student volunteers and professional sailors who crewed the mission's hospital boats were injured and killed by machinery, loose rigging, falls and drowning.[90] On 1 November 1908, Captain John Wesley Roberts of Twillingate, Newfoundland, was swept overboard as he commanded the Grenfell cargo schooner *Lorna Doone* on a routine supply run. While Roberts's body was never recovered, he was one of the few local people commemorated by the Grenfell mission, notably at the King George V Institute, where a room was named in his honour.[91]

These risks and injuries were an unavoidable – and indeed commendable – part of mission work, but not every risk was necessary or prudent. Elsewhere in this volume, Cameron Baldassarra argues that for middle-class men using canoes for recreation or adventure, risk was voluntary, appealing and even ennobling. The character-building mythology of the "frontier" had the same effect on urbanite Grenfell mission workers and leaders; indeed, some were likely inspired by Dillon Wallace's account of the death of American explorer Leonidas Hubbard (used by Baldassarra in his chapter). Mission workers' enthusiasm for sport hunting, for example, resulted in a surprising number of gunshot wounds.[92] But it was on the water that mission workers took some of their greatest risks, often acting against the advice of more experienced fishers and sailors. In the later summer of 1893, Grenfell sailed the tiny launch *Princess May* through heavy seas, fog, and uncharted waters to Okak in the far north of Labrador, an extremely dangerous journey that would have been beyond his ability were it not for the aid of an Inuit pilot.[93] Grenfell's expedition was not undertaken for any clear reason, and the experienced English crew of the *Albert*, stationed further south, "found his behaviour unnecessarily reckless and hoped that as time went on his good fortune would desert him long enough to show him the risks he took."[94] With similar bravado, Dr Mather Hare of Harrington Harbour hospital set out in severe weather to retrieve a patient, ignoring – with more than a hint of pride – the pleas of local fishers: "It was curious to hear the comments of the men as we came through the fleet anchored there, and more than one voice was raised in a hail advising us not to venture out into the wild smother of sea, rain and fog that were raising high carnival outside the headland; but get my patient to hospital I had to."[95] In this instance, as in many others, the professional authority of the doctor overruled the vernacular knowledge of fishers.

Because mission workers depended on local knowledge and expertise to travel over both sea and land, a decision to travel in hazardous conditions meant that risk was also extended to the people who made these journeys possible. Grenfell's famed 1893 voyage is the most obvious illustration of this, but Hare's account shows there were many similar tales. For example, when James T. Wiltsie, a mission worker from Columbia University, narrowly missed catching the coastal steamer *Prospero* in Newfoundland in 1912, he was forced into a hasty decision: "Shall we brave Notre Dame Bay" in the middle of a gale, Wiltsie wondered, "or give up the chase as too dangerous?"[96] Wiltsie chose to give chase, but as his small hired boat entered open water, the engineer "lost his footing and slipped down near the fly wheel where part of his shoe was torn away by the engine, his foot, in some way, miraculously escaping injury."[97]

Why did they do it? For Wiltsie, it may have been the same thirst for adventure on a remote "frontier" – the thrill of "the chase" – that attracted so many other urban Americans to the Grenfell mission.[98] Frontier imagery was routinely employed to recruit summer volunteers like Wiltsie, with Labrador's "invigorating climate" and "varied" opportunities for work and play promising a refreshing alternative to city life.[99] Grenfell himself, as Rafico Ruiz writes, was "seeking to embody and act out a form of muscular Christianity capable of modeling the corporeal potential white fisherfolk bodies held."[100] It was not enough for Grenfell to prove himself the equal of any mariner in Labrador: he had to be better. Despite his audacious voyages, however, not everyone accepted this image. After one schooner master implied that the *Strathcona* was a "pleasure yacht," for example, Grenfell wrote angrily that "the idea of the mission steamer being a 'pleasure yacht' grated on one's nerves."[101]

CONCLUSION

The structure of the Labrador fishery, and the use of credit rather than cash, was a source of frustration for Grenfell mission authorities. The mission believed that the credit system deprived the fisher of personal initiative: unable to escape his debts, he had become "so apathetic that he has found it hard to make any great headway."[102] But the fishery was also deemed badly organized and unnecessarily hazardous. Alexander MacKenzie, a mission volunteer from Cambridge, Massachusetts, wrote that the Labrador fishery needed more trained officers and regular vessel inspections, while Grenfell believed that cod traps risked fishers and vessels by compelling them to "race" to the fishing grounds "months earlier than necessary."[103] The Newfoundland and Labrador fisher would do well, he wrote, to emulate the enterprising schooner fishers of Gloucester and New England, men who chased the fish rather than waited for them and who did not believe "in fish being a failure."[104] The long-range banks fisheries of New England and the North Sea had the added advantage of distantly separating male and female fishing labour, although the occurrence of accident and injury in the latter fishery, as we have seen, was no less commonplace than in Labrador.

The Grenfell mission believed that more modern fishing methods and better regulation would improve the safety – or, at least, the morale – of fishers in Labrador. But local fishers were far more resourceful, and less fatalistic, than mission leaders believed, and their work was shaped by generations of accumulated knowledge concerning ecosystems, weather, and seamanship, and their own experience on the water began at a very early age. They were perfectly capable of assessing danger for themselves and, as Dr Hare's experience illustrates, willing to advise Grenfell mission workers accordingly. By the early twentieth century, fishers were also growing increasingly intolerant of unnecessary risk created by exploitative working conditions, particularly in the seal fishery. The *Greenland* disaster of 1898, Shannon Ryan argues, "became a turning point for Newfoundland society. For the first time people expressed their concern publicly over the risk to lives in the seal fishery. They were no longer satisfied with the view that disasters were "Acts of God for which no mortal was to blame."[105] Similarly, as Lynne D. Fitzhugh writes, residents of Labrador did not necessarily share Grenfell's view "that they led impoverished lives or required outside intervention. They had their own internal heroes and social safety nets, and they were proud of their homely medical accomplishments."[106] The Grenfell mission may have distrusted traditional remedies, balked at the involvement of women in fishing labour, and felt compelled to intervene in perceived social problems such as the consumption of alcohol, but it was a relative latecomer to a region where survival strategies and labour arrangements reflected generations of experience and the unique challenges of life in a subarctic climate.

NOTES

1 "Dr. Grenfell's Heroic Work," *Among the Deep Sea Fishers* (ADSF) 1, no. 1 (April 1903): 5.
2 "Grenfell mission" is not fully capitalized in this chapter. This is because the organization was managed under the auspices of the Royal National Mission to Deep Sea Fishers until 1914, when it was incorporated as the International Grenfell Association; "Dr. Grenfell's Heroic Work," 5.
3 Ibid.
4 Selby Jefferson, "A Mission Worker's Life in Labrador," *Toilers of the Deep*, February 1895, 56–7.
5 "Dr. Grenfell's Heroic Work," 5.
6 Rose, *No Right to Be Idle*, 2.
7 See Pickstone, "Production, Community and Consumption."
8 Ruiz, *Slow Disturbance*, 6.
9 Cooter and Luckin, introduction to *Accidents in History*, 7.
10 Bashford, "Medicine, Gender, and Empire," 117.
11 Ibid.
12 Junila, "Call of the Wild."
13 Connor, "American Aid, the International Grenfell Association, and Health Care in Newfoundland," 249–50.
14 Ibid., 251.
15 Connor, "'We Are Anglo-Saxons,'" 47.
16 Capes and Robinson, "Health and Safety in the British Deep-Sea Trawl Fisheries," 298.
17 Robinson, *Trawling*, 71.
18 Ibid., 77.
19 Friend, *Fishing for Souls*, xxxv.
20 Robinson, *Trawling*, 79.
21 Friend, *Fishing for Souls*, 142.
22 Ibid.

23 G.A. Hutchison, "Speech Given to the Annual Meeting of the Royal National Mission to Deep Sea Fishermen, Queen's Hall, London," ADSF 8, no. 2 (July 1910): 1–2.

24 Villiers, *Deep Sea Fishermen*, 94.

25 Hutchison, "Speech Given," 1; "The Annual Meeting, 1913," editorial, ADSF 11, no. 2 (July 1913): 4.

26 Rompkey, *Grenfell of Labrador*, 38.

27 Hiller, "Wilfred Grenfell and Newfoundland," 26.

28 Korneski, *Conflicted Colony*, 58.

29 Wilfred Grenfell, "Dr. Grenfell's Log," ADSF 7, no. 3 (October 1909): 18; Horton H. Heath, "The Summer Visitor in Labrador," ADSF 10, no. 2 (July 1912): 39.

30 Sister Bussell, "A Hospital Story," ADSF 1, no. 1 (April 1903): 12.

31 Ibid.

32 Crellin, *Home Medicine*, 240.

33 Wilfred Grenfell, "Log of the S.S. Strathcona," ADSF 1, no. 4 (January 1904): 11.

34 Wilfred Grenfell, "Doctor Grenfell's Log," ADSF 10, no. 3 (October 1912): 22.

35 "Battle Harbour Jottings," ADSF 7, no. 4 (January 1910): 18.

36 Rompkey, *Grenfell of Labrador*, 50.

37 Ibid.

38 Bui Tran, "Life and Death in the Building of the Victoria Bridge (1854–1860)," in this volume, 149–50.

39 Ethel Gordon Muir, "The People on the Labrador and Their Needs," ADSF 8, no. 2 (July 1910): 37.

40 Ibid.

41 Porter, "'She Was Skipper of the Shore Crew,'" 40.

42 Boyd, "Sunbonnets on the Beach," 33.

43 Ennis and Woodrow, eds., *Strong as the Ocean*, 36.

44 See Ryan, "Newfoundland Spring Sealing Disasters to 1914."

45 Ryan, *Ice Hunters*.

46 Squire, *Newfoundland Outport in the Making*, 77.

47 Ibid, 79.

48 Power, "Occupational Risks, Safety and Masculinity, 575.

49 Hall, *Towards an Encyclopedia of Local Knowledge*, 133, 161.

50 Carter, *Merchant Seamen's Health*, 6.

51 Connor, "American Aid," 254.

52 Smith, *Fifty-Two Years at the Labrador Fishery*, 120.

53 Untitled note, ADSF 7, no. 3 (October 1909): 4.

54 Rompkey, *Labrador Odyssey*, xix.

55 Rompkey, *Grenfell of Labrador*, 54.

56 Wilfred Grenfell, "Dr. Grenfell's Log," ADSF 7, no. 3 (October 1909): 11.

57 Korneski, *Conflicted Colony*, 106.

58 Goudie, *Woman of Labrador*, 64.

59 Ibid, 97.

60 "The Real Doctor Grenfell," ADSF 2, no. 4 (January 1905): 21.

61 Ibid.

62 Untitled note, ADSF 7, no. 4 (January 1910): 5.

63 Austin Reeve, "The Summer Hospital at Indian Harbour," ADSF 11, no. 1 (April 1913): 15.

64 John M. Little, "St. Anthony Hospital," ADSF 12, no. 3 (October 1914): 98.

65 Wilfred Grenfell, "Dr. Grenfell's Log," ADSF 7, no. 3 (October 1909): 18.

66 "Invisible labour" is used by Peter L. Twohig to describe the "groups of health care workers who have received relatively little attention from historians," such as Inuit nursing aides who worked with the Grenfell mission. Twohig, "'Everything Possible Is Being Done,'" 2.

67 International Grenfell Association, St Anthony Hospital Admission Records 06063 and 06058, St Anthony Hospital, NL. The author is indebted to Jennifer J. Connor, who kindly provided access to anonymized copies of these records.

68 Wilfred Grenfell, "Dr. Grenfell's Work in Labrador and Newfoundland," ADSF 2, no. 1 (April 1904): 10.

69 Wilfred Grenfell, "The Log of the S.S. Strathcona," ADSF 1, no. 3 (October 1903): 8.

70 Roy C. Philips, "Pilley's Island Hospital," ADSF 12, no. 1 (April 1914): 19.

71 A.W. Wakefield, "Forteau," ADSF 12, no. 2 (July 1914): 47.

72 Rose, *No Right to Be Idle*, 3, 8.

73 Ibid, 3.

74 Wilfred Grenfell, "Dr. Grenfell's Log," ADSF 9, no. 4 (January 1912): 21.

75 Wilfred Grenfell, "When I Was Worrying," ADSF 9, no. 1 (April 1911): 29.

76 Patrick J. Aylward, "The Friend of the Fisherman: Victim of a Terrible Accident," ADSF 2, no. 1 (April 1904): 3–4.

77 Ibid.

78 Wilfred Grenfell, "Why I Am Against Liquor," ADSF 5, no. 1 (April 1907): 18.

79 Ibid, 19.

80 Ibid.

81 Wilfred Grenfell, "The Close of Open Water," ADSF 4, no. 4 (January 1907): 9–10.

82 Anonymous, "The Sailors' Home," ADSF 9, no. 1 (April 1911): 8.

83 Ibid.

84 Grenfell, *Vikings of To-Day*, 55.

85 Ibid., 55.

86 Rompkey, *Labrador Odyssey*, 165.

87 Quoted in Hiller, "Wilfred Grenfell and Newfoundland," 26.

88 Rompkey, *Labrador Odyssey*, 165.

89 Edith Mayou, "Jottings from Harrington," ADSF 7, no. 2 (July 1909): 24.

90 See, for example, H. Mather Hare, "Jottings from the Harrington Harbour Hospital," ADSF 8, no. 1 (April 1910): 20.

91 E.E.W., "Items from the New England Grenfell Association," ADSF 11, no. 1 (April 1913): 20.

92 Wilfred Grenfell, "The Call to Service," ADSF 12, no. 3 (October 1914): 96.

93 Rompkey, *Grenfell of Labrador*, 63.
94 Ibid, 69.
95 Hare, "Jottings from the Harrington Harbour Hospital," 19.
96 James T. Wiltsie, "From St John's to St Anthony," ADSF 11, no. 1 (April 1913): 28.
97 Ibid.
98 Connor, "Putting the 'Grenfell Effect' in Its Place."
99 Quoted in Connor, "'We Are Anglo-Saxons,'" 65–6.
100 Ruiz, *Slow Disturbance*, 7.
101 Grenfell, "Close of Open Water," 10.
102 Lawrence Mott, "Sport and Charity in a Frozen Fairyland," ADSF 10, no. 1 (April 1912): 33.
103 Alexander McKenzie, "Our Side," ADSF 1, no. 2 (July 1903): 5; Wilfred Grenfell, "Dr. Grenfell's Log," ADSF 8, no. 3 (October 1910): 22.
104 Wilfred Grenfell, "Doctor Grenfell's Log," ADSF 8, no. 4 (January 1911): 17.
105 Ryan, "Newfoundland Spring Sealing Disasters to 1914," 37.
106 Fitzhugh, *Labradorians*, 49.

BIBLIOGRAPHY

Archives

Charles S. Curtis Memorial Hospital, St Anthony, NL.
Digital Archives Initiative, Memorial University of Newfoundland, St John's, NL.
Maritime History Archive, Memorial University of Newfoundland, St John's, NL.

Periodicals

Among the Deep Sea Fishers (ADSF) was the official organ of the International Grenfell Association, appearing approximately quarterly between 1903 and 1981. Initially published in Toronto, the magazine was relocated to New York City after the Grenfell mission was incorporated as the International Grenfell Association in 1914. This move reflected the growing importance of American contributors and volunteers to the work of the IGA. ADSF is available from Memorial University's Digital Archives Initiative at https://dai.mun.ca/digital/hs_fisher/.
Toilers of the Deep: A Monthly Record of Mission Work amongst Them. Published by the Royal National Mission to Deep Sea Fishermen in London.

Other Sources

Bashford, Alison. "Medicine, Gender, and Empire." In *Gender and Empire*, edited by Philippa Levine, 112–33. Oxford: Oxford University Press, 2004.

Boyd, Cynthia. "Sunbonnets on the Beach: The Occupational Folklore of Beach Women in Grand Bank, Newfoundland, 1880–1940." *Folk Life: Journal of Ethnological Studies* 56, no. 1 (2018): 25–39.

Capes, Susan, and Robb Robinson. "Health and Safety in the British Deep-Sea Trawl Fisheries during the Nineteenth and Twentieth Centuries." *Mariner's Mirror* 94, no. 3 (2008): 298–313.

Carter, Tim. *Merchant Seamen's Health, 1860–1960: Medicine, Technology, Shipowners and the State in Britain*. Woodbridge, UK: Boydell Press, 2014.

Connor, Jennifer J. "'We Are Anglo-Saxons': Grenfell, Race and Mission Movements." In *The Grenfell Medical Mission and American Support in Newfoundland and Labrador, 1890s–1940s*, edited by Jennifer J. Connor and Katherine Side, 45–68. Montreal: McGill-Queen's University Press, 2019.

Connor, J.T.H. "American Aid, the International Grenfell Association, and Health Care in Newfoundland." In Connor and Side, *Grenfell Medical Mission*, 245–66.

– "Putting the 'Grenfell Effect' in Its Place: Medical Tales and Autobiographical Narratives in Twentieth-Century Newfoundland and Labrador." *Papers of the Bibliographical Society of Canada* 48, no. 1 (Spring 2010): 77–118.

Cooter, Roger and Bill Luckin, eds. *Accidents in History: Injuries, Fatalities and Social Relations*. Boston: Rodopi, 1997.

Crellin, John K. *Home Medicine: The Newfoundland Experience*. Montreal: McGill-Queen's University Press, 1994.

Ennis, Frances, and Helen Woodrow, eds. *Strong as the Ocean: Women's Work in Newfoundland and Labrador Fisheries*. St John's, NL: Harris Press, 1996.

Fitzhugh, Lynne D. *The Labradorians: Voices from the Land of Cain*. St John's, NL: Breakwater Books, 1999.

Friend, Stephen. *Fishing for Souls: The Development and Impact of British Fishermen's Missions*. Cambridge: Letterworth Press, 2018.

Grenfell, Wilfred Thomason. *Vikings of To-Day: or, Life and Medical Work among the Fishermen of Labrador*. London: Marshall Bros, 1895.

Hall, Pam. *Towards an Encyclopedia of Local Knowledge: Excerpts from Chapters I and II*. St John's, NL: Breakwater Books, 2017.

Hiller, James K. "Wilfred Grenfell and Newfoundland." In Connor and Side, *Grenfell Medical Mission*, 23–44.

Junila, Marianne. "Call of the Wild: Public Health Nursing in Post-War Finland." In *Medicine in the Remote and Rural North, 1800–2000*, edited by J.T.H. Connor and Stephan Curtis, 215–35. London: Pickering & Chatto, 2011.

Korneski, Kurt. *Conflicted Colony: Critical Episodes in Nineteenth-Century Newfoundland and Labrador*. Montreal: McGill-Queen's University Press, 2016.

Pickstone, John, and Roger Cooter, eds. *Companion to Medicine in the Twentieth Century*. London and New York: Routledge, 2003.

Porter, Marilyn. "'She Was Skipper of the Shore Crew': Notes on the History of the Sexual Division of Labour in Newfoundland." In *Their Lives and Times: Women* in *Newfoundland and Labrador: A Collage*, edited by Carmelita McGrath, Barbara Neis, and Marilyn Porter, 33–47. St John's, NL: Killick Press, 1995.

Power, Nicole Gerarda. "Occupational Risks, Safety and Masculinity: Newfoundland Fish Harvesters' Experiences and Understandings of Fisheries Risks." *Health, Risk and Safety* 10, no. 6 (December 2008): 565–83.

Robinson, Robb. *Trawling: The Rise and Fall of the British Trawler Fishery*. Exeter: University of Exeter Press, 1996.

Rompkey, Ronald. *Grenfell of Labrador: A Biography*. Toronto: University of Toronto Press, 1991.

– ed. *Labrador Odyssey: The Journal and Photographs of Eliot Curwen on the Second Voyage of Wilfred Grenfell, 1893*. Montreal: McGill-Queen's University Press, 1996.

Rose, Sarah F. *No Right to Be Idle: The Invention of Disability, 1840s–1930s*. Chapel Hill: University of North Carolina Press, 2017.

Ruiz, Rafico. *Slow Disturbance: Infrastructural Mediation on the Settler Colonial Resource Frontier*. Durham: Duke University Press, 2021.

Ryan, Shannon. *The Ice Hunters: A History of Newfoundland Sealing to 1914*. St John's, NL: Breakwater Books, 1994.

Ryan, Shannon. "Newfoundland Spring Sealing Disasters to 1914." *Northern Mariner/La marin du nord* 3, no. 3 (1993): 14–58.

Squire, Harold. *A Newfoundland Outport in the Making: The Early History of Eastport, Together with an Eyewitness Account of the Greenland Disaster*. Eastport, NL: n.p., 1974.

Twohig, Peter L. "'Everything Possible Is Being Done': Labour, Mobility, and the Organization of Health Services in Mid-20th Century Newfoundland." *Canadian Bulletin of Medical History/Bulletin canadien d'histoire de la medicine* 36, no. 1 (2019): 1–26.

Villiers, Alan. *The Deep Sea Fishermen*. London: Hodder and Stoughton, 1970.

7

An Allowance for Accidents

Alberta's 1908 Workmen's Compensation Legislation

Ceilidh Auger-Day

Standing to speak in a Calgary school gym in February 1909, Alberta's attorney general, Charles Cross, received an anticipatory round of applause from his audience, a crowd so much larger than expected that extra chairs had to be brought in to accommodate everyone. He began his speech by telling the sombre story of a young widow who had come to him many years before. Her husband had been killed in a workplace accident, but no one had seen what had happened, and with no solid evidence of exactly what took place, there was no legal way to sue the employer for damages. Her husband had been the family wage earner, so the family was left not just grieving but impoverished, and within a few years her son was arrested and imprisoned for forgery. Implying a direct connection between events, Cross painted a bleak picture of what happened to working families after a workplace accident. His speech did not end on a tragic note, however, for his government had recently passed the 1908 Workmen's Compensation Act. Though it was too late for the family in question, Cross proudly proclaimed that, with this new legislation, the family left behind after such a workplace accident would have received $1,800 within half a week of the man's death. Working families would still grieve, but they were no longer to be left destitute. To this announcement, the room once again burst into applause.[1]

As Attorney-General Cross's enthusiastic audience realized, the new workmen's compensation legislation provided, for the first time, a reliable way to claim benefits in the case of a workplace accident, radically changing the financial effect of accidents on workers and workers' families.[2] In a broader context, Cross's speech reflected much more: a concern over industrial accidents, growing state interest in ways to keep the working poor out of poverty (and off municipal poor rolls), and a shift towards thinking statistically about both individuals and their actions. As the introduction to this volume emphasizes, a new statistical conception of risk, alongside growing concern and ambivalence over the place of danger on the job, caused western workers and state legislators alike to spotlight workplace accidents.[3] Although Sandlos's chapter on mining makes evident the flawed state responses to dangerous work sites, the late nineteenth and early twentieth centuries were nonetheless the start of a period of exploration around how to respond to work-related injuries. This search for solutions arose at least in part as a result of growing awareness of the magnitude and after-effects of industrial accidents and growing radicalism by workers unions.[4] Efforts to deal with on-the-job casualties involved many different interest groups and covered a large amount of ground: tort law, restrictions to tort defences, protective legislation, private and workplace-wide commercial insurance, workmen's compensation laws, and, eventually, the adoption of workmen's compensation boards.[5]

The story of workmen's compensation presented here is one in which Alberta played a leading role between 1908 and 1914, and it demonstrates the degree to which the Prairie provinces were drawing on international developments for inspiration and ideas. In a newly created province under its first leadership, the provincial elite were actively deciding what kind of place Alberta would be. Coming from Ontario or the Midwestern United States, Alberta's most influential citizens combined the cultural assumptions of their backgrounds – perhaps above all an inherent belief in Anglo-Saxon supremacy and the importance of civilizing others – with a regional pride that resulted in something more innovative than a simple attempt to replicate the areas from which they had come.[6] Boosters, as they were known, believed in the superiority of the British values established in Upper Canada, but they also insisted that Alberta was not destined to be merely a second Ontario. In drafting workmen's compensation, Alberta focused not only on developments in England and Eastern Canada but also on the younger, perhaps more flexible and inventive areas of the British Empire (joining other provinces in their interest in developments in New Zealand and Australia), and on any new innovation within other nations.

Alberta was also a place where industry was increasingly important but not yet fully established. As a writer in the *Edmonton Bulletin* noted in 1909, Alberta's early move towards industry (particularly coal mining) became an opportunity to do what other more established places could not – introduce legislation that employers could adjust to and grow up with, so to speak, before they were large enough to successfully fight the introduction of such laws.[7] British Columbia's slightly earlier and Manitoba's just later legislation both make sense according to this logic of the development of industry within the Western provinces.[8] Alberta then, was a unique place where an active "civilizing" energy, newly developing industry, and the need for a whole new body of legislation combined to put the province on the leading edge of the movement towards Workmen's Compensation legislation in 1908.

The history of Workmen's Compensation and the formation of Workmen's/Workers' Compensation Boards (wcbs) in Canada has received some consideration from historians. Eric Tucker's 1990 monograph on occupational health and safety in Ontario from the mid-nineteenth century to World War I, Robert Storey's many valuable publications on the subsequent history of worker safety in the province, and Magda Farni's study of Quebec's 1909 workers' compensation law all contribute to more nuanced conceptualization of how class relations, capital, Canadian law, and the state intersected in the creation of policy to compensate injured workers and their families.[9] Nevertheless, within much of the literature on the subject, there is an emphasis on the 1910–13 Ontario Workers' Compensation Commission carried out by William Meredith, attributing to him alone what in reality took many jurisdictions and many iterations to create.[10] Yet Ontario – and William Meredith's report – only registered on the radar late, and without nearly as much fanfare as it is now awarded in the history of Canadian wcbs. As I explore the development of workmen's compensation legislation in Alberta, I focus specifically on the 1908 legislation that, for the most part, removed workmen's compensation from the courts and applied it to a significant number of workers for the first time. Tracing this development in the provincial legislation re-centres the history of workmen's compensation away from the Meredith report and towards a more complex story of development. The 1908 Alberta legislation had a more significant impact on workers than did the 1918 changes to the system made in the wake of the Meredith report, which only indirectly made its way to Alberta in the years following its enactment in Ontario. The Meredith myth developed later, simplifying an otherwise complex history and celebrating the role of WCBs rather than workmen's compensation more broadly. It became accepted in part because of the work it did in creating a more unified national system in Canadian minds – a system that moreover honours rather than questions our supposedly British roots.

The complexity comes in part from the combination of local circumstances with international trends in the development of welfare states. Individual states were creating laws that reflected their own needs and suited their own cultural agendas. Historian Julia Moses compares, for instance, the way that Germany used socialist-style government coverage of workers' compensation to quiet labour unrest and maintain government control, to the focus on individual rights in Britain that facilitated the development of private insurance contracts. Italy fell somewhere in between, charting a path that balanced traditional solutions with attempts to build credibility within a new government both internally and internationally.[11] However, many western countries were facing similar issues and experiences in a world increasingly affected by mass industrialization, and were also actively aware of and drawing on each other in finding solutions. Through this process, new ideas of risk and an increasingly statistical approach took hold and spread through most of these nations, causing them to change in similar ways.[12] Individual influences on each region were complex, and shifts were often overlapping, making it difficult to pinpoint clearly the origins of these programs in any particular jurisdiction. Yet despite the local circumstances, the end results often paralleled modifications in other places, creating an overall sense of a sudden unified movement.

Historians working on topics related to workmen's compensation and accidents emphasize that the development of workmen's compensation schemes was attended by a complex array of disparate players with different agendas and varying degrees of interest and power. Local governments exchanged opinions on how to respond to workplace accidents but also on ideas of risk and the statistical citizen more generally, and yet each region was also subject to its own local culture, power centres, and logic. Those writing internationally on the development of workers' compensation (in its many possible forms) sometimes emphasize the importance of different players, but many scholars also recognize that workers' compensation was successful because (and where) it had a broad range of support from different factions. Historians such as Price V. Fishback and Shawn Everett Kantor, John Fabian Witt, and Julia Moses emphasize how local cultural differences created a hodgepodge style of compensation policies with variations among countries, and with local regions or nations adopting or developing workmen's compensation as it suited their own needs and style of administration.[13] Regional solutions and local movements that focused on accident compensation legislation were therefore not always obviously predictable by simpler explanations that have sought to make sense of these developments on purely economic, political, or cultural grounds. Consequently, looking at how these systems developed in one Canadian province contributes as much and perhaps more than large overarching narratives to our overall understanding of how ideas and policies changed, and why, in the early twentieth century.

THE DEVELOPMENT OF 1908 WORKERS' COMPENSATION LEGISLATION IN ALBERTA

Early attention to workmen's compensation varied significantly by region within Canada, as the issue fell under provincial jurisdiction. However, by 1886 it was an important-enough topic that it became part of the broad remit of the federal government's Royal Commission on the Relations of Capital and Labour. The commission, which published its final report in 1889, did not address labour issues or industrial accidents in western Canada, and none of its recommendations were directly implemented, except for the creation of the federal Labour Day holiday. While the commission may have been a pre-election bid for votes more than a serious desire for political change, the detailed testimony of employers, employees, and social reformers appearing before the commission spoke directly to the working and living conditions under industrial capitalism. It also demonstrated the attention that both provincial and federal governments were paying to the issues relating to workers – including workmen's compensation – in the late nineteenth century, and the degree to which these issues were in fact widespread voter concerns.[14] As Jason Devine argues, the attention these issues garnered was largely a response to growing worker unrest and the movement towards unionization and militancy in certain industrial settings, but Tucker's analysis of Ontario's 1884 Factory Act indicates that it also reflected an acknowledgment by "a wide spectrum of the community" of the high cost that workers were paying in industrial jobs.[15]

In 1898, Canadian news outlets acknowledged the passing of a British workmen's compensation law, one that provided for "the right, namely to receive compensation upon a fixed scale in case of any accident not brought about by the 'serious helpful misconduct of the injured man himself.'"[16] In the Canadian prairies, still largely part of the Northwest Territories at the time, a bill passed in 1900 that essentially brought these areas in line with Ontario's 1886 law, limiting the defences an employer could use in a suit for compensation.[17] The Canadian system still functioned in the same way as before – injured employees or their families were obliged to sue employers for damages in the case of a workplace accident and were required to prove that the employer was somehow responsible – but the defence of common employment/the fellow-servant rule (if a fellow employee was responsible for the accident, then the employer was not) was eliminated. The Ordinance to Secure Compensation to Workmen, as the law was known, still allowed employers to argue that the accident had been at least partially the worker's fault (contributory negligence), or that the worker had known the job would be risky or that a specific hazard would or might exist (assumption of risk) in order to avoid financial responsibility for an injured worker.[18] But employers could no longer argue that a fellow worker's mistake meant that compensation for the accident was not the company's economic obligation.

Major industrial employers on the prairies were largely connected to railways and mining. These occupations involved constant communication between employees to move production forward, often under circumstances

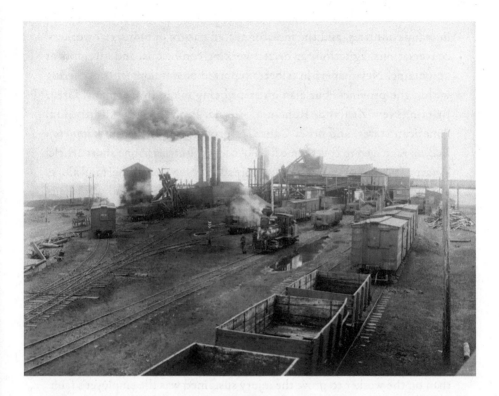

Fig. 7.1 *Galt Colliery, Lethbridge, Alberta*, ca. 1904–07. Major industrial employers on the prairies were largely related to railways and mining. Common hazards included poor visibility, flammable materials, and moving machinery.

that were not ideal; consequently, the numbers of accidents that resulted from a communication error were high.[19] Though contributory negligence and assumption of risk eliminated employer responsibility in many cases, the shift away from common employment as a defence was significant. Thus, brakeman Howard West, seeking damages of $4,000, took a case against CPR to the Supreme Court in 1901, alleging that the train accident he was injured in was caused by the carelessness of some of his co-workers.[20] The suit was not one that would have been possible before the 1900 limitations on employers' ability to elude responsibility.

The western provinces drew on many sources in their thinking about workmen's compensation, once again underscoring both the degree to which this was a worldwide movement under consideration by leaders in many countries, and the interconnected nature of industrial workers' conversations, agitation for better working conditions, and attempts at unionizing. Newspapers in Alberta reported on developments occurring within the province, but also on steps being taken in Germany, Great Britain, New Zealand, Romania, Russia, France, Serbia, individual American states, and other Canadian provinces. In 1911, the *Edmonton Bulletin* managed to cover almost all of these countries in one short article, "Wave of Progressive Legislation Spreads."[21] Nor were Albertans alone, of course, in their attention to external developments around workmen's compensation. When the British Columbia Compensation Act went into effect in May 1903, a writer who was against the bill blamed New Zealand for setting a poor example, stating that the British Columbia bill was "raw crude legislation, which looks like something copied bodily from the New Zealand statutes."[22]

The British Columbia law put the responsibility on the employer to pay for employee injuries in all cases except where the worker was solely responsible for his own injury or death. In a reversal from the previous situation, the onus was now on the employer to prove non-liability rather than on the worker to prove the injury sustained was the employer's fault. Financial responsibility was capped, however, at $1,500 – much lower than legal suits often demanded. This law received only moderate attention in the Prairie provinces at the time, and Alberta's laws remained those of limiting employer liability.

Only a few years later, however, the British Columbia law appeared more appealing to members of Alberta premier Alexander Rutherford's cabinet, as did pre-existing forms of compensation legislation from other jurisdictions. That was because miners in the newly formed province of Alberta started agitating for changes to working conditions, including an eight-hour day, better safety protections, and better financial compensation in case of an injury or death. In May 1907, the Alberta government bowed to activist pressure and created the Royal Commission on the Coal Mining Industry.[23] Then, in June, six men were killed at the Edmonton area Strathcona Mine in the largest mining disaster the region had ever experienced. Though it was later eclipsed by even bigger and more deadly mining disasters in the province – particularly the Bellevue Mine explosion in 1910

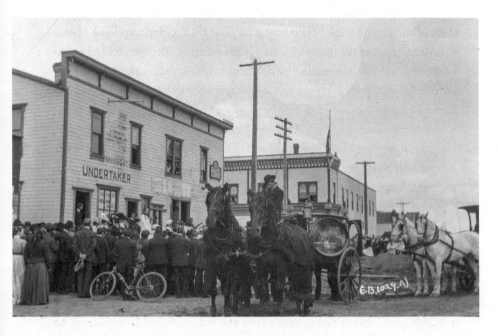

Fig. 7.2 Procession at funeral of victims of mine disaster at Strathcona, 1907.

and the Hillcrest Mine disaster of 1914, both in the Crowsnest Pass area – the Strathcona Mine explosion had a profound influence on early compensation legislation in Alberta for two reasons: the mining commission was still underway when it occurred, and one of the three co-owners of the mine was Premier Rutherford himself. Both details meant that the issue of accident compensation was suddenly and very publicly close to home. Throughout the month of June, newspapers were filled with reports of the Strathcona mining disaster, the royal commission, and extended analyses of the demands of miners.[24]

In the final report on 1 July 1907, the coal mining commission asserted that the laws in effect regarding compensation for accidents, though "fair in theory, are in practice useless."[25] The report supported the miners' concerns that it was "impossible in almost every case for any compensation to be recovered regardless of where the blame might rest" and recommended a "Special Compensation law" that sent the review of all accidents to a "Special Commission" with final say in determining damages.[26] Faced with the economic and social fallout of a large-scale accident, seeking to win votes and appease the miners causing labour unrest, Rutherford and members of his cabinet responded by drafting workmen's compensation legislation. An Act with Respect to Compensation to Workmen for Injuries Suffered in the Course of Their Employment, otherwise referred to as the Workmen's Compensation Act 1908, paid particular attention to miners and to mining but also covered Albertan industries more generally.[27] The proposed legislation led printing union member J.W. Adair to declare to a crowded opera house of mostly blue-collar workers that "an act of this nature was particularly needed in Alberta."[28]

The small Conservative opposition grumbled about some of the changes the Liberals had made from the model laws they were emulating. They were ostensibly worried about employers, but they also, conversely, suggested that if anything the law did not go far enough, and once or twice called it a "vote-catcher."[29] But there was little question it would pass. On 5 March 1908, almost two decades after the federal Royal Commission on the Relations of Capital and Labour that went nowhere, and two years after the expanded British compensation law it was modelled on, Alberta successfully passed its own workmen's compensation legislation.[30] The legislation followed the British workmen's compensation law in all but a few details.[31] It was also similar to that law in British Columbia, which in turn read almost exactly like that of New Zealand's still earlier law. Thus, Alberta drew from a tangled tradition but one in which it (like British Columbia) had a distinct advantage. As a writer in the *Edmonton Bulletin* explained, Alberta was just starting to develop industrially and had yet to become established enough to create powerful, employer-led political lobby groups; this meant it would be easier to pass work-related laws and integrate them into growing industries, without the political resistance or reorganization that might be required in an industrially established location.[32]

Alberta did make some small but significant changes to the British Columbia system, however. There was no cap on the maximum that one could receive in the case of permanent disability.[33] Fault was not considered under the Alberta law, unlike cases in British Columbia in which compensation was not awarded if the accident could be shown to be the worker's own fault.[34] These changes were well received. One journalist comparing the two provinces trumpeted the superiority of Alberta payments: "In British Columbia, the mecca of Socialism, the indemnity was only $1,500; in Alberta it was $1,800; in British Columbia the indemnity for a funeral was $100; in Alberta $200; in British Columbia the height of a building from which an accident must take place is 40 feet, in Alberta it is only 30 feet; in British Columbia the indemnity to miners is only $5 per week, in Alberta it is $7.50."[35] The *Edmonton Bulletin* reported in 1909 that "while it is true that nothing human is perfect, it would seem that the government of Alberta have put a measure upon the statue books in the Workmen's Compensation Act that comes as near doing justice to all parties concerned as can well be devised."[36] Even detractors such as the Reverend Arthur Murphy described the new act "as more advanced than the Compensation Act in force in England, Ontario or British Columbia."[37]

Despite the rhetoric, the 1908 Alberta workmen's compensation law did not remove recompense for work accidents entirely from the courts and from costly and unpredictable lawsuits for damages, although it did take steps in that direction. Miner Sam Wannak used the courts to sue the owners of the Bush Mine, for instance, but the issue revolved around whether Wannak had already been "discharged" at the time of his injury and whether he had ignored posted signage warning him not to enter the shaft where he was injured.[38] In the absence of such complicating factors, however, the new legislation simplified court work considerably. Recommended amounts of compensation were laid out for employers to follow (and employees to see and expect). Though not legally binding on this point, the law established a process of payment upon injury that was automatic – to replace one in which employers might wait to be sued to offer payment – and directed employers and employees who could not agree towards arbitration rather than lawsuit. Edmonton-area workers John Green and Edmond Pion, for instance, both won their compensation amounts through arbitration by a judge. Green had permanently injured an arm on a punching machine, and Pion had lost his left eye to a flying shard of steel.[39] The act also had much lower requirements for establishing the employer's negligence in causing the accident. A generally dangerous trade or work environment now placed the onus on the employer to pay for accidents that arose in the general pursuit of business.

Under Alberta's new Workmen's Compensation Act, accident insurance coverage for workers was now required, but employers arranged the details of coverage with their own choice of private insurer.[40] The details of these arrangements by large companies and municipal employers were often published in local papers. The *Red Deer News*, for instance, advertised that Red Deer firemen were covered by the London Guarantee and Accident Society, specifically noting that the insurance had been taken out in accordance with the new Workmen's Compensation Act. The town paid $3 per $1,000 worth of coverage, and each fireman was covered for $2,000 (i.e., the town would pay $6 per fireman, presumably annually, for accident insurance sufficient to cover their fire brigade). In the case of an accident, London Guarantee and Accident Society would compensate the town of Red Deer, which, in turn, would disburse the money to the injured fireman or his relative.[41]

In the early years following the law's enactment, employers shared widespread concerns about being able to insure completely against the risk of employee accidents.[42] When the Conservative opposition party leader Albert Robertson addressed the Alberta legislature in late January 1909, he suggested the new act "made employers liable to damage to workmen that they are unable to cover by insurance."[43] He argued that "the government should provide facilities for insurance" in order to lessen the burden on employers, and guarantee workers that employers would in fact have sufficient funds to cover their payments in the case of an accident. The act, he argued, "makes the employer liable for compensation, but takes no steps to insure [sic] that he shall have placed himself in a position to meet the liability imposed upon him."[44] A month later, the Conservatives again advertised their platform on labour legislation, calling on the Liberal majority government to put into place either a greater provision of private insurance for employers or a system of government insurance, or a combination of the two, in order to better protect both employers and workers under the new act.[45]

Not everyone was convinced that this was such an insurmountable obstacle. Edmonton's *Saturday News* dismissed employers' concerns around the availability of insurance, standing by Liberal reassurances. The *Saturday News* also lacked empathy for worried bosses, suggesting that the benefits of the act were great enough to outweigh any distress it caused to employers trying to adjust: "Employers may be put to some temporary inconvenience, and even loss, just as practically every radical change in the public interests requires someone should suffer, but the idea is a sound one and when the change is brought fully into effect, everyone concerned will be the better for it."[46] In March that year, two days after the Conservatives made another call for the government to make provisions for insurance, the *Raymond Rustler* published a British news article that was a "complete answer" to these concerns and featured an insurance company covering all risk on behalf of an English employer under the equivalent British act.[47] Journalists at the *Edmonton Bulletin* similarly concluded that there were only small premiums to pay for more than sufficient coverage.[48] In other words, news sources implied that insurance companies were perfectly able, and more than willing, to insure workplace accidents on behalf of employers. By December 1909, the government incorporated the Provincial Insurance Company, which offered accident insurance and coverage to employers for their liability under the Workmen's Compensation Act, curtailing further argument.[49]

THE SIGNIFICANCE OF 1908 LEGISLATION IN ALBERTA

Soon after the implementation of the 1908 act, a new narrative appeared in newspapers and speeches when discussing workplace accidents, one that made clear the "before" and "after" of workmen's compensation. Here we see the kind of sense-making of the accident that is evident elsewhere in this volume: in Samira Saramo's chapter on newspaper accounts of house fires in Canada's Finnish communities, and in Cameron Baldassarra's chapter on memorializing death on Ontario's Petawawa River. If the man in question had been injured in the present day instead of a few months or years ago, the stories commonly went, the Workmen's Compensation Act would have taken care of him. The men injured before the 1908 legislation was enacted, however, were unjustly left broken and destitute. The act, in other words, had a profound and immediate effect on how people thought of workplace accidents in Alberta.

The narrative was used for differing purposes: as political support, as celebration of the new act, or as a way of raising funds for someone whose

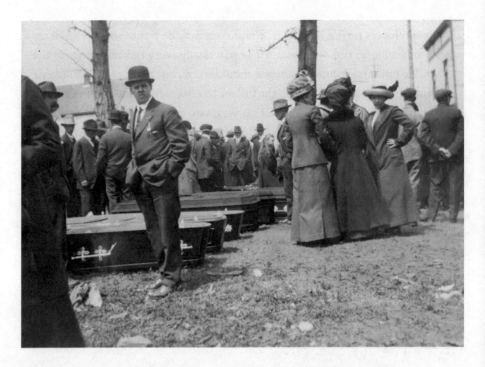

Fig. 7.3 Coffins ready for burial, after mining disaster at Hillcrest, Alberta. Accident legislation did not stop accidents from occurring, as this 1914 mining-disaster funeral attests. It did provide easier and surer access to financial stability in the wake of an accident.

injury happened before the act came into effect. All of these accounts began with someone whom the writer claimed would have been adequately taken care of without question under the act but, due to the misfortune of timing, had instead experienced ongoing suffering and destitution stemming from the moment of the accident. In one example, Travis Baker wrote to the *Edmonton Bulletin* after it printed a letter from two women calling attention to the plight of a community member injured in a railway accident: "Had this Fred Cross sustained his injuries today instead of three months ago," Baker wrote, "the government, with its Compensation Act, would be by his side soothing his sorrows and wiping tears from that grief-stricken and friendless wife and child."[30]

Although rarely directly referenced, gender, dependence, and disability underpin this emerging narrative of the introduction of workmen's compensation to Alberta. As the introduction to this volume sets out, men performed the labour in Canada's dangerous resource extraction and transportation industries, leaving women dealing with economic responsibilities, the healing work, and the emotional labour after the accident. The idea of workmen's compensation as the friend of a working man's wife and children was thus immediate and pervasive, and indeed dovetails with Tamara Myers and Megan Davies's analysis elsewhere in this volume of the maternalist state and its focus on children as a civic investment. Here, political rhetoric matched economic reality, for women (particularly married women, even if their husbands were home injured, or on reduced wages) had far fewer opportunities to earn a living and were likely to earn significantly less for the work they did, which was often piecemeal and part of the informal economy. In addition, they often had children at home whose care would remain their responsibility. Charity might be available if the family became desperate, but it varied in availability and was subject to the decision of community members of a different class to find the family worthy of pity. The reputation of workmen's compensation as a far less capricious force in saving wives and families was certainly deserved.

Theda Skocpol's groundbreaking 1992 argument that early federal state social provisions were aimed at soldiers and mothers rather than workers was helpful to historians grappling with early welfare state analysis.[51] It is helpful here because it allows us to see how the health and welfare state shored up traditional household power relations by supporting working men's power over their wives, especially as their success in maintaining control over the conditions of their work became less assured. In Alberta, this patriarchal focus is evident in the arguments made for workmen's compensation, especially the assumption that women were always completely reliant financially on their husbands. The following example is typical: "His family are absolutely dependent on his foresight and thrift to make provision for the hour of need. It only too frequently happens that the workman does not make such provision and when disablement or death comes suffering and destitution fall upon his wife and children."[52] Yet Alberta miners who testified during the Royal Commission on the Coal Mining Industry reported their incomes to vary wildly from month to month and to sometimes be incredibly low – far too low to support a family through this income alone. One man made between $8.75 and $127 a month, for instance, while another had made between $13 and $140 per paycheque, and a third brought home $132 in his best month but only $4.40 in his lowest-paying month.[53] This suggests that those among them who had families were already well versed in either surviving through frugality in the lean months or in creating alternative income sources (even without recourse to working-men's fraternities, churches, or other charitable income that might be available in the wake of an accident).

As the Workmen's Compensation Act was drawn up, however, Attorney-General Cross in particular consistently evoked this rhetoric of saving widows and orphans in his speeches and heard it echoed back by supportive labour men, even though many of them likely lived more complex realities at home. Cross used language he believed would garner the most support: "Widows and orphans would automatically receive adequate compensation when the bread-winners were suddenly taken off by fatal accident," and "Who would not pay that sum to protect the widows and orphans of the province?"[54] This language was also used by labourers during these political meetings and by concerned citizens in their calls for support of individual injured men. Vocal labourer Travis Barker referred to Fred Cross's post-accident situation as "nothing but desolation before that family."[55] While the man's wife was considered to be "consequently destitute," Cross's supporters also revealed in passing that since his wife's arrival in the country, she had been working in domestic service to support herself and their young child (and, presumably, her badly injured husband).[56] Officially and publicly, compensation was needed because an income-earning male head of household was vital to women's survival. The complete erasure of women's historical techniques for coping with financial hardship, either in the wake of an accident or to supplement low income from a "breadwinner" husband, and the lack of alternative possibilities for how to structure a family in any of these discussions, suggests that this was the only family dynamic considered acceptable (at least publicly) to men across the class spectrum.

Historian James Struthers draws on previous feminist analysis when he points out that "the welfare state itself is a gendered, two-tiered construct in which 'rights-based' social insurance programs, both in design and administration, typically serve a male wage-labour force. In contrast, discretionary 'needs-based' social assistance ... responds to the particular vulnerabilities and moral expectations surrounding women's dependence within the family."[57] Historian Nancy Forestell makes clear the degree to which women felt the need to reassure their injured man of his continued dominant role within the family. By making the consequences of accidents to working men less tragic, workmen's compensation helped justify a patriarchal family structure in which the woman's place was at home and the working man remained the income earner and head of house, even when injured and perhaps incapacitated.[58] That alternative strategies or other opportunities for women to find work in the wake of an accident were completely missing from the conversation suggests that in Alberta, as in other places, whether consciously or not, a patriarchal family structure was being reified and upheld by those who supported the act. For the most part, this patriarchal underbelly went unmentioned in discussion around financial support for women and children and as the ability of workmen's compensation to provide continued financial solvency within the confines of a traditional family structure was celebrated at face value.

After they passed their 1908 Workmen's Compensation Act, Albertans took great pride in reporting how many other places looked to Alberta's example to create their own laws. Alberta took credit for being an inspiration, and it is entirely possible that, directly or indirectly, it was. In 1909, the *Edmonton Bulletin* ran a lengthy summary of a bill under consideration in Quebec, beginning, "The Quebec Legislature is now considering a workmen's compensation bill along similar lines to the Alberta act" and assuming that readers would find a dissection of similarities and differences interesting.[59] In March 1910, the same newspaper declared that Nova Scotia was "Following Lead of Alberta" in introducing compensation for workers killed or permanently injured on the job.[60] And by 1911, the *Edmonton Capital* was scornful of the belated nature of "Ontario's awakening" and its plan to appoint a commission to look into the matter.[61] Far from imagining that the Ontario commission could be a useful or ground-breaking enterprise, or that it might build further on existing acts and laws in other provinces, the reporter maintained,

There is nothing left to do but to frame the act. And even in this Ontario should need no commission. By sending a stenographer to the nearest law library with instructions to take from the statutes of the province of Alberta the compensation act which was enacted by the legislature of this province, substituting only the name "Ontario" where the name "Alberta" occurs, Ontario would get the best compensation act on the continent of North America, or, for that matter, in the world. With the Alberta law to copy from, the Ontario commission is wasteful and ridiculous excess.[62]

During this period, workmen's compensation laws and systems for addressing the needs of injured workers were multiplying around the world. Germany had introduced collective government-run workmen's compensation in 1884. Britain had introduced the 1897 Chamberlain Act, which it expanded in 1906. By 1910, Belgium, Finland, Norway, Russia, Spain, and Sweden had mandated systems of employer responsibility for worker accidents. Similar responsibilities existed in New Zealand, Queensland, and South and West Australia. Austria, Hungary, Greece, and Luxembourg had systems in which responsibility was shared between employers and employees.[63] Alberta, Quebec, and British Columbia all had compensation acts on the books.[64] For the other Prairie provinces, laws in both Manitoba and Saskatchewan would come in 1911, the same year as in Nova Scotia.[65] In 1911, Alberta newspapers also noted the introduction of a state-collected form of workmen's compensation in Washington, and within another four years most American states had introduced some form of workmen's compensation.[66]

Finally, in 1913, William Meredith submitted his report in Ontario, essentially advocating for the German system of government-run, collectively assessed, no-fault compensation. It slowly wound its way into legislation by 1914 and was enacted the following year as Ontario's now much celebrated Workmen's Compensation Act. In 1916, though, Manitoba Legislature passed a law "[providing] the same scale of compensation payments as a similar act in Ontario" but without "[embodying] the principle of the state accident fund."[67] In other words, despite having the Meredith document and a newly established Workmen's Compensation Board in Ontario readily available as models, Manitoba did not in 1916 choose to establish a Workmen's Compensation Board or move to a system of collective liability as Ontario had, but rather elected to emulate other regions in important aspects of its system. However, British Columbia *was* interested and moved to a system of collective liability the following year. Once it took hold in the West, it seems to have garnered more serious attention from Alberta as a possibility that would completely remove from the courts the burden of deciding Workmen's Compensation cases, speed up resolution and payment, and better ensure the coverage of workers and the insurance status of employers by involving the government more directly in the process.[68] In the late 1910s, Alberta would become one of a number of provinces to create a Workmen's Compensation Board to oversee all workmen's compensation. The following years would bring a series of further amendments, but there was also a collective national effort starting in the 1920s to bring the provinces together under more uniform legislation.[69]

Lurking behind these administrative and policy machinations were deeper societal and cultural notions of masculinity, concerns about the breakdown of the family and impoverished childhoods, and stories of profound vulnerability and suffering. As a comparison with Anh-Dao Bui Tran's chapter on risk management in the mid-nineteenth century work site makes clear, responsibility for keeping workers safe and dealing with workplace accidents had shifted from the individual worker or the employer to the state. Nonetheless, both represent a patriarchal response to the spectre of the industrial accident.

CONCLUSION

In 1918, Alberta passed an act to create a Workmen's Compensation Board to run its now collectively assessed, government-overseen system, based on what was originally a German model. This was a significant shift away from the British system that legally mandated employers' responsibility for accidents but with employer insurance coverage provided for by commercial insurance companies. This bureaucratically meaningful change in approach received much less attention in the provincial press than the 1908 Alberta Workmen's Compensation Act of the decade before. The earlier act had generated extended news coverage and discussion, stretching from 1907 through 1910, often landing on newspapers' front pages. The responses differed because having a relatively comprehensive system of compensation for workers (versus not having one at all) had much greater significance for Alberta's employees and employers than any changes in specific details of how that system was run.

As a cultural change from a British to a German model, the leap that Meredith made was exceptionally open-minded. To have a Canadian precedent likely made it easier for other provinces to follow suit, although American states such as Washington had already made at least some elements of this leap and were receiving attention for it north of the border.[70] Perhaps more profoundly, the consequences of this shift changed the landscape for private accident companies; what initially looked like a golden opportunity for nation-wide insurance businesses was suddenly redirected in most provinces into a non-profit state board. Yet these changes were, on the whole, not life-altering ones for most workers. The 1908 act changed the compensation landscape *for workers* much more than the 1918 one, despite all the attention we now give to the latter.

Paying attention to the ways in which workmen's compensation first took shape allows us to return the emphasis to the workers themselves (and their families): to see the often profound consequences that more uniform and less fault-oriented compensation had on working-class lives years before the implementation of government-run boards. It also gives space for a more nuanced understanding of how initial approaches to early workmen's compensation developed out of larger shifts taking place around risk and societal responses to workplace accidents. The development of early workmen's compensation was made possible in part by philosophical changes happening in Western Europe and its colonial offspring, as nations became increasingly interested in the idea of gathering information about individuals and using it to create policy that would encourage productive citizens. Early workmen's compensation also had implications for how risk was understood and responded to. As historian Julia Moses notes, "The last third of the nineteenth century saw a radical reformulation of ideas about individual responsibility and social risk. It implied a new role for the state, and a novel understanding about the function of the law, in governing what were perceived as social problems."[71] The new field of statistics, in particular, would play an increasingly crucial role, making possible an expanding insurance industry and also allowing government to imagine new ways to intervene through policy and law. Risk, including the risk of workplace accidents, became something that increasingly could be predicted statistically and regulated through policy or otherwise controlled, or at least insured against.[72]

Alberta, as a new political region lead by a fiercely proud elite, turned out to be well suited to become an earlier adopter of new laws protecting labourers. Workmen's compensation legislation in Alberta was significantly imbued with both regional factors (such as the dominance of mining within Alberta industry and provincial miners' organizing strength) on the one hand and by transnational influence (in the form of existing international models and growing response to worker's safety needs) on the other. The extensive trans-provincial debate, both before and after the 1908 act passed in Alberta, meant that legislation was developed with an eye on other provinces and was felt to be both on the leading edge within Canada and founded on solid international examples. In the end, what was originally implemented in the province was designed to be suited to local needs while also in large part replicating almost exactly already existing legislations, particularly those in Britain.

Initially, only a few male-dominated industries were protected by workmen's compensation, but this coverage grew exponentially. In all workplaces where it applied, legislation profoundly altered the impact of job-related accidents on workers and their families. But with workman's compensation came implications around gender, disability, ethnicity and other rich topics for historians. Some of the import for women and for early twentieth-century cultural understandings of masculinity have been barely touched on here, as workmen's compensation shored up patriarchal notions of a household supported by a male breadwinner. Additionally, as Roger Cooter and Bill Luckin note in writing in the field of accident history more generally, workers' compensation allowed capitalist systems to naturalize work accidents without calling attention to the degree to which accidents fell along class or racial lines, obscuring the mark of race and class on the distribution of accidents within society.[73] A disability lens is likewise absent in this chapter, but no less important, nor have I tackled the connection, highly relevant to Alberta, between colonial development and the paternalistic health and welfare state. There is much more to be explored, in other words, than I have been able to cover here.

Ultimately, as the example of Alberta shows, paying attention to the ways in which workmen's compensation developed prior to the Meredith report gives us a much more nuanced understanding of the lives of workers and the significance of workplace accidents in early twentieth-century Canada. It allows us to see the ways in which responses to workplace accidents were changing, not because of the national adoption of a single innovation but as an ongoing and piecemeal response to a complex, internationally shared process: a shifting understanding of risk – and an adoption of statistics as the primary way to make sense of and contain risk – that was applied uniquely at the regional level according to local logic and culture. The result was a network of national, provincial, or state workmen's compensation systems that eventually largely arrived in similar places via different avenues and influences. In Alberta, the real moment of change in worker's lives came not in the wake of the later creation of a provincial board but in 1908 with the enactment of provincial workmen's compensation legislation that first guaranteed workers and their families access to financial compensation based not on fault but simply on the fact of their having been injured on the job.

ACKNOWLEDGMENTS

This article was supported by doctoral completion funding through Associated Medical Services (AMS). It benefited from the generous collaboration and editing skills of Megan Davies and Dian Day. Thank you to Erika Dyck, Laura Larsen, David Mitchell, Rebecca Pratt, Amy Procter, David Smith, and Gary Weber, and to digitization staff at the Provincial Archives of Alberta and the archives of University of Calgary and University of Alberta.

NOTES

1 Big Meeting in Separate School – Mr. Cross Heartily Applauded," *Edmonton Bulletin*, 3 February 1909.

2 Moses, *First Modern Risk*, 6.

3 Rodgers, *Atlantic Crossings*, 209–10; Alborn, *Regulated Lives*, 3.

4 Witt, *Accidental Republic*, 5–6. Witt is discussing the United States, but his observation here applies to Canada as well.

5 Klein, *For All These Rights*, 4; Rodgers, *Atlantic Crossings*, 218–19.

6 Francis, "Rural Ontario West," 125–31.

7 "How the Compensation Act Protects the Worker," *Edmonton Bulletin*, 13 January 1909.

8 Saskatchewan remained almost entirely agriculturally focused and did not have the population or the industry base needed to make workmen's compensation a priority.

9 Tucker, *Administering Danger in the Workplace*; Storey, "Social Assistance or a Worker's Right"; Storey, "They Have All Been Faithful Workers"; Fahrni, "Victimes de la tâche journalière." Political scientist Andrew Stritch has also published on workers' compensation in Quebec; see Stritch, "Power Resources, Institutions, and Policy Learning." For western Canada, see Devine, "'In an Equitable and Sympathetic Manner.'" Additional secondary literature includes two (in-house) histories of provincial WCBS (Saskatchewan and British Columbia, the latter by Anjan Chaklader), one chapter (by Robert Babcock) in an edited collection, two articles (by Andrew Stritch and Michael Piva), and a handful of dissertations, of which Jason Devine's on Alberta is the most relevant.

10 See, for example, the Association of Workers' Compensation Boards of Canada (AWCBC), *"Canadian Workers' Compensation History,"* https://awcbc.org/en/about/workers-compensation/, or the Canadian Association of Workers' Advisors and Advocates (CAWAA), "The Meredith Principals," https://cawaa.org/pages/the-meredith-principals.

11 Moses, *First Modern Risk*, 260.

12 Ibid, 3.

13 Fishback and Kantor, *Prelude to the Welfare State*, 198–9; Moses, *First Modern Risk*, 255–60; Witt, *Accidental Republic*, 9–10, 209–11.

14 Kealey, *Canada Investigates Industrialism*, xx.

15 Devine, "'In an Equitable and Sympathetic Manner,'" 1, 3, 8–9, 10, 30; Tucker, *Administering Danger in the Workplace*, 76.

16 "Our London Letter," *Calgary Weekly Herald*, 11 August 1898, 7.

17 An Ordinance to Secure Compensation to Workmen, ONWT (1900), chap. 13.

18 See, for example, Saskatchewan Workers' Compensation Board, *Story of Workers' Compensation*, 6–8.

19 See "Hurt by Cars Result Fatal," *Frank Paper*, 21 January 1909, for just one example, in which the engineer "thought he got a signal from [the man killed] but could not see him for steam and he could not be certain who gave the signal."

20 "Tuesday's News," *Calgary Weekly Herald*, 21 February 1901.

21 "Wave of Progressive Legislation Spreads," *Edmonton Bulletin*, 18 December 1911.

22 "More Radical Mining Legislation," *Outcrop*, 26 February 1903.

23 Arthur L. Sifton, *Report of the Royal Commission on the Coal Mining Industry in the Province of Alberta 1907* (Edmonton: Jas. E. Richards, Government Printer, 1907), 5–7. The Government of Alberta website credits the 1906 Lethbridge Strike specifically for leading to government action. Alberta Culture and Tourism website, n.d. "Coal: Triumphs and Tragedies: Labour Revolution," http://history.alberta.ca/energyheritage/coal/triumphs-and-tragedies-1914-1930/labour/default.aspx.

24 See in particular *Strathcona Evening Chronicle* and *Edmonton Bulletin* for related coverage.

25 Arthur L. Sifton, *Report of the Royal Commission*, 13.

26 Ibid.

27 "Chapter 12: An Act with Respect to Compensation to Workmen for Injuries Suffered in the Course of Their Employment," in *Statutes of the Province of Alberta* (Edmonton: Jas. E. Richards, Government Printer, 1908), 39.

28 "Compensation Act Criticized," *Edmonton Bulletin*, 20 February 1908.

29 "The Working Man Will Get Benefit," *Edmonton Bulletin*, 15 February 1908.

30 The British law was originally enacted in 1897 and expanded in 1906.

31 "Employees' Compensation," *Taber Free Press*, 13 February 1908; "Compensation Bill Is In," *Frank Paper*, 13 February 1908. *Taber Free Press* called the British and Alberta laws "practically identical," and *Frank Paper* used similar wording.

32 "How the Compensation Act Protects the Worker," *Edmonton Bulletin*, 13 January 1909.

33 "Insurance under the Workmen's Act," *Edmonton Bulletin*, 19 February 1909. It was this lack of cap that would have Alberta employers crying to government about not being able to insure sufficiently.

34 "Compensation Act Will Stand," *Edmonton Bulletin*, 8 January 1909.

35 "Calgary Only Place Where Sectional Cry Is Raised," *Edmonton Bulletin*, 10 March 1909.

36 "Insurance under the Workmen's Act," *Edmonton Bulletin*, 19 February 1909. Employers against the act, on the other hand, were advocating for its repeal "before it goes broadcast throughout the country." "Employers Ask Repeal of Act," *Edmonton Bulletin*, 7 January 1909.

37 "Compensation Act Will Stand," *Edmonton Bulletin*, 8 January 1909.

38 "Around the City: Applies for Compensation," *Edmonton Bulletin*, 13 October 1910.

39 "Two Cases in Court under Workmen's Compensation Act," *Edmonton Bulletin*, 8 November 1910.

40 "Mr. Robertson's Address in Debate on the Speech from the Throne. Omissions of Compensation Act," *Red Deer News*, 27 January 1909; "The Working Man Will Get Benefit," *Edmonton Bulletin*, 15 February 1908. Opposition leader Albert Robertson referred to accident insurance as "a virtual necessity" for employers under the terms of the new law, and Attorney-General Cross agreed.

41 "The Town Council: Insurance for Firemen," *Red Deer News*, 17 February 1909.

42 "Employers Demand Repeal of the Compensation Act," *Edmonton Bulletin*, 6 January 1909; "Employers Ask Repeal of Act," *Edmonton Bulletin*, 7 January 1909; "Compensation Act Will Stand," *Edmonton Bulletin*, 8 January 1909; John MacDonald, "Correspondence – Workmen's Compensation Act," *Edmonton Bulletin*, 3 March 1909; "Price of Coal Jumps to $5.50 – Other Difficulties," *Edmonton Bulletin*, 9 January 1909. A number of companies were also supposedly put out of business by the act, though the *Edmonton Bulletin* notes (with sarcastic humour) that some of these were subsequently seen conducting business as usual.

43 "Mr. Robertson's Address in Debate on the Speech from the Throne: Omissions of Compensation Act," *Red Deer News*, 27 January 1909.

44 Ibid.

45 "Conservative Platform. Labour Legislation," *Red Deer News*, 3 March 1909.

46 "Note and Comment," *Edmonton Saturday News*, 16 January 1909.

47 No title, *Raymond Rustler*, 5 March 1909, 4.

48 "Insurance under the Workmen's Act," *Edmonton Bulletin*, 19 February 1909; see also a journalist's interview with insurers, "Compensation Act Will Stand," under "The Insurance Men," *Edmonton Bulletin*, 8 January 1909.

49 "Of General Interest," *Western Globe*, 12 January 1910; "Notice," *Edmonton Bulletin* (5:00 p.m. edn), 12 January 1910.

50 Travis Barker, "Correspondence – Who Will Help?", *Edmonton Bulletin*, 29 January 1909.

51 Skocpol, *Protecting Soldiers and Mothers*, 525. For an earlier monograph on the development of the Canadian welfare state, see also Morton and Wright, *Winning the Second Battle*.

52 "Two Measures for the Workingmen," *Edmonton Bulletin*, 17 February 1908.

53 "Bellevue Miners' Evidence," *Strathcona Chronicle*, 7 June 1907.

54 "Compensation Act Will Stand," *Edmonton Bulletin*, 29 January 1909; "Trying to Arouse Business Men," under "East End Voters Endorse New Act," *Edmonton Bulletin*, 19 January 1909.

55 Travis Barker, "Who Will Help?", Correspondence, *Edmonton Bulletin*, 29 January 1909.

56 The fundraising was for the wife to return with her child to England, as the company was only willing to repatriate Fred. Even this offhand mention of the woman's work is surprising; it is the only mention of a woman working or finding means other than the compensation act or charity to support her family in all of the newspaper articles between 1907 and 1909 on workmen's compensation and work accidents that I reviewed. Tellingly, the fact of her paid work does not change any of her fundraisers' language or assumptions that without a male breadwinner (or his compensation through the act, once it passed), a woman was financially destitute without outside support. Mary Adelaid Barrow and Maud Richardson, "Who Will Help?," Correspondence, *Edmonton Bulletin*, 29 January 1909.

57 Struthers, *Limits of Affluence*, 4. Struthers draws on Linda Gordon, Barbara Nelson, and Nancy Fraser.

58 Forestell, "'And I Feel Like I'm Dying,'" 80.

59   "Quebec Compensation Bill," *Edmonton Bulletin*, 1 April 1909.

60   "Following Lead of Alberta," *Edmonton Bulletin*, 11 March 1910.

61   "The Ontario System of Making a Law," *Edmonton Capital*, 25 October 1911.

62   Ibid.

63   "Manitoba Royal Commission on Workmen's Compensation: Report, 1910," *Sessional Papers of Manitoba* (no. 24), 643.

64   Ibid, 649.

65   Saskatchewan Workers' Compensation Board, *Story of Workers' Compensation*, 21.

66   "Washington Has a Compensation Law," *Edmonton Bulletin* (morning edition), 3 October 1911. While Alberta shared with the American Midwest a general progressive ideology at this time, movement in Canada towards workmen's compensation largely preceded most American initiatives; there was some movement towards workmen's compensation in the United States prior to 1911, but the few laws passed were quickly declared unconstitutional and struck down. For American initiatives, see Fishback and Kantor, *Prelude to the Welfare State*, 103; Witt, *Accidental Republic*, 4; Fisher, "Field of Workmen's Compensation in the United States," 221–78.

67   "Manitoba's Legislative Program – In Aid of Labor [sic]," *Grain Growers' Guide*, 29 March 1916.

68   "Govt. Commission Asks Special Board Administer Proposed Compensation Act," *Edmonton Bulletin*, 24 January 1918.

69   The project of unifying the various provincial programs is ongoing and AWCBC and CAWAA are both involved.

70   "Washington Has a Compensation Law," *Edmonton Bulletin* (morning edition), 3 October 1911.

71   Julia Moses, *First Modern Risk*, 255.

72   Cooter and Luckin, "Accidents in History," 3–5; Bouk, *How Our Days Became Numbered*, 210.

73   Cooter and Luckin, "Accidents in History," 5–7; Green, *Risk and Misfortune*, 8.

BIBLIOGRAPHY

Archives

Glenbow Library and Archives, University of Calgary
Provincial Archives of Alberta
Peel's Prairie Provinces collection of digitized materials, University of Alberta

Newspapers and Periodicals

Calgary Weekly Herald
Edmonton Bulletin

Edmonton Capital
Edmonton Saturday News
Frank Paper (Frank, Crowsnest Pass, AB)
Grain Growers' Guide
Outcrop (Canterbury, BC)
Raymond Rustler
Red Deer News
Strathcona Chronicle
Strathcona Evening Chronicle
Taber Free Press
Western Globe (Lacombe, AB)

Other Sources

Alborn, Timothy. *Regulated Lives: Life Insurance and British Society, 1800–1914.* Toronto: University of Toronto, 2009.

Bouk, Daniel B. *How Our Days Became Numbered: Risk and the Rise of the Statistical Individual.* Chicago: University of Chicago Press, 2015.

Cooter, Roger, and Bill Luckin. "Accidents in History: An Introduction." In *Accidents in History: Injuries, Fatalities and Social Relations,* edited by Roger Cooter and Bill Luckin, 1–16. Atlanta: Rodopi, 1997.

Devine, Jason Corey. "'In an Equitable and Sympathetic Manner': Alberta's Workmen's Compensation and the United Mine Workers of America, District 18's Welfare Fund." Master's thesis, University of Calgary, 2011.

Fahrni, Magda. "'Victimes de la Tâche Journalière': La Gestion des Accidents du Travail au Québec Pendant la Grande Guerre." In *1914–1918: Mains-d'Oeuvre en Guerre,* edited by Laure Machu, Isabelle Lespinet-Moret, and Vincent Viet, 296–306. Paris: La Documentation Française, 2018.

Fishback, Price V., and Shawn Everett Kantor. *A Prelude to the Welfare State: The Origins of Workers' Compensation.* Chicago: University of Chicago, 2000.

Fisher, Willard C. "The Field of Workmen's Compensation in the United States." *American Economic Review* 5, no. 2 (June 1915): 221–78.

Forestell, Nancy M. "'And I Feel Like I'm Dying from Mining for Gold': Disability, Gender, and the Mining Community, 1920–1950." *Labor: Studies in Working-Class History of the Americas* 3, no. 3 (2006): 77–93.

Francis, R. Douglas. "'Rural Ontario West': Ontarians in Alberta." In *Peoples of Alberta: Portraits of Cultural Diversity,* edited by Howard Palmer and Tamara Palmer, 123–42. Saskatoon: Western Producer Prairie Books, 1985.

Green, Judith. *Risk and Misfortune: A Social Construction of Accidents.* New York: Routledge 2003.

Kealey, Greg, ed. *Canada Investigates Industrialism.* Toronto: University of Toronto Press, 1973.

Klein, Jennifer. *For All These Rights: Business, Labour, and the Shaping of America's Public-Private Welfare State*. Princeton: Princeton University Press, 2003.

Morton, Desmond, and Glenn Wright. *Winning the Second Battle: Canadian Veterans and the Return to Civilian Life, 1915–1930*. Toronto: University of Toronto Press, 1987.

Moses, Julia. *The First Modern Risk: Workplace Accidents and the Origins of European Social States*. New York: Cambridge University Press, 2018.

Rodgers, Daniel T. *Atlantic Crossings: Social Politics in a Progressive Age*. Cambridge, MA: Harvard University Press, 1998.

Saskatchewan Workers' Compensation Board. *The Story of Workers' Compensation in Saskatchewan*. Regina: Houghton Boston, 1997.

Skocpol, Theda. *Protecting Soldiers and Mothers: The Political Origins of Social Policy in the United States*. Cambridge, MA: Belknap, 1992.

Storey, Robert. "'They Have All Been Faithful Workers': Injured Workers, Truth, and Workers' Compensation in Ontario, 1970–2008." *Journal of Canadian Studies* 43, no. 1 (2009): 154–85.

– "Social Assistance or a Worker's Right: Workmen's Compensation and the Struggle of Injured Workers in Ontario, 1970–1985." *Studies in Political Economy* 78, no. 1 (2006): 67–91.

Stritch, Andrew. "Power Resources, Institutions, and Policy Learning: The Origins of Workers Compensation in Quebec." *Canadian Journal of Political Science* 38, no. 3 (2005): 549–79.

Struthers, James. *The Limits of Affluence: Welfare in Ontario, 1920–1970*. Toronto: University of Toronto Press, 1994.

Tucker, Eric. *Administering Danger in the Workplace: The Law and Politics of Occupational Health and Safety Regulation in Ontario, 1850–1914*. Toronto: University of Toronto Press, 1990.

Witt, John Fabian. *The Accidental Republic: Crippled Workingmen, Destitute Widows, and the Remaking of American Law*. Cambridge, MA: Harvard University Press, 2004.

8

"Don't Shoot Crooked Chute"

Memorializing Death and Mediating Risk on Ontario's Petawawa River

Cameron Baldassarra

On 12 May 1968, the editor of *Maclean's* magazine, Blair Fraser, drowned in Rollway Rapids on Algonquin Park's Petawawa River.[1] Fraser was not the first canoeist to die in the turbulent waters of the Petawawa, nor would he be the last. The manner in which he drowned was not unique: he and his partner missed a portage obscured by the high waters of spring runoff and lost control of their boat in rough waves.[2] Fraser's autopsy stated that the mechanism of death was drowning, but there was also evidence that he had hit his head: he was not wearing a helmet, a practice now common in whitewater canoeing. What is unique about his accident is how it was reported and written about. Fraser's case is an important marker of a cultural shift in the discursive and practical responses to accidents, particularly fatalities, that occurred along the Petawawa River and in the broader world of postwar outdoor recreation. His death is also emblematic of the era's deindustrialization of the riverine environment – many working-class foresters and loggers drowned in the Petawawa in the century before Fraser's fatal trip – and how the shift to recreational use of the river brought with it changes in the perception and memorialization of accidents in Algonquin Park.

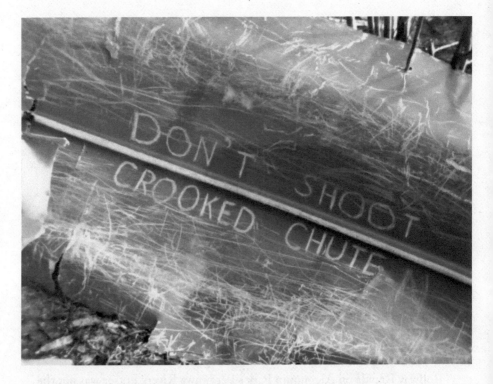

Fig. 8.1 Wrecked canoe, with cautionary note. Crooked Chute on the Petawawa River, well known to canoeists as a dangerous stretch of rapids, has wrecked many canoes.

Fraser's craft of choice was the canoe, a boat of national significance that has played a central role in many accident-ridden adventures throughout Canada's past. In their introduction to *The Politics of the Canoe*, Bruce Erickson and Sarak Wylie Krotz state that the canoe's "mythic legacy as a national vehicle" came to prominence at the turn of the nineteenth century, serving to reinforce colonial ideals of masculinity and a burgeoning sense of Canadian national identity.[3] The technological innovations and economic boom that followed World War II also resulted in a rapid expansion in wilderness travel that brought middle-class professionals like Fraser to outdoor recreational areas such as Algonquin Park. Where Fraser and his fellow paddlers differed from Victorian era explorers and glory seekers was in applying a risk-mitigating approach to their wilderness travel, similar to the measured risk taking described by Christopher Dummit in his examination of middle-class Vancouverites' postwar penchant for (safe) mountaineering.[4] Central to Dummitt's thesis is the concept of the "Manly Modern" – middle-class men recreating in the wilderness as a way to reinforce their masculinity – which Dummitt suggests was perceived as being threatened by the comfort of suburban life.[5] In their meta-analysis of the concept of risk in recent tourism literature, Anna-Maria Gstaettner, Diane Lee, and Kate Rodger conclude that risk is perceived as a "central and positive element of the outdoor experience. Anticipated positive outcomes were frequently cited as motivation for, and benefit of, risky outdoor activity participation."[6] The pursuit of masculine recreation, escape from the urban (or suburban) environment and search for "positive outcomes" of risky recreational activities might explain how Blair Fraser found himself on the Petawawa River during the elevated water levels of the spring melt.

In spite of its known danger, the Petawawa River continues to be a popular destination for white-water canoe trippers and has long held primacy of place among park visitors, canoeists, anglers, and residents.[7] The river runs from near the western boundary of Ontario's Algonquin Provincial Park 190 kilometres to the east, where it joins the Ottawa River. The park section is a well-travelled route, popular with canoeists and famous within that community for its challenging rapids. Prior to European colonization, Indigenous peoples considered most of the river to be a significant navigational challenge, though the lower, calmer sections near its confluence with the Ottawa were important locations for catching staple food fish such as sturgeon and eels.[8] Skip Ross, an Algonquin elder and long-time resident of Petawawa, explained that "our people used it, but the only problem is that it is too rough, too many portages, so they started goin' up the Mattawa, and another little river that goes into Cedar Lake."[9] The names of the rapids indicate the river's history as a dangerous space for Indigenous peoples, European surveyors, recreational canoeists, and the lumbermen who drove logs down its length for well over a century: Devil's Cellar, Devil's Chute, Beelzebub's Whirlpool, Dracula, Fury, and The Keeper, among others.[10] Tommy Cloutier, a forestry contractor with a long family history of both logging and recreating along the Petawawa, confirmed the sometimes intimidating nature of the rapids when sharing his memory of lending his son a canoe: "Lotta people are a little anxious when it comes to those rapids. My son brought my [aluminum] canoe back like an accordion – never did float the same!"[11] These same turbulent waters attracted paddlers like Fraser, with the improved gear and easier access available in the postwar period, to attempt the challenging descent.

Cloutier's tale is one of seven oral histories used in this chapter, drawn from two general groups of land users: those with experience in the forestry industry (loggers, forestry company owners, contractors), and those who work or participate in recreational canoeing (canoe trippers, recreational fishing, campers), or recreation-adjacent jobs (park rangers, river guides). The participants' life experiences cover the 1930s to the 1990s, an era that saw the decline of forestry on the Petawawa River and the rise of recreation as the predominant human activity along the watershed. The lived experiences and memories of the research participants in this study demonstrate an attitudinal shift from the acceptance of logging accidents as a daily part of life towards a risk-averse culture of canoe tripping that dominated the accidental history of the Petawawa River from the 1960s onward. The findings in this chapter parallel the theories of masculinity put forward by Dummit. His suggestion that shifting perceptions of masculinity in the modern era promoted "the social significance of risk management for men" is clearly supported by the response to and memorialization of Blair Fraser's accidental death, particularly the characterization of Fraser as cautious.[12] This shifting perception of risk revealed through the oral histories in this book parallels the similar shift from acceptable risk to risk aversion demonstrated in my literary analysis of the memories of early twentieth-century explorers, the public discourse regarding Fraser's death, and the broader body of popular canoe literature – especially guidebooks – covered in this chapter.

In her 1997 book *Risk and Misfortune: The Social Construction of Accidents*, health sociologist Judith Green lays out a clear argument for the "dramatic transformation of how accidents are classified, discussed and managed" in the twentieth century, a temporal range that mirrors the scope of this study and reflects the shifting perceptions of risk found in my research data.[13] Green suggests that the rise of modernity and scientific thinking caused a cultural shift in the conceptualization of accidents from being viewed as unfortunate events resulting from bad luck, fate, or misfortune to being seen as avoidable incidents largely the fault of those involved.[14] Simultaneously, her discussion of mountaineering accidents and mountain rescue organizations clearly suggests that 1990s era outdoor recreation participants and organizations perceived risk and accidents as phenomena that could be managed or avoided. The interviews in this chapter support this claim, with a number of Algonquin park rangers and recreational canoeists laying the fault for canoe accidents squarely on paddlers.

I begin this study of the history of accidents on the Petawawa River with a comparison of the discourse surrounding Blair Fraser's 1968 drowning with the romanticized narratives of early twentieth-century adventure-mishap memoirs, illustrating a shift from romanticizing failures in judgment and skill to regarding mishaps and fatalities as a source of important risk-management lessons.[15] I go on to explore how the perception of accidents has changed from a widely accepted and rarely memorialized risk of participation in the industrial logging operations that dominated the river in the early half of the twentieth century, to the later perception of accidents as an avoidable outcome of ill-preparedness or incompetence on what had become a space dominated by recreation and leisure. This evolution from accepted risk in the industrial context to unacceptable risk in the leisure context demonstrates how perceptions of risk shifted independently in those two disparate worlds.

FROM HEROIC MISFORTUNE TO CALCULATED RISK: NARRATIVES OF THE CANOE ACCIDENT

Tales of accidental deaths or near misses in the remote Canadian wilderness have long captivated readers and continue to add interest to recreational canoeing guidebooks such as those available for the Petawawa River.[16] These narratives found their first expression in early canoe-adventure memoirs such as Dillon Wallace's *The Lure of the Labrador Wild*. First published in 1905, it recounts an attempted canoe expedition that was meant to cross the Labrador Peninsula from the Atlantic Ocean to Ungava Bay.[17] Wallace presents his navigational errors, his partner's death, and his own near-starvation as a character-building experience that steeled his resolve and brought him closer to God.[18] He profited significantly from the publication of his book, which became a bestseller and remains in print. Another oft-repeated narrative of canoe adventures gone wrong is John "Jack" Hornby's ill-fated 1927 canoeing adventure on the Thelon River in what is now Nunavut. Romanticized notions of serious accidents on canoe trips are apparent throughout the many works detailing the series of gross miscalculations that led to the 1927 death by starvation of Hornby's entire canoeing party.[19] Authors such as George Whalley valorized the suffering and struggle for survival of the expedition's members by sharing "Hornby's feats of strength and endurance" and observing that though his "name is now overshadowed by the manner of his death, he lives still in the long Northern memory."[20] Whalley's emphasis on "feats of strength and endurance" speaks to the prevalence of performative masculinity in early twentieth century Canadian canoe culture. Bruce Erickson describes the canoe expeditions of that era as being a space dominated by white men attracted to the disciplinary power of leisure: "These men sought out wild spaces to build their authority as masculine subjects in the face of the changing social relations brought on by industrial capitalism, urbanization and the rise of immigration."[21]

Unlike would-be explorers such as Wallace and Hornby, Blair Fraser was an urban professional participating in short-term recreational trips. A writer, journalist, and editor, he paddled with prominent authors and highly placed politicians like Pierre Elliot Trudeau. Thus, it was no surprise to find that the details of his fatal mishap appeared on the front page of the *Globe and Mail* and in a full article in the nationally distributed weekly news magazine *Maclean's*.[22] Fraser's accidental death has also had a lingering impact on popular canoe literature. The most recent example is Roy McGregor's 2015 non-fiction *Canoe Country*, which follows the Fraser family on a 2013 canoe trip down the Petawawa to repair a damaged memorial at the site of their father's death.[23] In stark contrast to the glorification of accidents and failures in the early half of the century, postwar Canadianists and popular historians such as McGregor and James Raffan have contributed to the canoe-accident literature by revisiting and re-evaluating canoe mishaps; Raffan analyzed the 1978 Lake Temiskaming tragedy where twelve students and a teacher died of hypothermia after their canoes capsized in high winds.[24]

While neither McGregor nor Raffan romanticizes the circumstances leading to their subjects' accidental deaths, both celebrate the courage of rescuers and focus on the canoe as a positive symbol of Canadianness. The popular nature of their work and the wide readership it finds among paddlers has likely influenced the manner in which recreational canoeists now view approaches to canoe tripping. Raffan, a noted contributor to the Royal Canadian Geographic Society, is an outdoor educator who has spoken about and taught risk management for summer camps and paddling organizations across Ontario.[25] Writers revisiting the adventure narratives of the Victorian age now do so with a more critical eye, frequently acknowledging the hubris that led to the mishaps in the wilderness of the likes of Wallace and Hornby. Clive Powell-Williams pointed this out in no uncertain terms in his 2002 examination of the Hornby expedition: "A myth, once established is hard to break down, particularly when it confirms the wishful thinking of an entire class. Jack's [Hornby] irrationality, which appeared with such clarity to the professionals [trappers and guides] who had known him in the north, and which is even more apparent today, was perfectly opaque to anyone predisposed to his heroism."[26]

While the pursuit of fame, poor planning, ego, and overconfidence were at the root of Hornby's and Hubbard's eventual demise by starvation, the accidental nature of their deaths was based on a slow accumulation of risk factors that crept further and further out of their control. Raffan has a novel approach to evaluating risk and assessing the likelihood of an avoidable accident – what he calls the "lemon theory" of risk management, based on slot-machine gambling.[27] We can apply this to Hornby's and Hubbard's poor judgment: individual risk factors such as bad weather, exhaustion, dehydration – aka lemons – kept accumulating until their trips turned completely sour: no single accident killed them. The cumulative impact of minor mistakes such as packing insufficient food, over-reliance on hunting abilities, and lack of proper winter clothing all played a role in both men's deaths.[28] The mechanism – starvation – allowed them to be cast as heroes fighting a losing battle against their own demise.

In contrast, the majority of accidents faced by canoeists like Fraser on the Petawawa were the result of comparatively straightforward, individual, and immediate mechanisms: slips, trips, falls, capsized canoes, burst dams, and errant sparks setting fires, causing instantaneous injury or death. Similarly, the memoirs of long-time park residents and former rangers such as Ralph Bice reinforce the immediacy of river accidents; there is no suggestion of romanticism or heroism in the matter-of-fact recounting of incidents such as the 1923 accidental drowning of an Algonquin Park resident: "He went out across the ice, and on his way back they told him 'that ice isn't going to carry you back George, it is going fast'. But he tried it and he drowned only a couple hundred yards from his camp."[29] Bice offers no further comment or discussion of George's death.

For recreational users, a capsized canoe in challenging rapids was the most commonly stated mode of accident or injury recounted by the research participants interviewed for this chapter. The emphasis on capsized canoes is reflected in the many written accounts of long-time park residents, former rangers, amateur historians, and guidebook authors whose works make up the body of literature dealing with accidents along the Petawawa River. The revered Canadian canoeist, author, and filmmaker Paul Mason committed a section of his instructional book *Path of the Paddle* to the challenges of the Petawawa, the ever-present possibility of capsizing, and the tools and skills required to avoid that fate.[30] George Drought's *Petawawa River Whitewater Guide*, in print since 1993, is peppered with references to rapids that can "swamp or dump" a canoe and to strong currents "that would almost certainly take you over the falls."[31] His description of Crooked Chute drives the point home: "The Chute itself should not be run. Many wrecked canoes both in the Chute and scattered at the bottom attest to the fact that many people's skills are not high enough."[32]

Perhaps the most unfortunate aspect of the accidents suffered by recreational visitors to Algonquin Park in the postwar era is that in many cases, as with the expeditions of Hornby and Wallace, they were avoidable. The canoe routes throughout what is now Algonquin were used by Indigenous peoples, surveyors, and loggers prior to the 1893 creation of the park, and have been well maintained for recreational canoeing ever since.[33] The routes and their hazards have been thoroughly written about, with clear, detailed warnings of potential dangers and how to avoid them. Many organizations and professional guides have been available throughout the park's history to help recreational visitors learn the skills to conduct safe, independent trips or to lead inexperienced canoeists safely down the river. Skip Ross's oral history of his time on the Petawawa states that professional guides were commonly hired, even by canoe tripping-oriented youth camps, through the 1940s and '50s.[34] Jim Coffey, the operator of Esprit Rafting on the Ottawa River, has been running guided trips on some of the most dangerous sections of the Petawawa since 1984; his clients benefit from advances in safety gear, boat-building technology, and local knowledge of the river's hazards.[35] Hornby, Wallace, and other self-styled early twentieth-century explorers did not have the benefit of industry-leading professional guides like Coffey whose career has extended from the 1980s to today, or to instructional classics such as Mason's *Path of the Paddle* or C.E.S. Franks's *The Canoe and Whitewater*, both published in 1977.[36] Available since 1993 at most Algonquin Park offices and reputable outfitters are detailed Petawawa River and Algonquin Park guidebooks by park veterans such as George Drought and Donald Lloyd, who are both explicit in their warnings to canoeists with the aim of reducing the possibility of accidents and injuries.[37]

No written guidebooks existed for the Thelon River or the Labrador's George River watershed, a circumstance that added to Wallace and Hornby's interest in a region largely perceived to be unexplored by Europeans. Seeking out the unknown is the perceptual dividing line between the ethos and goals of recreational canoeists who head out on trips, guidebooks in hand, and the aims of the adventure seekers and explorers of the early twentieth century. The two groups of paddlers are similarly split in the retellings of their trips and especially their perception of accidents. Canoe authors such as Raffan and McGregor are risk averse, forgoing literary celebrations of masculine suffering in the face of disaster. Dummit's contention that modern masculinity is performed through the application of technical skill or knowledge to carefully negate risk is reinforced by the management approach favoured by Raffan, McGregor, and their contemporaries.[38] Similarly, the guidebook authors of the 1970s such as Franks and Mason offered paddlers visiting the Petawawa a wealth of risk-mitigating canoe-tripping techniques, including clear instructions on first aid and rescue.[39] The postwar discursive shift towards risk-averse canoe narratives and canoe safety literature is mirrored in Judith Green's broader observation of North American society's transition to a safety culture.[40]

MEMORALIZATION AND RISK TOLERANCE:
INDUSTRIAL VERSUS RECREATIONAL ACCIDENTS
ON THE PETAWAWA

The response to Fraser's drowning, both official and literary, indicates a significant contrast to the almost non-existent records on the many forestry workers who lost their lives labouring on the log drives that dominated the watershed from the 1830s to the 1940s. In addition to the write-ups in the *Ottawa Herald*, *Globe and Mail*, and *MacLean's*, Fraser's death was memorialized by an inscribed cross placed above Rollway Rapids, and the seemingly simple bureaucratic step of a coroner's report.[41] River drivers who died doing the dangerous work of running logs – like twenty-nine-year-old Emile Huard, who drowned in Surprise Rapids during the 1905 drive – usually received a quick in-situ burial and a makeshift wooden cross noting basic biographical information.[42] Sometimes they didn't even get a cross. Frank Knappen, a professor of forestry at Algonquin College, recreational canoeist, and Pembroke resident, confirmed the ad-hoc manner in which the lumbermen who died in work-related accidents were buried and memorialized on the Petawawa: "People wouldn't have material to make crosses, so they'd put boots up in trees – I saw them. You'd come across a portage and there's the old caulked boots in a tree and you'd go, 'Oh, there's a grave nearby.'"[43]

The discursive difference between the treatment of Huard and Blair is twofold: Fraser was a member of Ottawa's political class who went on canoe trips with future prime minister Pierre Elliot Trudeau and Sigurd F. Olson, a noted American naturalist and author of *The Lonely Land*.[44] Fraser had access to power and was memorialized because of it. He died while engaged in a recreational pastime, his participation in it not predicated on an expectation of the possibility of death or severe accident. He was a cautious paddler, and his death was a surprise.

Huard's situation was much different. Severe injury and fatalities were very much a possibility in his field, and the 1910s were the deadliest era to be an industrial worker in the province: workplace deaths hit a peak of thirty per hundred thousand workers in 1918.[45] Salisbury et al. stress the exceptionally dangerous nature of logging work, indicating that even as late as 1986, poor training, inexperience, and lack of regulation led to forestry workers having "the highest rate of lost time injury" in Canada.[46]

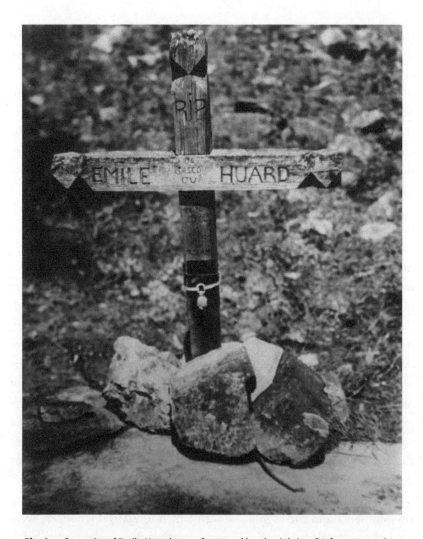

Fig. 8.2 Gravesite of Emile Huard, one of many ad hoc burial sites for forestry workers who lost their lives driving logs down the Petawawa River.

Huard worked in a less regulated era, exposed himself to far greater risk, and was forty years too early for provincial, federal, and employer benefits such as hospital and unemployment insurance in the event of injury.[47] Given these factors, his 1905 drowning was likely not much of a surprise to those labouring around him. Anh-Bao Bui Tran's chapter "Life and Death in the Building of the Victoria Bridge" in this book supports the argument that the deaths of industrial workers like Huard were often treated as inevitable. Following Bui Tran's argument, we can conclude that the deaths of loggers were seen as an unfortunate but expected part of the job. John Matchim's chapter reinforces the dangerous, masculine nature of industrial work in Canada around the end of the nineteenth century. Deaths and accidents of working men were so commonplace in the fishing industry that a boat (like a log drive) would continue with its work even after losing two crew members to fatal accidents.

Ralph Bice recalls in his 1980 autobiography the frequency with which foresters died in the Petawawa's rapids: "During the many years logs had been driven down the Petawawa, many of the river drivers had been drowned when jams broke suddenly, or a misstep caused a fall into fastwater ... there are graves at the foot of many of the falls and chutes."[48] Many of the gravesites noted by Bice are no longer obvious or clearly marked, their existence lost to decay and overgrowth. Huard is known to history because his grave marker, placed off the portage trail near the rapid where he drowned, survived long enough to be photographed and recorded in the archives of Algonquin Provincial Park.[49] His gravesite is now a point of historical interest, marked on park maps and noted in guidebooks. Fraser's privileged position in society allowed his accidental death to be mourned and memorialized and its nature and impact to publicly re-examined over the decades. Huard's working-class background and lack of privilege rendered his death little more than an interesting historical footnote.

Arthur F. McEvoy's investigation of the ecology of working environments and the regularity with which industrial labourers were injured on the job supports the conclusion that the accidents that befell loggers on the Petawawa were considered to be mundane hazards of the job.[50] Bud Doering, a former forester for Consolidated Lumber and longtime resident of Brent, a former railway town in the upper reaches of the Petawawa watershed, remembered the frequency with which logging accidents occurred during his childhood in in the 1930s and '40s. One accident he recalled – a mass casualty incident – would have been frontpage news by current media standards: "At the dam on Cedar Lake, a whole boatload of 'em went over and they all got drowned."[51] Bud made no mention of how many forestry accidents he was aware of, and it is unlikely that accurate data are available. Donald L. Lloyd, past director of the Friends of Algonquin Park and author of the classic guidebook *Canoeing Algonquin Park*, quotes a former park ranger, Mark Robinson, in his chapter on the Petawawa River: "It may be hearsay but the figure of 1300 men killed logging on the Petawawa system in the 100 years between 1830 and 1930 is sometimes cited."[52] The accuracy of the statement is impossible to confirm, but a comparison to the provincial statistics gathered by the Lumbermen's Safety Association, the predecessor of the current organization Workplace Safety North, indicate that a figure of 1,300 log drive deaths in one hundred years is not beyond the realm of reality.[53]

Ceilidh Auger-Day's chapter on the expansion of workers compensation and workers rights in western Canada reinforces the dangers faced by workers in the 1900s, but also suggests that both politicians and workers were beginning to be less accepting of the assumed dangers of industrial jobs. Even so, forestry accidents in the Petawawa region do not seem to have received the same bad press as the mining disasters and railroad accidents that caught the attention of Alberta legislators. Even in newspapers of local logging towns like Pembroke, Renfrew, and Arnprior, logging accidents were rarely noted. News items covering non-industrial accidents and deaths were common, albeit brief and filed among other daily tidbits from the region such as the trapping of a rare white muskrat and any number of community announcements of weddings and illnesses.[54]

In contrast, recreational accidents were of high interest, especially from a risk-reduction viewpoint. The *Arnprior Chronicle's* front-page article on 4 June 1936 revealed the community's concern in reducing accidental drownings. The intention of the local swimming club to hold a meeting is presented in detail, supported by arguments indicating that the "number of drowning accidents are less where swimming clubs are operated and children taught to swim."[55] Far from being a community devoid of concern for accidental deaths in the local waterways, the actions of the swimming club and primacy of place of the article indicate that preventing recreational accidents was important to Ottawa Valley citizens. Concern for risk-education in outdoor recreation would only increase as participation in leisure activities crept up in the postwar era.

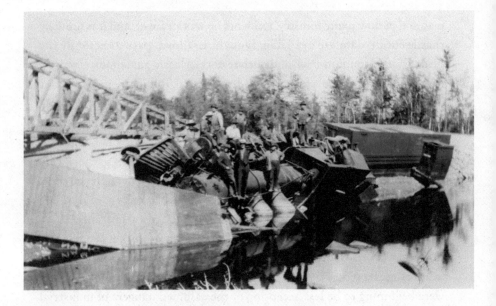

Fig. 8.3 Railroad accident at Cedar Lake.

Thirty years later, at the time of Fraser's accidental death, outdoor recreation in Canada was in a boom period. Provincial parks, remote areas, and wild rivers had all become more accessible following the postwar adoption of car culture, expansion of the highway network, and the burgeoning professional and middle classes with access to money and leisure time.[56] Where once prospective outdoor enthusiasts were dependent on local trains, they now had the freedom and independence of accessing the backcountry from their own vehicle. Early in the park's history, recreational visitors frequented hotels and lodges located along rail lines that intersected the park. Logging baron J.R. Booth's family lodge, the Turtle Club, was situated near the tracks at the confluence of the Petawawa River and Lake Travers.[57] As road networks were expanded, the primacy of rail as an entryway into the park began to decline, simultaneously allowing adventurous visitors to extend their trips beyond railway-adjacent waterways. By the end of the 1970s, most of the remaining hotels and lodges such as Whitefish Lodge, Nominigan Lodge, and Booth's Turtle Club had all shut down.[58]

Following the end of World War II, the use of the Petawawa and all watersheds in Algonquin Park shifted away from forestry and became dominated by the influx of car-borne recreational users. At the same time, postwar improvements in trucking and the expansion and improvement of Algonquin Park's internal road network reduced costs and improved access for the forestry industry.[59] Expensive, time-consuming, and dangerous log drives were no longer necessary, with those operations ceasing on the Petawawa by 1962.[60] The end of the drives left the park's waterways solely to the recreational inclinations of visiting canoeists and anglers.

The shift of the forestry industry in the Petawawa and hinterland of Algonquin Park from waterways and watercraft to land-based operations began slowly after the 1915 opening of the Canadian National Railway (CNR)'s Algonquin Route.[61] The new line through the park ran along most of the length of the Petawawa River from its junction with the Barron River to the village of Brent on Cedar Lake, connecting Ottawa to North Bay and points further afield. The route was a new source of accidents, the most common being derailments and fires, though in some instances near-misses with careless canoeists also occurred. Larry Cobb recalls a significant incident in 1986 when a CNR freight train derailed in the vicinity of the Achray Campground, located on the Barron River, a right tributary of the Petawawa proper. While no injuries occurred, the accident required the attention of park rangers to help safeguard the consumer goods from curious campers.[62]

To the CNR's credit, railroad workers also made contributions to preventing accidents along the river. Warren Walker, a former camper in the 1960s at Camp Ahmek on Canoe Lake, remembers getting help on portages along the Petawawa from railway workers.[63] Ralph Bice and Donald Lloyd also tell stories in their respective books about the role the CNR played in helping to prevent accidents. Lloyd shares a story of a CNR crew using a jigger (a handcar manually driven on tracks) to help campers avoid a long portage around a dangerous rapid.[64] Bice recalls working for the CNR on a brush gang as a summer job during high school. The gang's role was to help prevent forest fires by cutting back brush along densely wooded sections of tracks to reduce the risk of detritus being ignited by sparks from the trains.

The interactions between paddlers and train operators were not always positive – often owing to reckless behaviour by canoeists or the improper use of the railway lines as alternatives to portage trails. Tommy Cloutier recounted a near miss with a train, as he, his brother Hec, and some friends used the line as an easier portage up the river to a fishing spot:

> We put our two canoes on a trailer on the track. Hec says, "Geez that's a different kinda sound." Looks around the corner, and I said, "The train's coming! We gotta get the canoes off!" so we flipped 'em off and jumped. Two of my chums, they climbed them rocks, I dunno how they did it, straight up! And the train, he put the binders on [brakes], he thought he'd killed us, eh. And I'm holding the canoes, 'cause the wind keep pushing them out, and the wheel [of the trailer] kept hitting the train, cause we're right there and you only have that much space [shows about a 30cm distance with his hands]. Once [the conductor] stopped, he backs up and he says, "I thought I killed ya, what's yer name?" So I said "Jaques Demers" [an NHL player at the time – Tommy laughed as he recounted this detail], and he says, "You haven't heard the last of this." Well, he didn't even see my other two chums, they were way the hell up the rocks. He thought it was just the two of us, kept saying, "You have no business being on these tracks." Anyway, he kept goin' and we headed up to the Crow River to fish.[65]

Tommy Cloutier and his party's choices show the type of trouble recreational users of the Petawawa could get themselves into through individual decision-making. Their run-in with the train came at time when recreational and industrial uses of the river overlapped; by the mid-1990s, CNR had ceased operating on the line parallel to the Petawawa. This effectively ended the last remaining industrial activity in proximity to the waterway and removed a significant source of risk.

With changes in patterns of use came changes in the nature of accidents that occurred along the river. Instead of high numbers of annual injuries and deaths during the log drive, the far less common and generally less severe accidents suffered by recreational users took primacy of place. As the Petawawa's rapids had taken their toll on loggers for over a century, drowning remained the primary cause of death in the rare event of fatal recreational accidents, but as with Tommy and his brother, paddlers tended to survive their mistakes and were often able to self-rescue.[66] With improvements in safety equipment and more established search-and-rescue practices, many canoeists who got into trouble and were unable to extricate themselves could reasonably expect assistance from first responders.

Unlike Bud Doering's recounting of fighting forest fires in the 1940s, or Bice's observations of the frequency of fatalities among loggers during his pre-war time as a guide and ranger, Larry Cobb's recollections of accidents in the postwar era primarily focused on recreational incidents involving canoeists. Cobb, a former park ranger, recalls conducting a number of rescues throughout his time on the Petawawa in the 1980s and '90s and suggests that recreational fatalities were rare and often related to poor decision making: "In all these years, I think I've done two fatalities on the Pet. They didn't know what they were doing on Crooked [a notorious rapid]. No experience, group of four people just going down the river following the river guide, spend all the money on gear but weren't wearing their PFD [personal flotation device]."[67] Jessica Poff, a former park worker who sold camping permits and helped park visitors with route planning and campsite reservations in the 1980s and '90s, observed that "people'd rent canoes and be facing each other [incorrect seating positions], it'd happen all the time."[68] She also noted that "the sheer volume of people who have no experience who are going into the interior of Algonquin Park was always shocking – dangerously shocking – to me."[69]

Bud Doering, who grew up in the park in the 1930s and the '40s, worked as a forest-fire fighter in the area. He was direct in his recollection of the limited ability to provide rapid help to those suffering accidents in the park (whether recreational or industrial) at the time. He pulled no punches in describing the frequent outcome of mishaps in the inter-war years, saying that he "never had to do search or rescue, but had to go pick up a corpse once."[70] Cloutier, in addition to his somewhat reckless run-in with the train, also recalled that the CNR played an important role in accident response – but only if you were in a spot near the railroad and lucky enough to have a train come by at a time of need.[71] His recollection is supported by Larry Cobb's memory of the assistance that paddlers and rangers sometimes received from the CNR before the advent of satellite-based communication technologies: "People on the Petawawa River got stranded, they flagged the train down and got help, I remember that happened. Also a fatality outside the park near Pembroke. They flagged the train and brought the body to Achray. CN didn't like gettin' flagged much, but they always helped. They were pretty quick to let us know if they saw guys where they weren't supposed to be too."[72]

Cobb's memory of the nature of the accidental deaths he encountered, as well as their infrequency, reflects a sea change in the types of accidents that occurred along the Petawawa after the log-drive era. Instead of the unpredictable danger of working with log booms, canoeists suffered the consequences of poor risk-management decisions such as not wearing life jackets, or momentary lapses in skill or judgment, such as missing a portage take-out at high water. Recreational canoeists, regardless of period, made the choice to be on a river known to be difficult, in order to pursue their preferred leisure activity. Any choices to ignore potentially life-saving safety standards such as the use of personal flotation devices were also their own. In contrast, forestry workers had to be on the water driving logs to earn a living. The economic and social pressures of the work environment made it difficult, if not impossible, to refuse to carry out tasks. This difference is important in relation to the responses of the different users to accidents and risk. Recreational users, although aware of the risks, and (as stated in both Dummitt and Bye's research) interested in pursuing risky activities, would not have an expectation of death or injury.[73] In contrast, serious injury and death, as observed by Bud Doering, and reinforced by Silvestre's study of industrial accidents in Ontario and Hak's history of labour movements in the BC forestry industry, were an accepted part of life in the pre-war, industrial era of Algonquin Park.[74]

CONCLUSION

The rugged landscape of the Petawawa River has contributed to thousands of accidents that have occurred throughout the human history of the waterway. Individual judgment, social pressure, economic forces, ego, and the manner in which visitors have chosen to interact with the physical space are the most accurate indication as to whether their use of the river had a heightened likelihood of accidents occurring. While privileged visitors with access to leisure time, such as canoeists, could choose to add or remove risk by opting to portage a rapid or don the appropriate safety equipment, forestry workers faced the non-choice of engaging in dangerous work. This divide in privilege and class not only affected the frequency and severity of the accidents that occurred on the Petawawa but also how they were responded to and memorialized.

Popular literature and guidebooks of the 1970s onwards portrayed a risk-averse approach to canoeing on the river. The historical trend towards a safety-conscious attitude to risky recreation is supported by Green's observations of a twentieth-century shift towards the perception of risk and accidents being of the utmost concern. Her statement that an accident happening "demonstrates that risks have been inadequately managed"[75] is strongly supported by the oral histories of Jessica Poff, Jim Coffey, and Larry Cobb, who all worked in the outdoor recreation industry and took issue with lack of preparedness on the part of many paddlers on the Petawawa. This same concern about competence, or clear risk aversion, was not apparent in the oral histories contributed by the older generation of forestry workers such as Bud Doering and Tommy Cloutier, old-timers whose identities were wrapped up in the dangerous work of cutting and transporting timber.

In contrast to the culture of risk-averse recreation that developed in the postwar era, the accidents that befell Jack Hornby's ill-fated expedition up the Thelon River, or Wallace's companion Leonidas Hubbard on the banks of Goose Creek in Labrador, differ greatly and were perceived differently from the accidents experienced by recreational canoeists on the Petawawa.[76] The romanticized masculinity and celebration of heroic suffering diverges even further from the lived realities of the generations of loggers who daily faced the potential of accidental death in the course of their work on the Petawawa. Beyond social and cultural changes in the perception and celebration of risk that have altered the manner in which accidents are portrayed in current discourse, the mechanism and location of accidental injuries and deaths, as well as characteristics of the actors such as class, privilege, gender and ethno-cultural identity, all influence their portrayal in popular literature. Hubbard, Hornby, and Wallace – all white men, all wealthy, chose to "explore" the North in acts of what geographer Bryan Grimwood refers to as "the production of a particular, albeit hegemonic, Canadian nationalistic identity and imagination that is gendered, is colonial and perpetuates class distinctions."[77]

Unlike Blair Fraser, most recreational canoeists who drowned on the Petawawa in the modern era were neither publicly celebrated nor memorialized. No canoeist in the postwar era who survived an incident on Crooked Chute or a mishap in Beelzebub's Whirlpool appears to have sought public aggrandizement as Wallace did upon his return from his failed expedition. Members of canoeing parties may have written trip reports, and rangers and park employees like Jessica Poff and Larry Cobb who responded to accidents may remember them, but postwar leisure-class paddlers were not out to find fame and celebrity through their canoe-tripping exploits. Thus their errors, accidents, and in some cases deaths were not memorialized or critiqued for a broad audience – even less so the loggers who lost their lives. This obscurity stands in stark contrast to the romantic light in which Victorian and early twentieth-century adventurers' misfortunes were often portrayed.

Fraser's drowning, though widely reported and written about due to his public stature, was addressed very differently from the exploits and failures of the Hornbys and Wallaces of the previous era. He was not celebrated as heroic, nor was his mishap characterized as some form of the ultimate masculine or colonial sacrifice. Instead, he was remembered for his work as a journalist and for his love of the outdoor recreational opportunities that Canada offered. One of the most significant discursive differences in the literary treatment of his accidental death was that his caution and skill were noted by those memorializing him. He was remembered as a "sensible, safe canoeist ... never for a moment intending to risk Rollway in the spring high water."[78] His risk-averse approach to recreational adventure was indicative of the paradigm shift in the world of outdoor recreation occurring at the time.

Published or not, the shared memories of local residents like Bud Doering and Tommy Cloutier are testament to a general awareness of the long history of accidental deaths of forestry workers. The Petawawa has

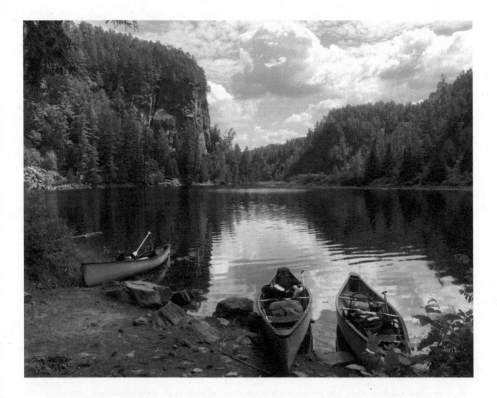

Fig. 8.4 The Natch, 2017, a popular stopping point for paddlers. This dramatic series of cliffs and rapids along the Petawawa continues to draw canoeists, despite risks.

rightly earned a reputation as a dangerous river worthy of respect. Not all visitors perceive or approach those dangers in the same way. While for some the turbulent waters of Crooked Chute or Rollway Rapids give rise to trepidation and fear, for others the river is still the crown jewel of whitewater canoe tripping. The river's long history as the site of thousands of often tragic industrial and recreational accidents now contributes to the sense of history felt and sought out by visiting tourists. Every rapid has a story behind its name and a gravesite along its length. Memorials like Emile Huard's grave or Blair Fraser's cross serve to provide paddlers with a sense of connection to the past. The Petawawa's accidental history is certainly tragic, but far from acting as a deterrent, it is one of the characteristics that makes the river unique in the eyes of canoeists.

ACKNOWLEDGMENTS

I gratefully acknowledge the generosity of the research participants who graciously contributed their time, recollections, and oral histories to this project: Tommy Cloutier, Larry Cobb, Jim Coffey, John "Bud" Doering, Frank Knappen, Jessica Poff, Skip Ross, and Warren Walker.

NOTES

1 Marshall, "Last Journey of Blair Fraser, Canadian."
2 Ibid.
3 Erickson and Krotz, introduction to *Politics of the Canoe*, 5.
4 Dummitt, *Manly Modern*, 78.
5 Ibid.
6 Gstaettner, Lee, and Rodger, "Concept of Risk in Nature-Based Tourism and Recreation," 11.
7 John "Bud" Doering, interview with author, 17 March 2018, Renfrew, ON; author's collection.
8 Skip Ross, interview with author, 1 December 2017, Petawawa, ON; author's collection.
9 Skip Ross interview.
10 Drought, *Petawawa River Whitewater Guide*, 39–60.
11 Tommy Cloutier, interview with author, 16 March 2018, Pembroke, ON; author's collection.
12 Dummit, *Manly Modern*, 3.
13 Green, *Risk and Misfortune*, 12.
14 Ibid.
15 Raffan, *Deep Waters*.
16 Lloyd, *Canoeing Algonquin Park*, 265–302.
17 Wallace, *Lure of the Labrador Wild*, 215–18.
18 Ibid., 218.
19 Stuart, "John Hornby," 184–5.
20 Whalley, *Legend of John Hornby*, 7–9.
21 Erickson, "Canoe Nation, 183.
22 Marshall, "Last Journey of Blair Fraser," 20–39.
23 McGregor, *Canoe Country*.
24 Raffan, *Deep Waters*, 1.
25 Matt Cruchet, "Risk Management," accessed 2 July 2021, https://paddlingmag.com/stories/risk-management-squeezing-the-lemons/; "Cold Water Paddling," RACCC – Ottawa's Canoe Camping Club, accessed 2 July 2021, www.raccc.ca/trips/safety/69-first-aid-and-rescue/219-cold-water-paddling.

26 Powell-Williams, *Cold Burial*, 250.

27 James Raffan, "Wilderness Crisis Management," accessed 14 August 2021. https://jamesraffan.ca/wilderness-crisis-management/.

28 Wallace, *Lure of the Labrador Wild*, 193.

29 Bice, *Along the Trail in Algonquin Park*, 74.

30 Bill Mason, *Path of the Paddle*, 138.

31 Drought, *Petawawa River Whitewater Guide*, 46, 52.

32 Ibid., 66.

33 Callan, *Top 60 Canoe Routes of Ontario*, 82.

34 Skip Ross interview.

35 Jim Coffey, interview with author, 1 December 2017, Waltham, PQ; author's collection.

36 Franks, *Canoe and Whitewater*; Mason, *Path of the Paddle*.

37 Drought, *Petawawa River Whitewater Guide*.

38 Dummit, *Manly Modern*, 131–2.

39 Mason, *Path of the Paddle*, 146.

40 Green, *Risk and Misfortune*.

41 McGregor, *Canoe Country*, 134–42.

42 Lloyd, *Canoeing Algonquin Park*, 269.

43 Frank Knappen, interview with author, 4 January 2018, Pembroke, ON; author's collection.

44 Olson, *Lonely Land*.

45 Silvestre, "Improving Workplace Safety," 533.

46 Salisbury et al., "Fatalities among British Columbia Fallers," 32.

47 Hak, *Capital and Labour in the British Columbia Forest Industry*, 6.

48 Bice, *Along the Trail in Algonquin Park*, 105.

49 Algonquin Park Archives Online, accessed 28 July 2021, https://algonquinpark.pastperfectonline.com/photo/BAA65B7C-0C3F-4B0D-B0A6-283640220190.

50 McEvoy, "Working Environments," 69.

51 Doering interview, 2018.

52 Lloyd, *Canoeing Algonquin Park*, 269.

53 Workplace Safety North, accessed 2 July 2021, https://www.workplacesafetynorth.ca/news/news-post/taming-deadliest-professions-ontario-wilderness.

54 Ibid.

55 "Arnprior Swimming Club to Hold Organizational Meeting," *Arnprior Chronicle*, 4 June 1936.

56 Bice, *Along the Trail in Algonquin Park*, 15; Killan, "Ontario's Provincial Parks," 38–41.

57 Lloyd, *Canoeing Algonquin Park*, 287.

58 MacKay, *Chonology of Algonquin Provincial Park*, 16–17.

59 Knappen interview, 2018.

60 Place, *Seventy-Five Years of Research in the Woods*, 15.

61 McKey, "Canadian National Railway's (CNR) 'Algonquin Route,'" 25.

62 Larry Cobb, interview with author, 28 January 2018, Cobden, ON; author's collection.

63 Warren Walker, retired chartered accountant, former camper at Camp Ahmek and recreational canoeist in Algonquin Park, in conversation with author, 25 February 2018, Big Gull Lake, ON.

64 Lloyd, *Canoeing Algonquin Park*, 285.

65 Cloutier interview, 2018.

66 Cobb interview, 2018.

67 Ibid.

68 Jessica Poff, interview with author, 3 January 2018, Whitney, ON; author's collection.

69 Poff interview, 2018.

70 Doering interview, 2018.

71 Cloutier interview, 2018.

72 Cobb interview, 2018.

73 Dummitt, *Manly Modern*, 78–80.

74 Silvestre, "Improving Workplace Safety," 533; Hak, *Capital and Labour*, 6.

75 Green, *Risk and Misfortune*, 119.

76 Wallace, *Lure of the Labrador Wild*, 153–63.

77 Grimwood, "'Thinking outside the Gunnels,'" 52.

78 MacGregor, *Canoe Country*, 143.

BIBLIOGRAPHY

Archives

Algonquin Provincial Park Archives and Collection, Algonquin Park Visitor Centre

Newspapers and Periodicals

Arnprior Chronicle
Maclean's Magazine

Other Sources

Bice, Ralph. *Along the Trail in Algonquin Park*. Toronto: Natural Heritage/ Natural History, 1993.

Callan, Kevin. *Top 60 Canoe Routes of Ontario*. Buffalo: Firefly Books, 2019.

Drought, George. *Petawawa River Whitewater Guide, Algonquin Provincial Park*. Whitney: Friends of Algonquin Park, 1993.

Dummitt, Christopher. *The Manly Modern: Masculinity in Postwar Canada*. Vancouver: UBC Press, 2007.

Erickson, Bruce. "Canoe Nation: Canoes and the Shifting Production of Space through White Canadian Masculinities." *Antipode* 40, no. 1 (January 2008): 182–4.

Erickson, Bruce, and Sarah Wylie Krotz. Introduction to *The Politics of the Canoe*, edited by Bruce Erickson and Sarah Wylie Krotz, 1–23. Winnipeg: University of Manitoba Press, 2021.

Franks, C.E.S. *The Canoe and Whitewater*. Toronto: University of Toronto Press, 1977.

Green, Judith. *Risk and Misfortune: A Social Construction of Accidents*. London: UCL Press, 1997.

Grimwood, Bryan S.R. "'Thinking outside the Gunnels': Considering Natures and the Moral Terrains of Canoe Travel." *Leisure/Loisir* 35, no. 1 (February 2011): 49–69.

Gstaettner, Anna-Maria, Diane Lee, and Kate Rodger. "The Concept of Risk in Nature-Based Tourism and Recreation – A Systematic Literature Review." *Current Issues in Tourism* 21, no. 15 (2018): 1784–1809.

Hak, Gordon. *Capital and Labour in the British Columbia Forest Industry, 1934–74*. Vancouver: UBC Press, 2007.

Killan, Gerald. "Ontario's Provincial Parks and Changing Conceptions of Protected Places." In *Changing Parks*, edited by John S. Marsh and Bruce W. Hodgins, 34–49. Toronto: Natural Heritage/Natural History, 1998.

Lloyd, Donald. *Canoeing Algonquin Park*. Toronto: Hushion House, 2000.

MacKay, Rory. *A Chonology of Algonquin Provincial Park*. Algonquin Park Technical Bulletin no. 8. Whitney: Friends of Algonquin Park, 1988.

Marshall, Douglas. "The Last Journey of Blair Fraser, Canadian." *Maclean's*, 1 August 1968.

Mason, Bill. *Path of the Paddle*. Gloucester, UK: Cordee, 1977.

McEvoy, Arthur F. "Working Environments: An Ecological Approach to Industrial Health and Safety." In *Accidents in History: Injuries Fatalities and Social Relations*, edited by Bill Luckin and Roger Cooter, 59–89. Atlanta: Rodolpi, 1997.

McGregor, Roy. *Canoe Country*. Toronto: Random House Canada, 2015.

McKey, Doug. "The Canadian National Railway's (CNR) 'Algonquin Route,' 1915–1995." In *Social Science Research in Parks and Protected Areas*, 25–9. Waterloo: Parks Research Forum of Ontario, 2003.

Olson, Sigurd F. *The Lonely Land*. Toronto: McClelland & Stewart, 1961.

Place, Ian C. M. *Seventy-Five Years of Research in the Woods: A History of the Petawawa Forest Experiment Station and Petawawa National Forestry Institute*. Burnstown, ON: General Store Publishing, 2002.

Powell-Williams, Clive. *Cold Burial*. New York: St Martin's Press, 2002.

Raffan, James. *Deep Waters*. Toronto: HarperCollins, 2002.

Salisbury, D.A., R. Brubaker, C. Hertzman, and G.R. Loeb, "Fatalities among British Columbia Fallers and Buckers." *Canadian Journal of Public Health* 82, no. 1 (January/February 1991): 32–7.

Silvestre, Javier. "Improving Workplace Safety in the Ontario Manufacturing Industry, 1914–1939." *Business History Review* 84, no. 3 (Autumn 2010): 527–50.

Stuart, Hugh. "John Hornby, 1880–1927." *Arctic* 37, no. 2 (June 1984): 184–5.

Wallace, Dillon. *The Lure of the Labrador Wild*. Halifax: Nimbus Publishing, 1990.

Whalley, George. *The Legend of John Hornby*. Toronto: MacMillan Canada, 1962.

PART THREE | NARRATIVES

9

Wind, Error, and Providence

Shipwrecks in New France

Colin M. Coates

Governor Louis de Buade de Frontenac deemed his first voyage to Canada rather fortunate (*assez heureux*) when he wrote his report to the minister of the marine a few months after he landed at Quebec. He had arrived on the seventy-first day of his journey, and his ship had only come close to sinking as it passed Baie Sainte-Marie, when it grounded twelve or fifteen times.[1] Frontenac went on to assure the minister of the relative safety of navigation to the colony. His nonchalant inclusion of the near-accident highlights the reality of shipwrecks for many of those who ventured onto an ocean-going vessel between France and New France.

The French word for shipwreck, *naufrage*, according to the Académie française, was "used for all ships which perish by misfortune at sea, and the men who are on them."[2] Shipwrecks were, by definition, accidents, and in contrast to the smaller-scale incidents involving ocean and river risks described in this volume by John Matchim and Cameron Baldassarra, they were usually on a large scale. As Cynthia A. Kierner argues, shipwrecks became the archetype for the category of "disaster" in eighteenth-century North America.[3] These disasters were indeed collective accidents, but they were also individual at the same time. While all passengers and crew risked perishing in these accidents, in some cases individuals or even everyone aboard might survive. Shipwrecks often elicited chaotic responses, and subsequent written and pictorial representations attempted to create order out of the chaos. Matchim and Baldassarra analyze the explanatory focus on personal risk-taking among fishers off the Newfoundland and Labrador coasts and canoeists on the Petawawa River: as they show in their chapters, state officials, survivors, and their relatives made efforts to attribute meaning and blame to the unfortunate events.

For accidents in the early modern period, historians emphasize the explanatory role of Providence, or the will of God, and they point to the shift to more secular and scientific understandings in the eighteenth century. Some historians of shipwrecks in North America argue for a change to Enlightenment-era explanations of such tragedies and attempts to avoid them through deploying scientific knowledge.[4] The evidence for New France complicates this trajectory. French explanations of colonial shipwrecks in the seventeenth and eighteenth centuries combine the approaches: accounts of the shipwrecks blamed practical circumstances related to wind and human error, while survivors' narratives invoked the role of Providence and individuals' abilities to endure the aftermath of the accident.

In New France, those who recorded accounts of shipwrecks understood them through the lens of culture and religion, but they tended to emphasize empirical considerations within or beyond human control. Shipwrecks were laden with theological and cultural significances, and narratives provided necessary meaning to the series of unfortunate events. Even if human decisions created the preconditions that made a shipwreck more likely, most accounts stressed the effects of wind and visibility. Shipwrecks made up the key type of accidents that individuals feared in New France, and they posed existential questions related to the distance between the colony and France, the fragility of life, humans' lack of control over their environment, and in some cases the intercession of Providence in delivering individuals to safety.

The contrast between shipwreck narratives in New France and New England is striking. Referring to influential writers Cotton Mather and James Janeway in New England, Kierner argues, "These pious purveyors of early shipwreck stories … understood shipwrecks not as disasters that could be prevented or ameliorated but rather as providential judgments or messages from God, who orchestrated these harrowing episodes to proffer sinners opportunities for personal reflection and reformation."⁵ Although pious French Catholic clergy might occasionally offer similar rhetoric, as we will see, shipwreck narratives from New France rely less on Providence than do those from the English colonies to the south. Wind and human error played key explanatory roles.

THE ORDINARINESS OF THE SHIPWRECK

Shipwrecks were an essential product of colonialism. Steve Mentz writes concerning the phenomenon in the early modern era, "There is no global expansion without catastrophe."⁶ Imperial expansion was predicated on the relative reliability of ocean-going vessels, but that left room for many accidents along the way. For Europeans, the colonial presence in northern North America depended on maritime connections.⁷ The ocean and the rivers provided the routes for communication, not just with metropolitan France but also between the spread-out French settlements in North America, at least during the seasons when it was practical to travel by water. Settlers and key consumer goods arrived by ship, and the lucrative trade in beaver and other furs exported overseas provided the economic justification for the French presence. Kenneth Banks insists that water-borne navigation remained a standard and routine way to travel to and through New France, and that its perils can be overstated.⁸ Throughout the history of the colony, the most efficient way to travel during navigation season involved the use of watercraft. But even if accidents were objectively rare, danger always loomed.

As Karl Figlio states, an accident represents an "unforeseen event which is also expected."⁹ While passengers and crew certainly wished to avoid a shipwreck, they were all too aware of the possibility that one might occur. In New France, wills typically began with a recognition of the "certainty of death and the uncertainty of its timing."¹⁰ Any prospective settler leaving France for the colony was certainly aware of one thing: the unpleasant danger posed by the Atlantic crossing. Contagious diseases often spread on the lengthy journey, and other perils like storms, pirates, and icebergs could threaten the lives and the possessions of the passengers and crew. Once past the open ocean en route to Quebec, ships braved the obstacles of the St Lawrence River – the shoals, reefs, currents, and tides that might conspire with adverse winds to render the vessels vulnerable. The danger of colliding with another ship also framed crews' concerns.[11] Even on the narrower stretches of the St Lawrence River between Quebec and Montreal, canoes or smaller boats could capsize and imperil the lives of the passengers. The small ship ("*barque*") carrying the new governor of Trois-Rivières, Duplessis de Kerbodot, sank at Cap à l'Arbre in November 1651. It had hit some rocks, probably close to shore, as the governor was able to escape.[12]

Charles Vianney Campeau provides a compilation of some 3,700 ships known to have sailed to and from the French colony up to 1759. Reflecting genealogical interests in large part, this list focuses on passenger ships and does not attempt to include all of the many fishing vessels that crossed the Atlantic every year.[13] Using this online resource, it is possible to identify some ninety shipwrecks between 1660 and 1759. For this calculation, I excluded the few English vessels included on Campeau's website as well as those shipwrecks that occurred as a result of military action, since those were, by definition, not accidental. In most years, at least one shipwreck occurred, often leading to a loss of life or of cargo, or both. In the worst years, the list records four shipwrecks, usually a small proportion of the ships travelling between France and New France.

But only in a few rare stretches of five or more years were there no shipwrecks at all. Figure 9.1 shows that, for the people sailing to or living in New France, shipwrecks would have always been within recent memory. However, an increasing number of vessels crossing the ocean during the period of French control did not lead to more accidents. In other North Atlantic contexts, historians have proposed proportions of disasters. Jean-François Brière calculates that of the more than four thousand ships sailing from Saint-Malo for the Newfoundland cod fisheries from 1725 to 1792, 2.2 per cent ended in shipwreck; from the port of Granville from 1732 to 1792, the proportion was 1.5 per cent of some 3,567 ships. Taking a broader geographical perspective, Amy Mitchell-Cook stresses the regularity of shipwrecks, advancing a figure of 4 to 5 per cent of North Atlantic voyages between the seventeenth and early nineteenth centuries.[14] However, statistics alone of vessels that sank do not convey their cultural or economic significance.

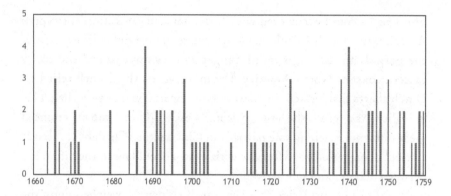

Fig. 9.1 Number of shipwrecks per year, New France, 1660–1759.
Compiled from https://naviresnouvellefrance.net/.

In any case, perceptions could be faulty and misleading predictors of the future. In August 1693, Governor Frontenac wrote optimistically to the minister in France that this was the first year in a long time that so many handsome vessels had arrived without accidents, unlike in the preceding year.[15] He undoubtedly was thinking of *La Providence*, a ship that sank in the supposed safety of the harbour at Quebec in 1692. Nonetheless, Frontenac's letter was followed a few months later by the loss of the king's ship *Le Carossol* at Sept-Îles, and *L'impertinent* in the Lower St Lawrence.[16]

The list indicates that very few ships sank in the open ocean. Most accidents occurred as ships neared land on either side of the Atlantic and were largely a product of the uncertainties and difficulties of navigation in coastal areas and on the St Lawrence River. Sailing through the St Lawrence relied on expert knowledge and pilotage, and the French colonial authorities, sometimes with support from their superiors in France, placed much effort on acquiring reliable navigational information and jealously guarding it from their European rivals.[17] As Margaret Schotte has explained, the French made important advances in navigational science in the seventeenth century.[18] Even with this knowledge, as we will see, seasoned captains could make impetuous mistakes and endanger their ships. Gilles Proulx concludes that the more closely ships approached Quebec, the more likely it was that human error lay behind a shipwreck.[19]

Shipwrecks could occur even within the harbours of Europe or North America. Accurately calculating longitude remained difficult throughout the period, and so ships faced danger as they approached the rocky eastern coast of North America. For many years, the French relied on Dutch charts that located the coast of Nova Scotia further west than it lay in reality. As a result, the large-scale naval expedition of 1746 experienced great difficulty reaching safe harbour in Chibouctou (Chedabucto) Bay.[20] Careful pilotage and good fortune with weather could mean the difference between disaster and safe arrival.

It is thus not surprising that the fear of shipwreck weighed upon the minds of travellers. Just as Governor Frontenac recounted his near-miss experience on his first voyage to New France, Marie de l'Incarnation, founder of the Ursuline order of nuns in New France, recorded the travails of her travels in 1639. Because of storms, the ship that carried her across the Atlantic had to cover more than 2,000 leagues instead of the usual 1,300: "We found ourselves within a hairsbreadth of sinking (*deux doigts du naufrage*), but He who commands the winds and the sea preserved us by his all-powerful hand (*son doigt tout puissant*)."[21] Noting that he had been shipwrecked three times in 1698, Claude-Charles Bacqueville de la Potherie reported, "There is no navigation more dangerous than the [St Lawrence] River, and however experienced the pilots who commonly ply those waters, they have a great deal of difficulty in getting out of trouble. The shoals of Manikouagan on the north coast are to be feared."[22] Granting the point that travellers had little reason to record an uneventful journey across the Atlantic, a range of writers commented on accidents or their fears thereof. Some notable shipwrecks led to detailed narratives.

SHIPWRECK NARRATIVES

In Euro-Christian tradition, shipwrecks hold particular metaphorical weight. For the English colonies to the south, historians have interpreted shipwreck narratives as justifications of the settler-colonial occupation of the territory, with Providence assuring the colonists that they were destined to occupy the North American lands.[23] The extant narratives of shipwrecks in New France do not reflect this perspective to the same extent.

The clearest evocation of divine intervention in accounting for shipwrecks lay in the explanations of the fate of the Anglo-American invasion fleet led by Admiral Sir Hovenden Walker. Eight ships of the flotilla
sank when, beset by a storm, they attempted to sail past Île aux Œufs on
22 August 1711. This disaster led Walker to abandon the large-scale invasion
and return to Massachusetts in disgrace. Not surprisingly, Catholic clergy
welcomed divine intervention against this Protestant attack. Jesuit Joseph
Germain invoked "God's protection of the nascent [Catholic] Church"
in the colony.[24] But, writing some decades later, Jesuit historian Pierre-
François-Xavier de Charlevoix provided a more dispassionate explanation
when he explained that human error had caused the loss of ships and the
lives of nearly one thousand crew members. The admiral had hubristically
refused to listen to the wise counsel of a French prisoner who was serving as navigator. Surprised by a sudden strong southeast wind, the ships
crashed against the island. Wrote Charlevoix, "The English admiral had
no one but himself to blame for the misfortune of his fleet."[25] In 1756, army
officer Louis-Antoine de Bougainville reflected on the military advantages
that the perils of the St Lawrence offered the colony: "This river bristling
with reefs and unparalleled for danger and difficulty of navigation, this is
Quebec's most effective rampart."[26]

More typically, narratives of shipwrecks related the practical reasons
behind the accidents. Récollet priest Emmanuel Crespel's 1742 book is the
key contribution from New France to the tradition of shipwreck narratives.
It fits well with a developing genre that took form soon after the publication of Daniel Defoe's extraordinarily popular shipwreck novel, *Robinson
Crusoe*, in 1719; a translation appeared in Governor Philippe de Rigaud de
Vaudreuil's personal library within a few years of its release.[27] Using the
epistolary style common in the eighteenth century, Crespel wrote an extended description of his shipwreck off Anticosti Island and his difficult
survival over the harsh winter months. With two editions in French (in
1742 and 1757), his book was also translated into German in 1751 and into
English in 1797, evidence of the European appetite for such depictions of
trial and survival.[28]

Crespel carefully wove foreshadowing into his narrative, mentioning
his embarkation for New France on the king's ship *Le Chameau* in 1723.

Some French readers might have known that the vessel would tragically sink off Cape Breton (Île Royale) only two years later. After some years in the Great Lakes region and on Lake Champlain, Crespel was recalled to France in 1736, and on his voyage to Quebec came close to perishing in the Sainte-Thérèse rapids. He was explicit in warning his readers of the dangers that lay ahead: "Prepare your heart for compassion and sorrow."[29]

At Quebec, Crespel was offered two possibilities for the transatlantic voyage: the king's ship *Le Héros* or the private vessel *La Renommée*, on which he could serve as chaplain. He chose *La Renommée*, a new and well-equipped sailing ship, which left Quebec on 3 November, along with a number of other vessels. Eleven days later, the ship with its fifty-four passengers passed to the south of Anticosti Island. As they were propelled by a small wind from the north, the captain shared his concern about an incoming storm. A shift to a south-southwest wind endangered the vessel, and the crew attempted to head for Anticosti. A quarter-league from the island's south shore, the ship grounded on a rocky shoal. The hull breached, and water poured into the ship.

Knowing that the large island was inhospitable and believing it to be uninhabited, crew members clambered aboard a longboat (*chaloupe*) and a canoe (*canot*) in the rough seas. The gunner had the foresight to save some biscuits, guns, a barrel of powder, and a case of powder bags. The narrative conveys the minute-by-minute danger in which they found themselves in their attempt to reach shore: "No rudder, no strength, a horrible wind, a continual downpour, an enraged and ebbing sea: could we hope for anything more than a quick death?"[30] (The obvious fact that Crespel had survived to write the account would lessen the reader's anxiety, of course.) Crespel gave the crew a general absolution of their sins, and they prayed furiously. At the moment when the priest abandoned hope and hid his head in his coat to avoid seeing their destruction, a fortuitous gust of wind pushed the longboat to shore. The lesson was clear to Crespel: God had saved them all from death.

This was only the beginning of their tribulations, however, and these form the major part of the narrative. Those who had made it to shore were aware that no other ship would pass by for many months and the large island and winter's harsh weather would make it difficult for them to survive. The deep snowpack, lack of food, and fevers spreading among them increased their despair. While twenty-four men remained in makeshift cabins they had constructed near the shipwreck, the others embarked in the longboat and canoe on a perilous journey to find help. The two vessels became separated, and those in the canoe perished. When the survivors lost their optimism once a storm drove away their longboat from its position at anchor, Crespel did not hesitate to blame his companions for past crimes for which God was surely punishing them. Perhaps unconvincingly, he reassured them in theological terms: "What thanks must you render to the Lord for giving you this shipwreck as a way of easing your arrival at the Gates of Salvation!"[31]

Many succumbed to cold, malnutrition, and disease, but a small group of the hardiest set out to reach the French post of Mingan on the north shore of the St Lawrence, across the strait from Anticosti Island. The Indigenous people they encountered fled, fearing the diseases that the French men might bring them. Finally, an elder helped Crespel and his two surviving companions reach the French post. Fortified with provisions and a more reliable vessel, he returned to the island to find only a few survivors among his shipmates who had remained near the shipwreck. Four had managed to stave off starvation through eating the animal-skin clothing that had belonged to their crewmates, but one died in his weakened state after drinking eau-de-vie. Only five of all those who had been on the ship survived their ordeal on Anticosti. In June of the following year, Crespel returned to Quebec, served as a parish priest at Soulange for a year, and then sailed with much less drama for France. He eventually returned to the St Lawrence Valley for the remainder of his career.[32]

Crespel's is a narrative of hardship and survival, with gory and detailed descriptions to captivate his European readers. It is informed by a belief in Providence, but also by empirical accounts of weather, disease, and encounters with Indigenous people, providing satisfying specifics to enliven the story and render it intelligible and intriguing to readers. In that sense, it builds on the traditions of shipwreck literature in French (and English): emphasis on the corporeal experience of the accident and its aftermath, the shipwreck as a precursor to the act of survival.[33] The success of Crespel's work points to the appeal of the literary trope of the shipwreck, a metaphor that could build on connotations of the "ship of state," offer an allegory for the challenges of life itself, and perhaps most strikingly, become the basis for a story of invention and redemption,[34] as in Shakespeare's *Tempest* or Dafoe's *Robinson Crusoe*.

A second lengthy shipwreck story by military officer and merchant Saint-Luc de la Corne, although lacking the limited literary qualities of Crespel's account, conveys a similar narrative of a journey of survival. In late September 1761, la Corne sailed for France after the surrender of the French authorities in the colony. British Governor James Murray prepared the ship *L'Auguste* for this group of officers, soldiers, and their families. La Corne complained that the captain was not a proficient pilot, but the governor dismissed his concerns. As in Crespel's account, foreshadowing precedes the ultimate disaster. Near Île aux Coudres, the currents grew stronger, and while the ship moored and waited for better conditions, its big anchor broke. They barely avoided a shipwreck at this point (*Nous fumes à deux doigts du naufrage*); la Corne commented that in retrospect that would have been beneficial, as they were still in Canadian waters.[35] He recounted the shifts in the prevailing winds and the pleasant crossing they were expecting, until they encountered a violent (*impétueux*) northeast wind on 4 October. The storm raged for two days; the passengers prayed fervently, and God protected them. Fires broke out three times during meal preparations, but the crew managed to douse them. After a respite of a few days, another fierce wind, this time from the east, pushed them towards Newfoundland. They managed to catch some two hundred codfish, making up for the provisions that they had lost, when another easterly drove them towards Cape Breton. Unable to navigate according to the stars, the captain did not know their position. On 14 and 15 October, they saw land, but could not tell where they were: "We drifted at the whim of the winds and the storm."[36] The crew was exhausted, and the captain and his second-in-command were unable to force them to continue their efforts even by beating them; the likelihood of shipwreck had destroyed the crew's will. The captain headed for the mouth of a river in hope of safe harbour. When the ship grounded on a sandbar about 120 to 150 feet from land, they cut the masts, but violent waves turned the ship on its side. One longboat was lost to the waves, and some of the passengers and crew tried to scramble aboard the other one. Some threw themselves into the sea, only to drown. Those who remained on the ship were no more fortunate: that afternoon it broke apart. Only seven survived the wreck; 114 bodies washed ashore. None of the women or children aboard were saved.

Saint-Luc de la Corne's narrative conveys the embodied experience of the shipwreck and the great death toll, and then proceeds with a lengthy account of his scramble over the rocky coast and through dense forests and the struggle to survive the snowy winter on Cape Breton. As had happened with Crespin, Indigenous inhabitants rescued the small party and directed them to Louisbourg. Eventually, la Corne returned to Quebec on 23 February, where he related his story to Governor Murray. His long and difficult peregrination of over 550 leagues back to the St Lawrence Valley even overshadowed some of the horror of the shipwreck: "It would be hard to recount the sorrows and the strains that I experienced. The difficulties that I encountered in returning to my homeland lessened the idea of the shipwreck. I admit that the more I retell the circumstances of my shipwreck and my survival, the more astonished I am."[37] While la Corne's account drew inspiration from other shipwreck narratives in its form and motivations, he recognized its lack of the usual rhetorical flourishes: "I have recounted evenly and without embellishment all the circumstances; thus I do not claim to be an author. The truth has no need of being dressed up."[38]

ESTABLISHING REASONS FOR THE ACCIDENTS

If some published accounts embraced the cultural narratives of the period, shipwrecks were more than metaphors. In the ninety shipwrecks that occurred in New France, many lost their lives or at least experienced existential danger. Official accounts of shipwreck accidents tended to favour empirical explanations for the unfortunate events.

Incidents involving the kings' ships created more archival records than did the accidents of privately owned vessels. In one of the most consequential shipwrecks in the history of New France, the king's ship *Le Chameau* broke apart a short distance from Louisbourg, on Cape Breton, on the night of 27–28 August 1725. Jacques-Ange Le Normant de Mézy, the king's chief civil official at Louisbourg, travelled three leagues to the shore near the disaster on 29 August and immediately prepared a report for the minister in France. At the Côte de la Baleine, a great quantity of debris had washed ashore, the fleur-de-lys insignias proving that this was indeed the remnants of the king's ship. De Mézy and his companions found the bodies of the officers and passengers "naked in their shirts." The dead included the incoming intendant of New France Guillaume de Chazel, the pilot Chaviteau, and the son of the governor of the Montreal district. The inventory of the debris stressed the material consequences of the event: it included barrels, partitions, planks, broken masts, clothes, linens, and other fabrics, and many drowned pigs, cows, sheep, ducks, and other fowls.[39]

This report and other correspondence recorded the reasons for the wreck. The ship had been lost against the small island of Portnove. Local fishers reported a dreadful (*épouvantable*) gust from the southeast, which crushed the ship against a rocky coast (*une côte très ferrée*).[40] The more formal letter de Mézy wrote to the minister on 6 September repeated the explanation of the strong southeast wind, as did another letter written by Intendant Michel Bégon de la Picardière from Quebec a few weeks later.[41] Bégon sent two soldiers to dive into the waters of the cove to try (without success) to rescue the cannons and the colonial money supply lying on the bottom. The reports of the disaster focused on efforts to save as much as possible from the wreck, as in addition to ending the lives of so many prominent individuals, the accident created severe financial complications for the colony. Recognizing the difficulties inherent in navigation, Father Charlevoix, who had himself sailed on *Le Chameau* in 1720, concluded that in 1725 the same pilot had misjudged his ship's location by seventy leagues, causing the mortal accident.[42]

Jean Doublet's shipwreck story of 1667 also stressed the practical reasons for the accident before describing the corporeal sensations of shipwreck. Writing after 1707, Doublet, who had a distinguished career as a privateer, recounted his fateful return trip to France with his father. Soon after leaving Quebec early in the season on 8 May 1667, their voyage was interrupted when the ship was caught in the ice off the coast of Newfoundland: "A number of ice mountains floating on the water surrounded us and did not allow us to escape." Despite the fervour of their prayers and vows, and their efforts to use cables to protect them from the icebergs, after nine days their ship precipitously sank. Crew and passengers scrambled onto an iceberg, made a tent with two sails, and used panels and hatches from the ship as flooring to protect themselves from the cold. Unable to start a fire, they resorted to eating raw seal and seabird flesh and drinking the animals' blood. They vigorously hailed a passing ship, which nearly sailed away from the menace of the icebergs before they attracted its attention. The ship sent a boat and rescued Doublet, his father, the captain, and the others. Eight men had died on the iceberg, and three later succumbed from eating too much biscuit too quickly.[43] Like Crespel, Doublet emphasized the practical reasons for the shipwreck and the embodied, fruitless attempts to avoid disaster.

A third set of shipwreck accounts, on the sinking of the king's ship *L'Éléphant*, is a particularly interesting case, with alternative perspectives nuancing and complicating interpretation of the incident. As Thomas Wien notes, the official report downplayed suggestions of human error and focused on the heroic effort of saving the cargo.[44] In contrast, two other accounts point out the captain's and pilot's misjudgments.

Officially, the incoming colonial financial commissary Gilles Hocquart, who was himself aboard the ship, informed the minister that *L'Éléphant* had been wrecked the night of 1–2 September 1729 on a shoal off Cap-Brûlé, about ten to twelve leagues (fifty kilometres) downriver from Quebec. Unlike *Le Chameau*, this ship did not take its passengers with it when it foundered. In their official correspondence and an accompanying map, the colonial officials praised the ship's officers and those of the colony in saving not only the passengers but also most of the goods aboard. The report explained that the pilot Jacques Chaviteau had asked the captain at 8:00 p.m. to raise sail, as they were anchored in eighteen fathoms (*brasses d'eau*) in an area with many rocks that might sever their cables. Winds were from the north, and it was a clear moonlit night. Around 11:00 p.m., the pilot mistook some lights in the distance as being high up on shore in the forest rather than on a nearby vessel. He changed the ship's trajectory based on that assumption. At midnight, *L'Éléphant* hit bottom in three fathoms of water and the ship came to rest on its starboard side. Captain Louis-Philippe de Rigaud de Vaudreuil evacuated the passengers in

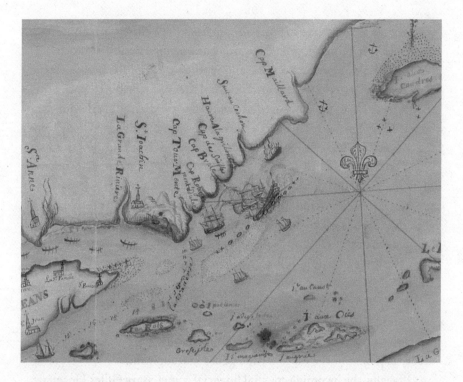

Fig. 9.2 *Carte figurative du promt secours envoyé, par l'ordres de Monseigneur le Mr de Beauharnois ... le 2 Septembre 1729.* Detail from map showing the shipwreck of *L'Éléphant* and the rescue operation.

longboats. At daybreak, he toured the ship at low tide and decided in conjunction with his officers to cut the masts in order to save the cargo. Over the next nine days, the goods were unloaded, but one longboat was lost, and the schooner of the port's captain sank as well. The officials reported that a carpenter from Quebec drowned in this risky and "ill-fated adventure" (*funeste avanture*). The gunpowder and bread on board had been soaked at the first tide, but the rest of the goods were saved.[45]

Officials provided a map to show the speed with which they sent help to *L'Éléphant* and to demonstrate the distances from Quebec's busy harbour (figure 9.2). As Wien argues, the official documents glossed over the captain's error in judgment. He was, after all, a member of a prominent colonial family, the Vaudreuils. The king's officials celebrated their own efficacy.[46] At the same time, they reassured the king that his vessel was not an entire loss, unlike *Le Chameau*, which had sunk only four years previously.

Unusually for colonial shipwrecks, contrasting evidence exists in this case. The author and libertine Claude Le Beau recorded the event in his book written on his time in New France, one of the few parts of his narrative not plagiarized from other sources.[47] He provided a counternarrative, meting out responsibility somewhat differently. About sixteen or seventeen leagues from Quebec, according to his account, some clergy – the new bishop was on board – demanded that Captain Vaudreuil not stop for the evening but continue to sail for Quebec. (A Sulpician priest, Pierre-Thomas Ruffin de la Maraudière, provided yet another version of the event, claiming that everyone aboard, not merely the clergy, urged the captain to keep sailing toward Quebec.[48]) At that time, a light northeast wind provided reassurance, as did the starlit night sky. But the wind became more violent, and during the evening the ship landed on a rock. The dreadful (*épouvantable*) shaking struck terror in the hearts of even the most experienced mariners. The crew attempted to save the ship by raising the sails and throwing out two anchors, but it spun on its cables and landed hard on another rock, breaking the keel. That was the moment of shipwreck.[49]

Both Le Beau and Ruffin de la Maraudière also blamed the pilots for mistaking the campfires of an Indigenous party in the forest for the lanterns of another ship. The choice to change course led them directly onto the rocks. Referencing Odysseus's difficult decision in steering between Scylla and Charybdis, Le Beau lamented, "In trying to avoid one danger, we fell into another." While the colonial officials' report and maps implied a degree of calm among the passengers, Le Beau described panic: "Each believed that he was approaching the end." Ruffin de la Maraudière agreed.[50] In the distance, the king's pilot, Richard Testu de la Richardière, mistook the intent of the cannon shots that appealed for assistance and only slowly made progress towards the ship.[51] Other ships, too, failed to come to the rescue of *L'Éléphant*. Le Beau claimed that more than 150 persons might have perished had the ship shifted two fathoms deeper. The longboat and canoe on the ship would have only saved one-quarter of those on board.

Le Beau then related not the selfless and successful salvage of the ship's cargo but the sailors' attempts to profit from the disaster by breaking

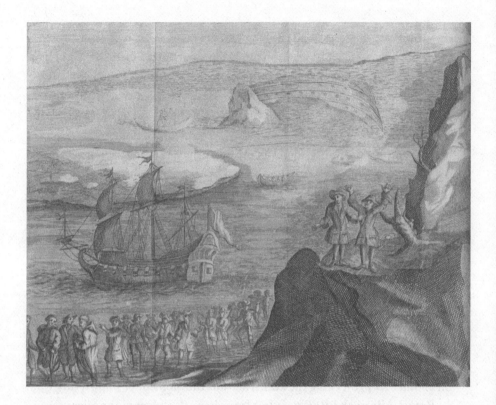

Fig. 9.3 Engraving of the shipwreck of *L'Éléphant*, from Le Beau, *Avantures du Sr. Le Beau*, between pages 50 and 51.

into the passengers' chests and plundering them. His and Ruffin de la Maraudière's accounts coincided with official ones in explaining how the passengers were evacuated to shore. Le Beau bemoaned that they had to make their way to Quebec on foot amid swarms of mosquitoes, and Ruffin de la Maraudière described their struggles through the mud and the lack of food along the way. Le Beau recalled the plaintive cries of a French merchant (*un Marchand forain*) who complained of the loss of his trinkets (*sa paquotille*): "I am lost; I am ruined; where am I here? What will become of me?" (*Je suis perdu; je suis ruiné; où suis-je ici? Que vais-je devenir?*)[52] For the merchant, the shipwreck had defeated the purpose of his voyage across the Atlantic, a similar existential question to the one that haunted Le Beau's longer plagiarized narrative.

Le Beau's book included an engraving of the shipwreck (figure 9.3), depicting the ship overturned against a rock in the St Lawrence and the longboat and canoe ferrying passengers to the safety of shore. Undoubtedly the two men on the right of the image are Le Beau and the merchant, the latter raising his arms in distress to heaven. The engraving does little more than reflect the content of the narrative, likely to provide some greater sense of verisimilitude to the account for the European reader.[53]

Like the shipwreck of L'Éléphant, the sinking of La Providence in 1718 occurred without loss of life, but it had serious financial implications. It had sailed from Quebec on 15 November, sinking the next day on a rocky shoal near Île aux Coudres after the bottom of the ship was punctured. The Compagnie d'Occident's shipment of 6,840 livres worth of coat (prepared) beaver pelts (castor gras) and 24,120 livres worth of unfinished (castor sec) pelts was at risk. Local inhabitants assisted in trying to dry and restore them to make them worth shipping to France.[54] Fearing that La Providence's companion ship, Le Cheval Marin, might also not have arrived in France, colonial officials gave duplicates of the letters to a passenger who had been aboard La Providence and granted him permission to travel via New England. In this way, colonial officials found ways to protect themselves against disaster: duplication of correspondence was a standard state information practice that provided assurances of reliable communication between the colony and metropolitan France. In that sense, it was analogous to insurance that protected the investments of those who owned ships.

THE ROLE OF PROVIDENCE

The writers discussed above did not evoke Providence in their accounts to explain the shipwrecks' occurrence, but they did so to explain the survival of shipwrecked individuals. The dei ex machina in such incidents were usually God and Sainte-Anne, patron saint of sailors and protector from storms. Many narratives pointed to the power of prayer. Jean Doublet and his companions prayed and made vows when they found themselves surrounded by icebergs off Newfoundland.[55] In escaping from La Renommée, Crespel and the ship's crew prayed to God and he recited the Miserere, the prayer asking for forgiveness for one's sins.[56] Claude Le Beau made no mention of God's intervention in explaining the passengers' survival of the shipwreck of *L'Éléphant*; however, his shipmate, the Sulpician priest Pierre-Thomas Ruffin de la Maraudière, did. He reported that everyone cried out, "Lord, have mercy on us, we are lost," and the ship's chaplain provided absolution to the passengers in case of a dire fate. Despite all the dangers involved in escaping the shipwreck, "God kept us safe."[57]

Other survivors, too, recounted their appeals to divine protection. The Jesuit missionary Charles Lalemant described his survival in a shipwreck in 1639 in particularly religious terms, but as with other stories, the cause of the accident was said to be natural: "What destroyed our vessel was a violent southwester, which arose when we were off the coast; it was so impetuous that, with all the care and diligence of our captain and crew, with all the vows and prayers which we could offer to avert the blow, we could not avoid being driven on the rocks."[58] Lalemant related that he owed his survival to being hailed by his companion Father Philibert Noyrot, who asked him to come up to the deck so that Lalemant could give him absolution, and Noyrot did the same for him. Strong waves broke the sides of the ship and swept Noyrot overboard, but Lalemant was able to cling to a plank and eventually make his way to land. While the shipwreck was a result of the fierce storm, Lalemant was clear in attributing his survival to God. The survivors managed with God's help to rescue provisions: "Providence sent us, in our want, five kegs of wine, ten pieces of pork, oil, bread, cheese, and a gun, and powder, which enabled us to strike a fire." Measuring his days by the saints, Lalemant recorded that the accident occurred on St Bartholomew's day (24 August) and the survivors were rescued by a Basque fishing boat on St Louis' day (25 August). The Basques pursued their fishing activities through to early October and then sailed with the survivors back to Europe. After a return voyage of forty days, beset by other violent storms, the fishing boat too was wrecked as they entered port near San Sebastian.[59] Providence played some role in explaining the initial shipwreck and its aftermath, though the reasons Lalemant gave for the accident focused primarily on the effects of shifting winds.

In another type of account of the experience of shipwrecks, ex-voto paintings provide the evidence that individuals prayed to God and the saints, particularly Sainte-Anne, and when they escaped their ordeal,

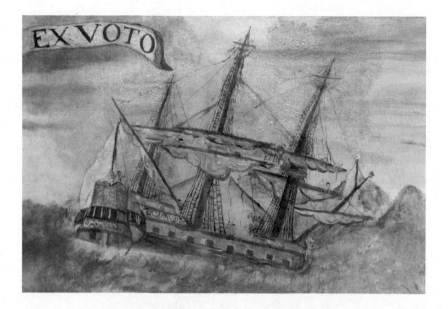

Fig. 9.4 Ex-voto, *Un navire dans la tourmente.* Offering for the safe arrival of a ship beset by rough waves, oil on wood, attributed to Paul Mallepart de Grand Maison, *dit* Beaucour (1700–1756).

might commission tableaux to convey their peril and give thanks for their salvation.[60] (These paintings are among the very few from the period of New France to convey images of landscapes and waterscapes.) Ex-voto paintings often portray the event that occasioned their production,[61] and therefore some depict shipwrecks or the fear of one occurring.

One ex-voto painting (figure 9.4), attributed to Paul Mallepart de Grand Maison, *dit* Beaucour, focused on the pitching ship beset by rough seas all around it. Tall mountains in the distance hint at the dangers of shores. The banner "Ex Voto" attached to a mast pointing towards heaven makes the purpose of the painting clear: the man who survived the difficult journey was offering thanks for his salvation.

The ex-voto recording the violent voyage of Captain Édouin's ship, *La Sainte-Anne*, in 1709 (figure 9.5) depicts clearly the challenge of the open ocean. On the trip from Newfoundland to Quebec, the ship was buffeted by a roiling sea. The painting prominently locates two religious figures on board: the priest Gaulin, reading his breviary and a Récollet priest, his

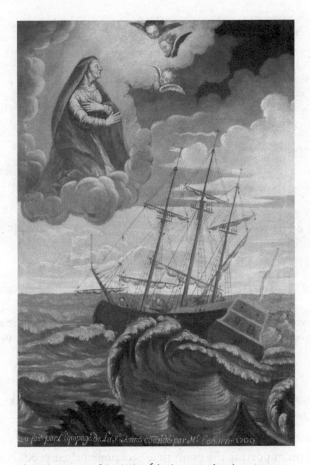

Fig. 9.5 Ex-voto of Capitaine Édouin, 1709, showing crew and passengers on the *Sainte-Anne* appealing to Sainte Anne to save their endangered ship.

arms outstretched in an appeal to Sainte Anne. Bathed in light and thus drawing the eye of the viewer, the saint looks towards three angel heads and gives her blessing to the ship as it battles the elements. Most likely painted by Michel Dessaillant, the large painting (163 cm × 112 cm) was donated to the church at Sainte-Anne de Beaupré.[62]

Not all ex-votos depict ships braving tumultuous open seas. Some focus on individuals who survived the incident, and therefore emphasize individual rather than collective danger. A third ex-voto (figure 9.6) shows

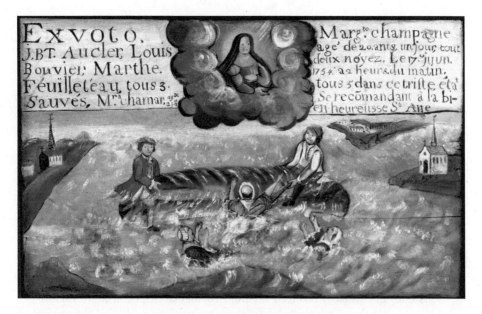

Ex voto.
J.BT. Aucler, Louis
Bouvier: Marthe.
Féuilleteau tous 3.
Sauvés, M.ᵉ chamar.

Marg.ᵗᵉ champagne
age' de 2.o.ans; un jour tout
deux noyez. Le 17. ᵈᵉ juin.
1754. a 2 heurs du matin.
tous 5 dans ce trifte éta'
Se recomandant à la bi-
en heureüsse S.ᵗᵉ Ane

Fig. 9.6 Ex-voto, 1754, showing overturned canoe, its five passengers praying to Sainte Anne to save them. Two men and a woman survived; two women did not.

the moment of salvation when a canoe was beset by heavy winds. Its five occupants were paddling on the St Lawrence early on a June morning in 1754 when the wind and waves turned rough, and the canoe capsized. The two men, both wearing red and therefore distinguished from the others in the painting, scrambled onto the overturned craft, but they only managed to save one of the women. The painting records the survivors' names for posterity: Jean Baptiste Aucler, Louis Bouvier, and Marthe Feuilleteau. It also commemorated Marguerite Chamart and Marguerite Champagne who, unable to cling to the capsized canoe, drowned in the waves. From the central-top position in the painting, Sainte Anne looks down benignly on the scene, and her image forms a triangle with the canoe. Two churches, one of them the Sainte-Anne shrine at Beaupré, hug the shore on either side of the St Lawrence.[63] Text on the painting makes it clear that all five canoeists prayed to Sainte Anne. Like textual narratives of shipwrecks, this ex-voto captures the corporeality of the accident: the viewer can imagine the terror of the women whose heavy dresses pulled them down into the water. Implying the cause of the accident in the rough waves in the fore-ground, the painting provides an explanation of the survival of three of the people in the canoe – the appeal to God and the saints. However, the image does not blame Providence for the misfortune.

CONCLUSION

Revealing the realities of life in the distant French colony as well as broader cultural and religious precepts, shipwrecks posed the existential issue of maintaining a French colony on the far side of the Atlantic. They repre-sented a danger that must have made it difficult to convince immigrants to sail for the colony and led some of those who made the trip across never to attempt to return to their homeland. The shipwrecks endangered the bodies and the goods the ships carried, and they exposed the fragility of existence in this early modern period. Providence helped account for sur-vival from shipwrecks, but it was sailing conditions, sometimes exacerbat-ed by human error, that explained the accidents in the first place. Winds, storms, shoals, and rocky shores imperilled ships, even if human decisions had led them at that moment to that specific spot. Praying to God and Sainte Anne, it was believed, might help deliver the individuals from the fate of drowning in rough seas.

In contrast to the historiography dealing with the English colonies to the south, where the primary explanation of the accidents was attributed to Providence, the study of shipwrecks in New France reveals that narra-tives largely focused on practical navigational considerations as the caus-es. Religious considerations came into play more directly in accounting for survival from the shipwrecks. Thus, to adopt the typology developed in the introduction to this volume, narratives of shipwreck accidents can be situ-ated on the boundary between cautionary tales and miracles. Passengers on the ships generally held no blame for the accidents, beyond the sinfulness of the human condition. Shipwrecks were collective; survival was individual.

Although rare in number, these accidents were significant crises, whether or not the passengers or crew survived them. They occasioned narratives to explain the embodied experience of the event, stories that survive in archives and published works and on church walls, reflecting moments in which settlers and crew faced individual and collective peril. It was worthwhile and necessary to fit the shipwrecks into a narrative, to account for the loss of human lives or goods and offer the edification of a story of survival. Vagaries of the wind and other conditions and sometimes navigator error lay at the root of the accidents, but not usually the stern hand of God. Rather, God and Sainte Anne helped account for survival from horrific accident. By not solely attributing the accidents to Providence, the French colonial Catholic attitude to shipwrecks encouraged practical approaches to understanding their causes.

ACKNOWLEDGMENTS

My thanks for their assistance to Alice Cameron, who transcribed many of the original documents, and Marie-Christine Pioffet, Margaret Schotte, Paul-André Dubois, Swann Paradis, the editors of this volume, and copy-editor Maureen Garvie. Translations are mine, with the exception of those sources already available in English.

NOTES

1 Frontenac au ministre, 2 November 1672, fols. 233–4, COL CIIA, vol. 3, Archives nationales d'outre-mer (France) (hereafter ANOM).
2 "Il se dit de tout vaisseau qui perit par fortune de mer, & des hommes qui sont dessus." *Le Dictionnaire de l'Académie françoise*, vol. 2, 112.
3 Kierner, *Inventing Disaster*, 38.
4 Porter, "Accidents in the Eighteenth Century"; Mitchell-Cook, *Sea of Misadventures*, 4; Spence, *Accidents and Violent Death in Early Modern London*, 19; Kierner, *Inventing Disaster*, 39.
5 Kierner, *Inventing Disaster*, 47.
6 Mentz, *Shipwreck Modernity*, xxiv; Blackmore, *Manifest Perdition*, xxi–xxiv.
7 Rainer Baehre in *Outrageous Seas*, 1, makes this point for British North America as a whole, and it applies of course to New France as well.
8 Banks, *Chasing Empire across the Sea*, 67.
9 Filgio, quoted in Campbell, "Philosophy and the Accidents," 27.
10 Cliche, *Les pratiques de dévotion en Nouvelle-France*, 239.
11 Proulx, *Between France and New France*, 64.
12 Lafrance, *Les Épaves du Saint-Laurent*, 35–8.

13 "Navires venus en Nouvelle-France: Gens de mer et passagers," accessed 7 December 2023, https://www.patrimoinequebec.ca/naviresnouvellefrance/. This website contains a wealth of data on the ships and people who sailed between France and New France, including passenger lists, ownership, and destinations.

14 Brière, "Safety of Navigation," 85; Mitchell-Cook, *Sea of Misadventures*, 30.

15 Frontenac au ministre, 14 August 1693, *Rapport de l'archiviste de la province de Québec* (hereafter RAPQ), vol. 8 (1927–28), 151.

16 Also available at https://web.archive.org/web/20220818004402/https://www.naviresnouvellefrance.net/html/pages16931694.html#pages16931694.

17 Furst, "La monarchie et l'environnement," 318–35.

18 Schotte, *Sailing School*, 90.

19 Proulx, *Between France and New France*, 159n22.

20 Pritchard, *Anatomy of a Naval Disaster*, 123–5.

21 Marie de l'Incarnation à l'un de ses Frères, 1 September 1639, letter 40, in Oury, *Marie de l'Incarnation, Correspondance*, 88–9.

22 Bacqueville de la Potherie, *Histoire de l'Amérique septentrionale*, vol. 1, 203: "Il n'y a point de navigation plus dangereuse que celle du Fleuve, & quelque experience que puissent avoir les Pilotes qui le frequentent, ils ont encore assez de peine à se tirer d'affaire. Les bâtures de Manikoüagan qui sont à la côte du Nord sont à craindre."

23 Sievers, "Drowned Pens and Shaking Hands," 743–76.

24 Germain, quoted in Pioffet, "Le désastre de l'île aux Œufs," 115–17.

25 "L'Amiral Anglois ne put guéres imputer qu'à lui seul le malheur de sa Flotte." Charlevoix, *Histoire et description générale de la Nouvelle France*, 361. A fresco depicting these shipwrecks can be seen at the Notre-Dame-des-Victoires church in Quebec City's Lower Town. Sébastien Couvrette, "Église Notre-Dame-des-Victoires à Québec," Québec d'hier à aujourd'hui, 2007, http://www.ameriquefrancaise.org/fr/article-587/%C3%89glise_Notre-Dame-des-Victoires_%C3%A0_Qu%C3%A9bec.html#.YP3dUY5Kg2w.

26 Bougainville, quoted in Proulx, *Between France and New France*, 77.

27 Inventaire après-décès de Philippe de Rigaud, Marquis de Vaudreuil, 19 June 1726, RAPQ, vol. 2 (1921–22), 248.

28 Pelletier, "Crespel, Emmanuel."

29 "Préparez votre cœur à l'attendrissement, & à la tristesse." Crespel, *Voiage du R.P. Emmanuel Crespel*, 42.

30 "Point de gouvernail, point de force, un Vent affreux, une Pluye continuelle, une Mer en fureur, & dans son reflus; que pouvions nous espérer qu'une fin prochaine?" Ibid., 52.

31 "Quelles graces n'avez-vous pas à rendre au Seigneur de vous avoir fourni par un Naufrage les plus surs moïens d'arriver au Port du Salut!" Ibid., 117.

32 Pelletier, "Crespel, Emmanuel."

33 Mentz, *Shipwreck Modernity*, xxv; Oliver, *Shipwreck in French Renaissance Writing*.

34 Oliver, *Shipwreck in French Renaissance Writing*, 3–4, 208.

35 La Corne, *Journal du voyage de M. Saint-Luc de la Corne*, 3.

36 "Nous voguions ainsi au gré des vents & de l'orage." Ibid., 12.

37 "Il seroit difficile de raconter les peines & les fatigues que j'ai essuyé; l'idée du naufrage se dissipoit par les difficultés que je rencontrois pour revoir ma Patrie. J'avoue que plus je me représente les circonstances de mon naufrage & de ma conservation, plus je m'étonne." Ibid., 37.

38 "J'ai raconté uniment & sans embellir toutes les circonstances; aussi je ne me donne point pour Auteur, la vérité n'a pas besoin d'être ornée." Ibid., 38.

39 "Nus En chemises." Monsieur de Mézy et autres, Procès-verbal de la perte du Chameau, 29 August 1725, fols. 213–15, COL CIIB, vol. 7, ANOM. Note that two pilots named Chaviteau were involved in separate shipwrecks: *Le Chameau* in 1725 and *L'Éléphant* in 1729. A few years earlier, the captain of *Le Chameau* complained about the inability of the two Chaviteau brothers, both pilots, to adjust their navigation plans when faced with new circumstances. Voutron au comte de Toulouse, 9 December 1720, fol. 281v, COL CIIA, vol. 42, ANOM.

40 De Mézy et autres, Procès-verbal, 29 August 1725, fols. 213–15, COL CIIB, vol. 7, ANOM.

41 De Mézy au ministre, 6 September 1725, fols. 221–2, COL CIIB, vol. 7, ANOM; Bégon au ministre, 28 September 1725, fols. 284–8v, COL CIIB, vol. 7, ANOM.

42 Charlevoix, *Journal d'un voyage*, vol. 3, 57, note a.

43 Bréard, *Journal du corsaire Jean Doublet de Honfleur*, 35–8, at 36: "Nous fusmes environnées d'une quantité de montagnes de glaces flotantes sur l'eau et nous enfermèrent sans pouvoir nous en décharger."

44 Wien, "*Rex in fabula*," 72.

45 Hocquart au ministre, 11 September 1729, fols. 186–7v, COL CIIA, vol. 51, ANOM; Procès-verbal du naufrage de l'*Éléphant* et du sauvetage de ses effets, 12 September 1729, fols. 237–9v, COL CIIA, vol. 51, ANOM.

46 Wien, "*Rex in fabula*," 72.

47 Andréanne Vallée provides a critical edition of Le Beau's work and identifies the sources he copied. Vallée, *Avantures du Sieur Le Beau*, 603–18.

48 Ruffin de la Maraudière, "Naufrage de 'l'Éléphant,'" 383.

49 Vallée, *Avantures du Sr. C. Le Beau*, 50–1.

50 "Voulant éviter un danger, nous tombâmes dans un autre;" "chacun croyait toucher à sa dernière fin," ibid., 53, 54; Ruffin de la Maraudière, "Naufrage de 'l'Éléphant,'" 384.

51 Le Beau incorrectly named Joseph Fleury de la Gorgendière as the king's pilot. Vallée, *Avantures du Sieur Le Beau*, 109n39.

52 Vallée, *Avantures du Sieur Le Beau*, 53–8.

53 Another illustration of a shipwreck in Bacqueville's *Histoire de l'Amérique septentrionale*, vol. 1, 100, shows the grounding of Captain Pierre Lemoyne d'Iberville's ship *Le Pélican* in Hudson Bay, but as this incident occurred in the context of a skirmish between English and French, it is not properly an accident.

54 Vaudreuil et Bégon au Conseil de Marine, 30 December 1718, fols. 118–21v, COL C11A, vol. 39, ANOM. This *La Providence* was a different ship from the one that sank off Quebec in 1692.
55 Bréard, *Journal du corsaire*, 36.
56 Crespel, *Voiage du R.P. Emmanuel Crespel*, 53.
57 "Mon Dieu, misericorde, nous sommes perdus"; "Dieu nous gardoit." Ruffin de la Maraudière, "Naufrage de 'l'Éléphant,'" 384, 386. Bishop Saint-Vallier explicitly forbade priests from offering extreme unction to Catholics facing imminent shipwreck, but it was possible to offer absolution. Saint-Vallier, *Rituel du diocèse de Québec*, 237.
58 Baehre, *Outrageous Seas*, 70.
59 Ibid., 72.
60 It is worth noting that crews regularly saluted Sainte Anne with cannon fire as they approached her shrine downriver from Quebec, nearing the end of a successful journey. Proulx, *Between France and New France*, 78.
61 Gagnon, *Premiers peintres de la Nouvelle-France*, vol. 2, 113.
62 Ibid., 119–20; Lukaitis, "Disassembling the Canvas," 30–1.
63 Lukaitis, "Disassembling the Canvas," 41–4.

BIBLIOGRAPHY

Bacqueville de la Potherie, Claude-Charles. *Histoire de l'Amérique septentrionale.* Vol. 1. Paris: Jean-Luc Nion et François Didot, 1722.

Baehre, Rainer, ed. *Outrageous Seas: Shipwreck and Survival in the Waters off Newfoundland, 1583–1893.* Montreal: McGill-Queen's University Press, 1999.

Banks, Kenneth. *Chasing Empire across the Sea: Communications and the State in the French Atlantic, 1713–1763.* Montreal: McGill-Queen's University Press, 2002.

Blackmore, Josiah. *Manifest Perdition: Shipwreck Narrative and the Disruption of Empire.* Minneapolis: University of Minnesota Press, 2002.

Bréard, Charles, ed. *Journal du corsaire Jean Doublet de Honfleur.* Paris: Charavay Frères éditeurs, 1884.

Brière, Jean-François. "The Safety of Navigation in the 18th century French Cod Fisheries." *Acadiensis* 16, no. 2 (Fall 1987): 85–94.

Campbell, Robert. "Philosophy and the Accidents." In Cooter and Luckin, *Accidents in History*, 17–34. Amsterdam: Rodopi, 1997.

Charlevoix, Pierre-François-Xavier de. *Histoire et description générale de la Nouvelle France.* Paris: la veuve Ganeau, 1744.

– *Journal d'un voyage fait par ordre du Roi dans l'Amérique septentrionale.* Vol. 3. Paris: Chez Rollin fils, 1744.

Cliche, Marie-Aimée. *Les pratiques de dévotion en Nouvelle-France: Comportements populaires et encadrement ecclésiastique.* Quebec: Presses de l'université Laval, 1988.

Cooter, Roger, and Bill Luckin, eds. *Accidents in History: Injuries, Fatalities and Social Relations*. Amsterdam: Rodopi, 1997.

Crespel, Emmanuel. *Voiage du R.P. Emmanuel Crespel, dans Le Canada et son naufrage en revenant en France*. Francfort sur le Meyn: n.p., 1742.

Le Dictionnaire de l'Académie françoise. Vol. 2. Chez la Veuve de Jean Baptiste Coignard et chez Jean Baptiste Coignard, 1694.

Furst, Benjamin. "La monarchie et l'environnement en Alsace et au Canada sous l'Ancien Régime: L'eau, politiques et représentations." PhD diss., Université de Montréal and Université de Haute-Alsace, 2017.

Gagnon, François-Marc. *Premiers peintres de la Nouvelle-France*. Vol. 2. Quebec: Ministère des Affaires culturelles du Québec, 1976.

Kierner, Cynthia A. *Inventing Disaster: The Culture of Calamity from the Jamestown Colony to the Johnstown Flood*. Chapel Hill: University of North Carolina Press, 2019.

La Corne, Saint-Luc de. *Journal du voyage de M. Saint-Luc de la Corne, Ecuyer, Dans le Navire l'Auguste, en l'an 1761*. Montreal: Fleury Mesplet, 1778.

Lafrance, Jean. *Les Épaves du Saint-Laurent (1650–1760)*. Montreal: Éditions de l'Homme, 1972.

Le Beau, Claude. *Avantures du Sr. C. Le Beau, Avocat en Parlement*. Amsterdam: Herman Uytwerf, 1738.

Lukaitis, Katrina Marie. "Disassembling the Canvas: A Visual Analysis of Marine Ex-Voto Images from Eighteenth Century Quebec and France." Master's thesis, Concordia University, 2010.

Mentz, Steve. *Shipwreck Modernity: Ecologies of Globalization, 1550–1719*. Minneapolis: University of Minnesota Press, 2015.

Mitchell-Cook, Amy. *A Sea of Misadventures: Shipwreck and Survival in Early America*. Columbia: University of South Carolina Press, 2013.

Navires venus en Nouvelle-France: Gens de mer et passagers. Database compiled by Charles Vianney Campeau. http://www.patrimoinequebec.ca/navires nouvellefrance/.

Oliver, Jennifer H. *Shipwreck in French Renaissance Writing: The Direful Spectacle*. Oxford: Oxford University Press, 2019.

Oury, Dom Guy, ed. *Marie de l'Incarnation, Correspondance*. Solesmes, France: Abbaye de Solesmes, 1971.

Pelletier, Jean-Guy. "Crespel, Emmanuel." In *Dictionary of Canadian Biography*. Vol. 4. University of Toronto/Université Laval, 2003. http://www.biographi.ca/en/bio/crespel_emmanuel_4E.html.

Pioffet, Marie-Christine. "Le désastre de l'île aux Œufs vu par les Hospitalières de Québec et de Montréal." *Littoral* 13 (Fall 2018): 115–17.

Porter, Roy. "Accidents in the Eighteenth Century." In Cooter and Luckin, *Accidents in History*, 90–106.

Pritchard, James S. *Anatomy of a Naval Disaster: The 1746 French Naval Expedition to North America*. Montreal: McGill-Queen's University Press, 1995.

Proulx, Gilles. *Between France and New France: Life aboard the Tall Sailing Ships*. Toronto: Dundurn Press, 1984.

Rapport de l'archiviste de la province de Québec. Vol. 2 (1921–1922). Quebec: Ls-A. Proulx, 1922.

Rapport de l'archiviste de la province de Québec. Vol. 8 (1927–1928). Quebec: L.-Amable Proulx, 1928.

Ruffin de la Maraudière, Pierre-Thomas. "Naufrage de 'l'Éléphant': Relation du voyage de Canada de l'année 1729," edited by A. Léo Leymarie. *Nova Francia* 5, no. 1 (January–February 1930): 370–94.

Saint-Vallier, Jean-Baptiste de La Croix de Chevrières de. *Rituel du diocèse de Québec, publié par l'ordre de Monseigneur L'Evêque de Québec*. Paris: Simon Langlois, 1703.

Schotte, Margaret E. *Sailing School: Navigating Science and Skill, 1550–1800*. Baltimore: Johns Hopkins University Press, 2019.

Sievers, Julie. "Drowned Pens and Shaking Hands: Sea Providence Narratives in Seventeenth-Century New England." *William and Mary Quarterly*, 3rd series, 63, no. 4 (October 2006): 743–76.

Spence, Craig. *Accidents and Violent Death in Early Modern London, 1650–1750*. Woodbridge, Suffolk: Boydell Press, 2016.

Vallée, Andréanne. *Avantures du Sieur Le Beau, avocat en Parlement, édition critique*. Quebec: Presses de l'Université Laval, 2011.

Wien, Thomas. "*Rex in fabula*: Travailler l'inquiétude dans la correspondance adressée aux autorités métropolitaines depuis le Canada (1700–1760)." *Outre-mers* 96, nos. 362–3 (2009): 65–85.

10

Accidental History and Manitoulin Island, ca. 1830–1960

Indigenous and Settler Experience

Geoffrey L. Hudson and Darrel Manitowabi

Settler colonization since the early nineteenth century on Manitoulin Island in Lake Huron provided the foundation for two significantly different yet coexisting perspectives on accidents and their possible meanings.[1] Settler and Indigenous peoples drowned in watercraft accidents, fell through the ice, experienced fires, and died or were injured in preparation for or during hunting. For Indigenous peoples, historical narratives embody stories of the lands and waters of Manitoulin Island and social relations with one another, and in turn the concept of an accident is a by-product of these relationships. With settler colonialism, the causes of accidents gradually changed with the advent of the church, colonial laws, and alcohol. For settlers, the memory of accidents, along with other significant family and community events, was central to the colonial project of turning settlers into settler-descendants, connecting newcomers to Manitoulin Island's agricultural spaces, the waters, and the forests. Settlers came, experienced accidents and misfortune, and persevered.

Centred on how accidents are understood in place, this chapter discusses the experience of accidents from both Indigenous and settler perspectives. It explores the ways in which accidents are constructed and produced from experience and mythologized over time by Indigenous peoples and settlers. As has been demonstrated across Turtle Island, both groups have vastly different worldviews, yet in occupying a shared geography, they also have shared experiences. We employ a "Two-Eyed Seeing" framework to regional history by presenting Indigenous and settler understandings of the history of accidents, drawing on Indigenous and Settler knowledge systems with a number of goals including improving mutual understanding.

The historical record of Indigenous accidents is limited, and existing data often obscures the accident by conflating it with a general category of violence and by relying on records created in the past by settler record keepers with settler perspectives. In his case study of Sioux Lookout, Ontario, T. Kue Young speculates that in pre-contact times, "accidents and violence likely contributed to a large proportion of overall mortality."[2] In the period 1944 to 1980, Young argues that accidents became a leading cause of mortality and in the years 1972 to 1981, represented 37.9 per cent, comprising railway, motor-vehicle, water transport, falls, fires, cold exposure, firearm, suicides, and homicides.[3] For British Columbia, Mary-Ellen Kelm argues that in 1943 Indigenous mortality due to accidents or violence was 131.7 per 100,000 compared to 69.6 for settler peoples, and that accidents were either environmental (e.g., drownings or landslides), related to fishing (e.g., infected fingers, dislocated shoulders), or related to alcohol (e.g., accidental shootings, drowning or violence).[4] Mary Jane Norris maintains that accidents, poisoning, and violence had replaced tuberculosis as a major threat to Indigenous health in Canada by the 1960s.[5]

Recent historical/epidemiological research by Jessica Kamckey on settler accidents on Manitoulin Island draws on death records for the periods 1870 to 1908 and 1921 to 1936.[6] Kamckey found that deaths resulting from physical injury contributed to 6 per cent of total deaths, with the majority a result of drowning involving young adults. Fires were also notable, primarily affecting children. She also identified a significant number of deaths attributable to "train derailments, boat fires and boat sinking," as well as accidental shotgun wounds involving young adults and adults. Alcohol was involved in a significant number of cases.[7]

This chapter in part explores Indigenous accidents on Manitoulin Island. The sources we analyze go beyond those used by Kamckey to include not only the Manitoulin Island death index but also relevant Library and Archives Canada records, the Wikwemikong Diary in the Wikwemikong Holy Cross Mission Archives, and local newspapers. We compare the Anishinaabek accidents on Manitoulin Island with the broader literature on the Anishinaabek accidents, situating Anishinaabek concepts of "accidents" and "history," which are not directly translatable to their Western equivalents. We then review the historical literature on Anishinaabek accidents and those on Manitoulin Island. Comparatively more sources for settler accidents are available, including Manitoulin Island settler newspapers, manuscripts in settler museums, local histories and websites that draw on these records, and oral histories shared by settler families and their descendants.

We begin with a joint brief geographical overview of the island and discussion of the Indigenous and settler background, followed by a section on the accident from the Indigenous perspective (written by Darrel), and then by a section (written by Geoff) on the settler perspective. Discussion of an important Indigenous-settler confrontation in the 1860s over resources that included an accidental component, jointly written, leads to a shared conclusion. By applying Two-Eyed Seeing to our case study, we advance "equitable power relationships between Indigenous and Western knowledges."[8] Two-Eyed Seeing originates with the Mi'kmaw elders Murdena and Albert Marshall, who propose this concept as integrating Indigenous and western knowledge systems to enhance learning, understanding, and relationship-building to leave "the world a better place." For the Indigenous lens, we emphasize the role of language and stories.[9] For the settler view, we rely on several scholarly perspectives, discussed in the settler accident section below. We come from different relevant backgrounds and write from our perspectives. In this process, we shared our research and discussed our findings, learning from each other.

The European settlement of Manitoulin Island was part of the great land rush and the commodification of nature, including the creation of new settler agrarian societies, which was common in North America and throughout the British Empire. Situated within broader histories of colonialism and of accidents in Canada, this chapter offers a microcosm of entanglements with the unforeseen in rural and remote locals. To see the island as rural and remote is to see through the relatively recent lens of arriving settlers; for the Anishinaabe, it is sacred and was inhabited for thousands of years prior to European arrival in the area. We also offer comparable perspectives to other chapters in this volume, including the importance of place and settler narrative creation (e.g., Davies and Myers), the cultural meaning of shipwreck and vessel accidents (e.g., Coates); and accident narratives and memory as articulated in local histories and other cultural projects (e.g., Mullally). This account, however, differs by seeing history through Two Eyes, settler and Anishinaabek, and further contributes to the global literature on settler colonialism with a focus on accidents.[10]

PLACE AND PEOPLE ON MANITOULIN ISLAND: ANISHINAABEK AND SETTLER BACKGROUND

Located in Lake Huron in northeastern Ontario, Manitoulin Island is the world's largest freshwater island, comprising over 4,400 square kilometres. In 2023, it has sixteen townships and six Indigenous reserves. Two maps (figures 10.1 and 10.2) show two perspectives of the island relevant to a Two-Eyed Seeing approach.

Since at least 9500 BP, Manitoulin Island has been home to Indigenous peoples.[11] The historical record shows it is the territory of the Ottawa (or Odawa) Anishinaabek.[12] According to Andrew Blackbird, the original name for Manitoulin is Ottawa Island. The Ottawa, who occupied this island before the arrival of Europeans, believed "the 'Great Master of Life' created their ancestors and set them down on the Manitoulin."[13] The first European on Manitoulin Island was the Catholic priest Father Joseph Antoine Poncet, who wintered there in 1648–49.[14]

In 1836, Father J.B. Proulx first visited Wiikwemkoong on the east end of Manitoulin Island and by 1838 set up a permanent residence there.[15] Within a year, Father Proulx had baptized seventy-eight people, forty-nine of them adults; these numbers give some insight into the Indigenous demography at the time of sustained Indigenous-European contact on the island.[16] Wiikwemkoong would become a central missionary post from

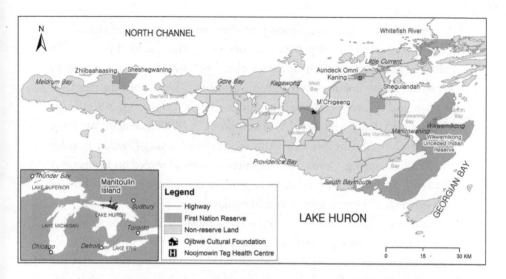

Fig. 10.1 Manitoulin Island, with Indigenous reserves and non-reserve land demarcated.

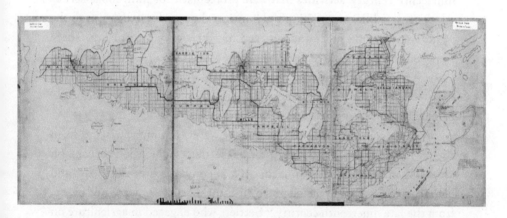

Fig. 10.2 Manitoulin Islands, Ontario Patent Map, demarcating townships and alienation of Crown lands.

which Jesuits would travel as far as Lake Nipissing, the north shore of Lake Huron, villages on Manitoulin, and Lake Superior.[17]

Manitoulin Island is subject to two treaties. The first, in 1836, aimed to relegate Indigenous peoples to a central location on the island, with a colonial establishment at Manitowaning.[18] This attempt failed, and a second treaty in 1862 carved the island into the current reserve settlements.[19]

Anishinaabek at Wiikwemkoong on the eastern portion of the island refused to sign this treaty, that land becoming the unceded portion. In 1880, six reserves existed: Sucker Lake, Sheguiandah, Sucker Creek, West Bay, Obidjewong, and Sheshigwaning.[20] The communities that remain today are Wiikwemkoong (formerly "Unceded portion of Manitoulin Island" and later "Wikwemikong"), M'Chigeeng (West Bay), Sheguiandah, Sheshegwaning, Aundeck Omni Kaning (Sucker Creek), and Zhiibaahaasing. Owing to the limited historical record on Indigenous accidents on Manitoulin Island, the reserve communities we profile are Obidjewong, Wiikwemkoong, and Sheguiandah.

Even before the treaties were agreed to by some Indigenous nations, mining licenses were granted, bringing settlers to Lake Huron and Lake Superior regions in general and Manitoulin Island in particular. At the same time, settlers fished the waters and logged the area from the mid-nineteenth century, activities that were problematic for Indigenous-settler relations. In addition to fishing and hunting, the peoples indigenous to the island made maple sugar and engaged in subsistence agriculture. There were roughly 1,364 Indigenous people on Manitoulin Island in the early 1860s. The 1862 treaty opened Manitoulin to settlers, and though initially they were slow to arrive, numbers increased, and the total population expanded to about 10,000 by the early 1890s.[21]

Steamships had started to traverse the waters around the island from the mid-1830s. From the 1860s and '70s, settler colonization focused on acquiring arable land. Farming changed in emphasis over time; oats and hay were replaced or supplemented by livestock, primarily cattle and sheep, from the late nineteenth century.[22] Settlers who engaged in agriculture on their new plots also worked in logging camps in the winter. The main source of transportation continued to be watercraft: boats, schooners, canoes, mackinaws, and steamships. Wood provided heat and building materials. Winter travel was over ice.[23] Tourism became a major industry by the 1880s, with people coming from the mainland and south to see the sights and to fish and hunt. Some resided over the summer.

By October 1918, the predominance of agriculture as the most important industry on the Island for settlers was confirmed in the politically significant Manitoulin by-election, when rural farmer settler men and newly enfranchised settler women (status Indians could not vote in Ontario elections until 1954) outvoted Manitoulin's more urban settlers to elect Ontario's first United Farmers member of the Legislature (MLA).[24] Key developments in the twentieth century facilitated rail and then car travel: a swing bridge in 1913 at Little Current allowed for trains and, from 1945, automobiles.[25]

For the Anishinaabek, fishing was important long before the arrival of settlers.[26] Farming became more common over the contact period, particularly at Wiikwemkoong by 1850, with the encouragement by Catholic priests. Indigenous economic livelihoods consisted of producing and selling maple syrup, and selling lumber to steamboats with local merchants in operation by the 1890s.[27] In common with settlers, Indigenous peoples also engaged in the timber and tourism industries.[28] By 1911, the first automobile arrived in Wiikwemkoong, marking a transition to modern transportation.[29]

"HISTORY" AND "ACCIDENT" IN ANISHINAABE WORLDVIEW

The Anishinaabek have no concise word for "accident" or "history." The anthropologist A. Irving Hallowell documents the concept of Anishinaabek history as more closely articulated through two types of stories.[30] The first is *tabatcamoin*, which he translates as "news or tidings" that consist of everyday events, some verging on being legends. The second is *atisokanak*, defined as "myths" or "sacred stories" told ritually during long winter nights and classified as living beings that have existed since time immemorial. According to Hallowell, "What we call myth is accepted by them as a true account of events in the past lives of living 'persons.'"[31]

William Jones, an Indigenous anthropologist who collected mythic stories among the Anishinaabek of Ontario and Minnesota, stated, "Myths are thought of as conscious beings, with powers of thought and action."[32] One myth collected by Jones has elements of an accident: in "The Death of Nanabushu's Nephew, the Wolf,"[33] the trickster Nanabushu dreams that his nephew, Wolf, drowns. Upon waking, Nanabushu pleads with Wolf always to use a stick to test brooks for water regardless of their appearing dry. Wolf does so for a time, but pursuing a moose, he falls while leaping across a seemingly dry brook and lands in the middle and drowns. Learning from the kingfisher that a manitou (spirit) caused the death, Nanabushu avenges Wolf's death by killing the manitou.[34] Anishinaabek on Manitoulin Island in modern times tell similar stories. The late elder William Trudeau told a story of dangerous water passages near Manitowaning Bay, where an underwater creature caused boats to capsize, drowning those on board.[35]

REVIEW OF ANISHINAABE RECORD OF ACCIDENTS

John Tanner, a child of settlers taken captive and raised by the Anishinaabek in Michigan and Manitoba, wrote an autobiography in 1830 with the assistance of the physician Edwin James. Tanner's memoir records several instances of accidents, including incidents of his bark dwellings catching fire.[36] In another, he and his brother fell through the ice; their clothing and moccasins froze, and they were unable to start a fire due to wet spunk wood. Facing the approach of death, Tanner persevered, found dry wood, and started a fire. After drying their clothes and surviving the night, they travelled home, meeting their mother partway bringing dry clothes and food. Tanner's mother anticipated they had fallen through the ice since they had not returned, and she walked all night to find them.[37] Other accidents that Tanner recounted include an accidental shooting, falling from a tree, a hunting accident, and injuries due to rough play while intoxicated.[38]

The German traveller Johann Kohl documented the way of life of the Anishinaabek of Lake Superior in the nineteenth century. According to Kohl, the Anishinaabek regarded "the smaller and greater accidents of life and melancholy events with much philosophy and admirable resignation."[39] In one instance, after a young man lay his gun down to play a game, his younger brother began fiddling with the gun hammer. The gun went off, killing the older brother. Following the burial, the younger brother fled to the forest, but his family pursued and consoled him, with no mention of the accident.[40]

Anthropological ethnographies are additional sources of information on Anishinaabe accidents. According to Hallowell's Anishinaabek informants, a balance existed between one's soul and body and in social relations, leading to the "Good Life."[41] Illness, misfortune, or death were not chance events but due to human sorcery and magic and had a psychological effect.[42] Hallowell calls this a "personalistic theory of causation," since persons cause events; accidents are thus caused by persons and are a consequence of one's behaviour. In an instance in 1940, when "a severe forest fire broke out at the mouth of the Berens River, no Indian would believe that lightning or any impersonal or accidental determinants were involved. *Somebody* must have been responsible."[43]

In his fieldwork among the Round Lake Ojibwa of northern Ontario, Edward S. Rogers noted that the environment and time of the year influenced the occurrence of an accident; westerly winds in summer, for example, often caused canoe accidents.[44] Rogers also documented the occurrence of accidental shootings among hunters, with one instance of a fatality.[45] Like Hallowell, he observed, "Practically all cases of illness, accident, and death are attributed to the sorcery of others."[46] A shaman could determine if an ailment or accident resulted from sorcery and then cure it.[47] Shamans had the power to invoke accidents through sorcery, while one shaman could curtail the power of another to prevent or eliminate accidents.

MANITOULIN ISLAND ANISHINAABEK ACCIDENTS

The Manitoulin Death Index provides some information on Manitoulin Island deaths from the late nineteenth to the mid-twentieth century. Deaths due to accidents listed in the index are attributed to causes including killed by a horse, logging accident, alcohol poisoning, drowning (most common), falling, burned to death, railway accident, hit by a falling tree, suicide, exposure due to intoxication, and murder by an intellectually challenged family member.[48] However, the index offers limited details of these accidents; below, we provide vignettes in the historical record to shed further light on accidents in Indigenous communities on the island.

Water Accidents

In a letter dated 30 September 1848, the Jesuit father Hanipaux details two drownings near Fort LaCloche on the north shore of Lake Huron near Manitoulin Island. At the time of his travels, frequent storms made water travel difficult. In another letter dated 5 November 1849, Hanipaux writes of his boat sinking. While he was travelling with a young Anishinaabe to baptize sick non-Christians, their boat was capsized by strong wind and waves, but both men found safety on large rocks nearby. The next day, they recovered and repaired their sunken boat and continued their journey.[49]

Hanipaux writes in a letter of 15 October 1857 about "a drunkard" who "fell from his boat into the water while holding a bottle to his mouth. His body is now at the bottom of the lake, or at least it has not been found."[50] The same incident recurred a year later: on 31 October 1858, Hanipaux writes of an Anishinaabe male visiting friends at Chibwaonaning (sic), who also drowned after falling from his canoe intoxicated.[51]

Accident at Obigewong

The Obigewong reserve existed from 1862 to 1927 and was home to a revered healer known as Jim Poquam.[52] His son, Kahgaygonaib, also known as Nobscot, excelled in using a bow and arrow. The Anishinaabek of Obigewong did not like Nobscot since he was known to be aggressive when consuming alcohol. One winter he died mysteriously, found face down in a waterhole on a trail. Speculation arose that an intoxicated Nobscot fell and drowned; foul play emerged as another theory. Without a formal investigation, the death remained a mystery.[53]

Industrial School Fire at Wikwemikong

On 20 January 1885, the Indian Office at Manitowaning reported the loss of the Boys Industrial School in Wikwemikong to a fire that started near the stove in the recreation room, "the exact cause ... unknown." No loss of life was reported, and there was no insurance in place.[54] On 22 January, the girls school also burned, starting about 5:00 p.m. The cause was said to be "a defective chimney," again with no record of loss of life and no insurance.[55] In further correspondence, the cause of both fires was "said to have been the result of accident."[56]

Fire broke out again at the girls school on 5 February 1911. This event, however, had different repercussions. The work of rebuilding began on 15 February 1911; by 16 May 1911, a dispute by the Indigenous workforce erupted over the rate of pay. By 7 June 1911, work had resumed, but on 10 June, it again stopped. On 15 July, the Montreal-based superior of the

Jesuits decreed that both the boys' and girls' schools were to move. The Lapointe farm in Spanish, Ontario, was chosen as the new location, and the work began on 20 September. By 1913, both schools had officially moved to Spanish, becoming the regional Catholic residential schools for generations of Manitoulin Anishinaabek.[57]

Accidents in the Wikwemikong Diary, Holy Cross Mission Archives

The Wikwemikong Diary provides the most in-depth profile of accidents in Wikwemikong and the region. Entries reference accidents between 1870 and 1954, the majority of them drownings (thirty-one). There are also four fires (three discussed above), and three accidents resulting in freezing to death. Alcohol consumption is linked to two drownings and in one death due to freezing (although there may be at least two, since one record refers to attendance at a dance the night before, possibly involving alcohol consumption).

Bearwalking

Given the Anishinaabek worldview of the connection between sorcery and accidents, bearwalking merits consideration for review. In the 30 August 1945 issue of the *Recorder*, a Manitoulin Island newspaper, a story featured James Nahwaikezhik of the Sheguiandah reserve killing his father who had put a curse on him.[58] A *Maclean's* magazine story of 1 August 1950 reported that the court record reveals Nahwaikezhik killed his father and intended to kill his mother since he believed both his parents put the bearwalk curse on him.[59] "According to superstition, the Bearwalk spirit is a malignant devil called out of the wilderness by an evil person, or witch. It enters the soul and body of the accursed, bringing every shape of misfortune, strange maladies and ultimate death."[60] Nahwaikezhik learned of the curse after consulting Laurence Toulouse, a medicine man who prescribed herbal medicine, but the headaches persisted, and the only cure was to kill the bearwalkers. After killing his father and attempting to kill his mother, who escaped to safety, Nahwaikezhik slept peacefully, his headache gone. Following a court debate over his sanity, Nahwaikezhik was declared sane and guilty of murder and sentenced to hang. His lawyer successfully appealed the death sentence, and he received a life sentence.[61]

In November 1951, Frank Debassige went on trial for the murder of Levi Bob. Peter Bob, Levi's brother, was married to Frank's sister and had died from an unknown cause. Levi accused Frank's mother and sister of bear-walking Peter. A quarrel arose between the two after alcohol consumption, leading to Frank shooting Levi. After a four-day trial, due to conflicting evidence, Frank Debassige was found not guilty.[62]

Analysis of Manitoulin Island Anishinaabek Accidents

The most common cause of historical Manitoulin Island Anishinaabek accidents is capsized watercrafts, often leading to drownings. Jesuit writings detail dangerous conditions on Lake Huron that made travel difficult. The cause of capsizing is not always apparent in the records, but some narratives point to alcohol as a cause. Freezing to death in winter is another cause of accidents in the historical record, as is fire, specifically concerning industrial schools. In these cases, there is room for interpretation. It may be that these fires were deliberately set, resulting in the move to Spanish.

The bearwalking incident in Sheguiandah, an instance of sorcery, is consistent with a cause of accidents in the comparative historical Anishinaabek record. Tanner, too, writes about bearwalking in his account, and both Hallowell and Rogers write about sorcery-caused accidents.[63] Bearwalking is not a conventional accident, but situated within Anishinaabek Seeing, it is equivalent to an accident as it is due to a person's actions.

Alcohol is often mentioned in both the historical Anishinaabek and Manitoulin Island records. Tanner, the Obidgewong account, and the Wikwemikong Diary contain entries on the problems arising from it and its role in accidents ranging from drowning to freezing. The Jesuit records highlight attempts to eradicate alcohol consumption by temperance movements.[64] Thus, Anishinaabek Seeing of accidents retain elements of continuity with accidents occurring before the arrival of settlers, though reoriented within the new structure of settler colonialism. In this reorientation, it is possible to see Hallowell's "personalistic theory of causation" as manifesting in new forms of accident causation in the shape of alcohol, missionaries, and law officers.

ACCIDENT IN SETTLER STORIES

Accidents loom large in Manitoulin Island settler stories. Sources are abundant and attest that accident stories were told and retold over generations. Farming, logging, sawmills, fires, water, ice, and, later, automobile travel were all hazardous. Accidents were and are framed and represented in a particular way in settler sources.[65] A discussion of these stories is a component of our Two-Eyed Seeing approach.[66] In this section we see through the settler lens, analyzing ways in which settlers on the island have represented their perspective and what the stories tell us about their lens on accidents – what they meant and mean to them. As in Sasha Mullally's discussion of rural accidents in her chapter in this book, local historians and settler institutions have an important role in the creation of settler accident narratives and memory.

Sources and the Settler Lens

Settler literature and sources include books, archive files, and online materials produced by the Manitoulin Genealogy Club, the latter based in the island community of Little Current.[67] The club makes available online a Death Index, an Obituaries Index, and a History Bites section.[68] The Death Index, roughly 570 pages in length, is based on provincial death records, memorial notices in the *Manitoulin Expositor*, and information provided by contemporary island settler descendants. The Manitoulin Obituaries are approximately 530 pages, and for our period, about ten pages mention accidents, drawn mainly from the *Manitoulin Expositor*, the *Recorder*, and settler stories. History Bites, covering 1877 to 2002 and 110 pages in length, contains many stories, most drawn from the *Manitoulin Expositor*. There are forty-four pages of relevant entries, largely focusing on 1880 to 1900. For settlers in rural areas and the near north, Manitoulin Island accidents were sought-after public news, and settler sources are both quantitatively and qualitatively rich, with significant detail included.

Genealogy Club materials again reflect the settler lens. This is evidenced by its support for the Early Settler, Pioneer, and Centennial Pioneer Certification Project "in their effort to record and preserve Early Manitoulin History."[69] "Early" history is settler history. Settler museums on the island provide a variety of relevant sources.[70] The online Genealogy

Club material draws on Manitoulin Island settler archives that state on their websites a commitment to settler history. An example of relevant archival material is the Diary of Thomas Simpson, from 1867 to 1872, included in a file the Gore Bay Museum. The museum file includes diary excerpts published in the *Manitoulin Expositor* as well as diary extracts written by Dr Simpson's grandson Brooke Claxton. Simpson was a nineteenth-century physician who practised on the Island and acted as coroner, Indian commissioner, and government surgeon to Indigenous inhabitants. He records in his diary several accidents from drowning and other causes.[71] The Gore Bay Museum also has a "History of Meldrum Bay" manuscript by Archie Wickett, written in January 1956. Wickett acknowledges sources that include older relatives; he writes about a number of accidents, including the story of two settlers who drown on their way to register a property claim in the 1860s. The story is also retold by Willis John McQuarrie in *True Tall Tales of Algoma-Manitoulin*.[72]

McQuarrie was a productive teller of settler stories. Publisher of Gore Bay's *Recorder* from the late 1960s, he also published the *Through the Years* booklet series from 1983 to 1997, with stories of bygone settler days.[73] He later drew on the *Through the Years* materials as well as a range of other sources in his *True Tall Tales of Manitoulin*, and it is to this book that we now turn before drawing on the Genealogy Club material to explore other aspects of the settler lens.

In his book's introduction McQuarrie states, "If we measure progress by how far we have come from what we were before, we have come a long ways from the days of the settlers. That was a benchmark of collective misery and misfortune. During the early days as the settlers moved into a new land, they were all prone to accidents as daily life was labour intensive."[74] McQuarrie's first chapter – in pride of place – is entitled "Accidents and Loss of Life: 'Tragic Events.'" In it he defines what an accident is, and in doing so highlights its importance to settlers' invention of tradition, an understanding of a people's pride in past accomplishments in the context of danger and hardship: "Accidents are a part of life. We all have them. Some might be avoidable while others are happenings thrust upon us, some innocuous while others with tragic results. All people are subject to them and in all walks of life."[75] This understanding of accidents is consistent with definitions in the literature about accidents in European-western societies of the nineteenth and twentieth centuries. In 1985 Karl Figlio defined the accident as an "unforeseen event which is also expected"; Roger Cooter and Bill Luckin discuss the paradox that "accidents may seem to be random and arbitrary, yet at the same time be expected or preordained."[76] The settler lens reflects western European developments in which the accident has been secularized since the medieval and early modern periods but chance and fortune continue to play a role.[77]

McQuarrie's stories are true in being accurate to the locally accepted settler understanding of them. They ring true to fellow settlers, yet are mythological in that they are not necessarily based in fact. McQuarrie writes, "If there is a story that might be somewhat separated from the absolute truth, you will certainly recognize it as simply a tall tale too good to not publish." He relies on stories gleaned from island newspapers and other sources including contributing settler descendants; his "book is written in memory of all those who lived and laboured in this region, often under some very adverse conditions, from the beginning to the present."[78] The settler lens is not necessarily objective (focused on "*interpretation* of concrete facts") in the sense that some scholars describe the western lens in Two-Eyed Seeing; rather, it can be, as on Manitoulin, community based, qualitative, emotional, and tied to a relationship to place, and in these ways share some traits with the Indigenous lens.[79]

McQuarrie gives representative examples of the range of settler accidents, most concerning marine mishaps, ice travel, shotguns, fire, and occupational accidents on the farm, in the sawmill, or fishing. One story concerning marine drownings, for example, took place in 1862 when the island was opened "to settlement of the White People following the signing of the treaty with the Indian Nations that year." Two recently arrived settlers drowned when their small boat turned over in rough water in the Mississauga Strait between Cockburn Island and Meldrum Bay on their way to register their land at the Land Registry office.[80] Early in the next decade, two brothers, having been granted eight hundred acres provided they built a mill, took on the task and were successful for nearly a decade. In 1882, however, one brother died when the ss *Manitoulin* burned and sank; five months later the other brother drowned in the sinking of the ss *Asia*, along with 122 other passengers and crew.[81] McQuarrie's settler story about the land registration accident following the 1862 treaty reveals a feature of the settler lens on accidents. Settler colonialism is about staying and building a future rather than coming, extracting, and leaving, as in other parts of the British Empire.[82] As in Coates's chapter in this volume, shipwrecks were collective significant events representing danger that exposed the "fragility of existence."[83] Registration and survey lines were essential to creating an agrarian settler society on the island. The shipwreck story is also a settler origin story: like the many other pioneer stories that involve accidents, these stories "validated newcomer claims to the environment."[84] Like other settler accident histories, they carry the transformative burden of turning settlers into settler descendants who know their origins.[85]

Settler Accidental Deaths

For island settlers, water or ice were the predominant modes of transportation for much of this period, and drowning deaths thus formed a significant number of accidents, along with those related to work. The Genealogy Club's online materials, like McQuarrie's work, include significant attention to accidents, and these tell us more about the settler lens on accidents. The Death Index, after all records post-1960s were eliminated, were searched for "accident," "drown," "fire," "shoot," producing a list of 147 settlers. Of these, eighty-four drowned (57 per cent of the total), seventeen were shot and died as a result, eight died in fires, two died in an automobile accident, thirteen died at work, six died in accidental falls, two died in childbirth, one perished in a train accident, and a child died by suffocation (bedding). Thirteen others died in unspecified "accidents." Some 70 per cent occurred prior to 1920, indicative of the Genealogy Club interest in the earlier periods of settlement.[86] A significant proportion of those drowned were under eighteen years of age, while most dying from shotgun accidents were just under or over eighteen. Those perishing in fires tended to be children, while those dying from falls were older adults. This representation of settler accidents correlates in several respects with Kamckey's historical epidemiological findings.

Settler Occupational Accidents

The settler lens reveals the types of accidents on the job that settlers high-lighted and for what period. Of the thirteen dying in occupationally related incidents in the Death Index, seven occurred from 1900 to 1919, four in saw-mill accidents. Post-1920, a couple of individuals drowned on the job (fishing, tugboat), another in lumbering, one on the farm, one while labouring (skull fracture). A missionary living on the island in the late nineteenth century commented on sawmill accidents: "In the mill, an accident may, and fre-quently does happen. One of the saws will split or some of the machinery give way and pieces of iron or steel are hurled with terrible force in every direction. Woe to the man whom such a piece may chance to strike."[87] As J.B. Bertrand notes in *Timber Wolves*, in logging "there were bound to be accidents ... These would include fractured limbs ... but rarely would there be a fatal accident in felling trees."[88] The fisheries, as McCullough and others indicate, could be even more dangerous, especially with spring and fall gales. Until 1920, most fishers worked in open boats, many in open water (for example, when gill-netting), where they would be particularly exposed to dangerous weather.[89]

Settler Accidents over the Long Term

The settler lens reveals the importance of accidents for settler understand-ings of time. Pioneers came, experienced accidents, and settled the island for themselves and their descendants. Obituaries emphasize the accident as part of a multi-generational settler family story. Isabel Baker died, aged eighty-seven, in 1912, successfully leaving nearly one hundred descendants. Her obituary emphasized accidents in her marital history. She married twice, her first husband dying building a railroad. After a few years she remarried, only to have her second husband also die on the job, "being drowned in the performance of his duty as lighthouse-keeper."[90] This obit-uary is consistent with the conclusions of Sarah Carter concerning the con-temporary emphasis on settler female reproduction and the male role as the economic subject in settlement.[91]

A History Bites story from 1934, "Settler Friends Recounting Tales of Youth," provides perspective on how accident stories are featured in the settler experience over time in sources other than obituaries. In the story, two friends meet after half a century of separation, with their accidental stories highlighted. One friend had lost his father on the ss *Asia*, and both friends had experienced a tragic accident working on the railway during construction of the "Soo branch." They were in a group of seven young men crossing the ice from the north shore when the ice gave way and one drowned. The rest were stranded on an island, killed and ate a dog, built a fire, and four days later "were rescued by Indians."[92] In this story, as with other settler stories from the island and other locales, Indigenous involvement takes the form of helping settlers deal with accidents, which may well have been interpreted as Indigenous acceptance of settlement.[93]

Settlers and Accident Prevention

History Bites contains more detail than Death Index material; the entries include consideration of accidental prevention and management. This focus is indicative of a shift in the western European and settler lens in the eighteenth and (especially) nineteenth centuries to fire and other forms of insurance, the use of statistics, and greater attention to accident prevention and preparedness, as discussed by Roy Porter and Craig Spence.[94] Mention is made of fire insurance at several times between 1884 and 1886 in the *Manitoulin Expositor*, which notes on nine occasions that "as usual, there was no insurance"[95] – a broad editorial hint to readers of the time! Other examples of settler concern with accident prevention are evidenced in 1885–86. These include references to life boats and life-saving stations, bystanders' roles in rescuing those falling through the ice, commissioners' reports on crew performance after maritime disasters, inhabitants' adequate preparation for winter journeys, domestic fire precautions, and fire-fighting effectiveness.[96] A train wreck in January 1910 at the Spanish River Crossing, resulting in thirty-nine deaths was reported at length, including a discussion of the inquest jury's recommendations for investigation by the CNR railway commissioners. Recommendations included additional men to keep the track in good condition given the "rigorous climate of New Ontario," roof openings for train cars, and boxes of emergency tools placed outside cars.[97] The role of alcohol in a number of accidents is reported as a matter of concern with respect to prevention. In 1885, two young women died from exposure during a trip in a winter storm, with teamster drunkenness leading

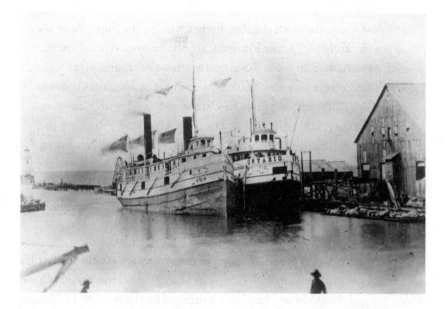

Fig. 10.3 ss *Asia* and ss *Ontario*, 1874.

to fatal results.[98] For Manitoulin, as on the remote BC island in Megan Davies and Tamara Myers's chapter in this book regarding health care, the colonial accident narrative illuminates how the dangers posed by place required prevention and management. On Manitoulin Island, the role of fate is also highlighted: not everything can be prevented or managed. In 1885, the *Expositor* observed that a Mr Proud was not "born under a lucky star," losing his thirteen-year-old daughter in a threshing-machine accident and a second child in the "burning of the [ss] *Manitoulin*." He had "since buried a third."[99]

1863 FISHERIES DISPUTE ACCIDENT:
SETTLER AND INDIGENOUS PERSPECTIVES

A significant incident involving an accident and culturally different settlers (Catholic French and Protestant English) took place after the second treaty. McQuarrie's discussion of the incident reveals a twenty-first-century settler perspective consistent with that of the 1860s. As McQuarrie tells the tale, a fisheries inspector, Mr Gibbard, had a violent encounter with the Rev. Father Kohler, the Superior of the Wikwemikong [sic] Jesuit Roman Catholic Priests. Armed constables were rushed in from Toronto to bring peace, and after what developed into a riot [by Wiikwemkoong Anishinaabek], it was agreed Mr. Gibbard would go to Ottawa to confer with Crown officials. At the meeting in Ottawa the Indians of Wikwemikong [sic] and the Priests lost their appeal [concerning Anishinaabek fishing rights] and history reveals that on Mr. Gibbard's return voyage to the Manitoulin, he was killed. Reports indicate that he disappeared and it was believed, but could not be proven, that he had been murdered when returning to the Manitoulin Island.[100]

McQuarrie's version is based on much of contemporary Anglo-Protestant settler and political opinion of the 1860s, including that of the *Toronto Globe*, which alleged that Gibbard had been murdered by the Jesuits. The Jesuits had a markedly different perspective, in which the accident plays an interesting role. A Father Carrez, writing in 1863 to his colleagues, denounced Gibbard's attempt to license fishing to settlers contrary to commitments made to the island's Indigenous peoples, maintaining that Gibbard was "severely reprimanded by the Toronto authorities for his brutal conduct." Carrez questioned what happened to Gibbard: "Did he fall by *accident*, or did he throw himself into the water out of spite and despair!" The allegations of murder were false, Carrez asserted.[101] In alleging accident or suicide, Father Carrez was taking a side in a very serious contemporary struggle over resources on the island between Indigenous peoples and settlers, one in which in one group of settlers – the Jesuits – resisted contemporary government settlement policy. The category of "settler" has a significant multicultural nature on Manitoulin Island, as elsewhere. The French Catholic Jesuits had been on the island longer than later settlers and had developed a distinctive relationship with the Wiikwemkoong Anishinaabek.[102]

Source material on the Indigenous view of the Gibbard incident is limited. An exception is the Witcher Report of 1863. The report states that the Wiikwemkoong people considered the fish reserves and Manitoulin and the surrounding islands to be their property and, in accordance with their own laws, expelled settler fishers from their waters and lands. They furthermore did not recognize the laws that Gibbard attempted to enforce. According to Ozawinimkee, who confronted Gibbard, he, Ozawinimakee, was "the Chief of this land. It is my ancestors', and they have been the proprietors up to this date." Due to this pressure, the settler fishers departed, as did Gibbard. While the settler historical record focuses on the death of Gibbard, the Indigenous focus is on defending sovereignty over land and fishery – an example of a Two-Eyed Seeing approach of accidents in history.[103]

CONCLUSION

Indigenous and settler perspectives combine in the 2008 video *Island of Great Spirit: The Legacy of Manitoulin.* The settler aspect includes the participation of Manitoulin museums and interviews with settler descendants and authors such as McQuarrie, who was proud to admit that he stretched the truth for a good tale. There are discussions of ice travel, fishing, and maritime accidents such as the sinkings of the ss *Manitoulin* and ss *Asia* in the late nineteenth century. Indeed, the video ends with a stirring rendition of "Asia Song."[104] The final minutes conclude with arguments that the old division between settlers and Indigenous peoples on the Island is not what it was, as demonstrated by the fact that half the team creating the video is Indigenous. They had gotten "along great," people on the Island "accept each other," and all Island long timers have a "spiritual connection" to the place.[105]

We argue instead, without denying the importance of a spiritual connection to the island, that the contrast between the understanding and significance of the accident for settlers and Indigenous peoples on Manitoulin Island is indicative of how far we need to go towards genuine understanding and acceptance.

For settlers, the telling and retelling of accident stories carries a "transformative burden" of turning settlers into settler descendants. It uses memory and creates a tradition to connect settlers and their descendants to Manitoulin Island's agricultural spaces, waters, and forests to which settlers came, experienced accidents, and persevered. In this storytelling, settlers possess and repossess Manitoulin Island in their imagination. The settler tie is an emotional one in which romanticism, settler myth and intergenerational ties are significant. On Manitoulin, the settler lens is community based, qualitative, emotional, and tied to place rather than objective and focused on the interpretation of facts, as some Two-Eyed Seeing scholars posit.

Dalley, in settler colonial reflections consistent with Two-Eyed Seeing, writes about his Australian settler ancestor and notes "there is a sense in which the difficulties that he experienced, surviving a shipwreck ... eclipse the horrors that colonisation wrought on Indigenous people ... In the Australian context, the sense of belonging, home and place enjoyed by the non-Indigenous subject—colonizer—migrant is based on the dispossession ... it mobilizes the legend of the pioneer, 'the battler,' in its self-legitimization" and "what is significant about my father's memory and family story is that it acted as a means of closing off a responsibility to Indigenous people."[106] Dalley also remarks that this settler memory is indeed across "what are relatively minute genealogical timespans" in Australia.[107] In the case of Manitoulin Island, this timespan is less than 170 years of 9,500 years of human habitation. Two-Eyed Seeing entails a reflection on self, openness to other perspectives, and "readiness to adjustment."[108] Dalley suggests that for himself and other settlers, it is time to reflect on the settler story, engage with Indigenous peoples in a new way, and start to rethink and reinterpret rather than to destroy or simply forget the past.[109]

For Manitoulin Island, settler and Indigenous peoples each mytholo-gized and experienced the same island and its vicinity in their own ways; they drowned in watercraft and in falls through the ice; they experienced fires and were injured or died during hunting, among other events. For Indigenous peoples, the mythic historical narrative is an embodiment through story of the lands and waters of Manitoulin Island and social re-lations with one another. Accidents gradually shift in focus in connection to settler colonialism, such as the church (industrial-school fires), the state (fishery act, courts in bearwalking), and alcohol consumption. In this chap-ter, our Two-Eyed Seeing approach to telling of the history of accidents on Manitoulin Island, balances Indigenous and settler views and experiences, offering a more comprehensive view of partial accident histories absent from settler imaginations. More discussion of how to research and write Two-Eyed Seeing history would not go amiss for future histories of Canada and elsewhere, for accidents and so much else besides.

ACKNOWLEDGMENTS

We thank the staff in the Museum, Archives and Libraries of Manitoulin Island, Algoma University, Archives of Ontario, and Libraries and Archives Canada for their generosity and good work.

NOTES

1 Settler colonialism has been defined as "an ongoing system of power" that "normalizes the continuous settler occupation, exploiting lands and resources to which indigenous peoples have genealogical relationships." Cox, "Settler Colonialism."

2 Young, *Health Care and Cultural Change*, 33.

3 Ibid., 47, 49, 55.

4 Kelm, *Colonizing Bodies*, 16–17.

5 Norris, "Demography of Aboriginal People in Canada," 51.

6 Jessica Grace Kamckey, "Manitoulin Island in Transition."

7 For accident details, see Kamckey, Physical Intervention Death Counts, table 4.23, 102.

8 Roher et al., "How Is Etuaptmumk/Two-Eyed Seeing Characterized?" 14. See also Wright et al., "Using Two-Eyed Seeing in Research with Indigenous Peoples"; Jeffery et al., "Two-Eyed Seeing," 321–5; Travers, "Seeing with Two Eyes."

9 Marshall et al., "Two-Eyed Seeing in Medicine," 46.

10 Literature on this is international in scope and includes Wolfe, *Settler Colonialism and the Transformation of Anthropology*; Veracini, *Settler Colonialism*; Laidlaw and Lester, *Indigenous Communities and Settler Colonialism*. For a recent overview of the debates and complexity in and concerning the field, see Carey and Silverstein, "Thinking with and beyond Settler Colonial Studies"; Weaver, *Great Land Rush*.

11 Julig, "Archaeological Conclusions from the Sheguiandah Site Research," 302.

12 In this chapter, we use the term Anishinaabek to refer to the original inhabitants of Manitoulin Island. The linguist Baraga defines Anishinaabe as "human being, man, woman or child ... also, Indian" and the suffix "g" denotes plural; see Baraga, *Dictionary of the Otchipwe Language*, 34–5. In the Manitoulin dialect, the suffix "k" is a variation of "g," and we thus use "Anishinaabek."

13 Blackbird, *History of the Ottawa and Chippewa Indians of Michigan*, 19; Major, *Manitoulin*, i.

14 Jones, "'8ENDAKE EHEN' or Old Huronia," 390–1.

15 Wikwemikong Diary, Holy Cross Mission, Jesuits in English Canada collection, administrative record series, Algoma University Archives, http://archives.algomau.ca/main/sites/default/files/2013-054_011_001.pdf.

16 Ibid., 1.

17 Cadieux, *Letters from the New Canada Mission, 1843–1852*, part 1, 49.

18 Canada, *Report on the Affairs*, 35.

19 Major, *Manitoulin*; Wightman, *Forever on the Fringe*.

20 Wightman, *Forever on the Fringe*, 81.

21 For discussions of the history of the island, see Wightman, *Forever on the Fringe*; Greene, *Wikwemikong First Nation*, 41–3; Pearen, *Four Voices*; Pearen, *Exploring Manitoulin*; Derry, *Manitoulin and Region*; McQuarrie, *True Tall Tales*; Kamckey, "Manitoulin Island in Transition."

22 McQuarrie, *True Tall Tales*; Pearen, *Exploring Manitoulin*; Derry, *Manitoulin and Region*; Pearen, *Four Voices*; Wightman, *Forever on the Fringe*; Greene, "Wikwemikong First Nation." For a discussion of the fisheries, see McCullough, *Commercial Fishery of the Canadian Great Lakes*.

23 Pearen, *Exploring Manitoulin*; Derry, *Manitoulin and Region*; McQuarrie, *True Tall Tales*; Wightman, *Forever on the Fringe*.

24 Griezic, "'Power to the People,'" 33–54.

25 Derry, *Manitoulin and Region*; Pearen, *Exploring Manitoulin*; Pearen, *Four Voices*; McQuarrie, *True Tall Tales*.

26 Derry, *Manitoulin and Region*, 194–218.

27 Wikwemikong Diary, 4–6, 13, 35.

28 Derry, *Manitoulin and Region*, 219–52.

29 Wikwemikong Diary, 51.

30 Baraga documents similar words to accident such as "frightful accident," "hurt," and "misfortune" (Baraga, *Dictionary of the Otchipwe Language*, 428), but there are no comparable words for "history" aside from *adisokan*, meaning "fable" (492). See also Hallowell et al., *Contributions to Ojibwe Studies*, 542. There are compilations of *aansookanak* on Manitoulin Island; see Smith, *Island of the Anishnaabeg*; Corbiere, *Gechi-Piitzijig Dbaajmowag*.

31 Hallowell et al., *Contributions to Ojibwe Studies*, 542–3.

32 Jones, *Ojibwa Texts*, part 2, 574n1.

33 Ibid., 89–100.

34 Ibid. In a letter dated 8 December 1848, this legend is remarkably similar to the experience of Fremoit at the Pigeon River, Lake Superior. Fremoit details while walking on ice, "Our guide, armed with a big stake, at each step struck this artificial surface [ice] that was frequently treacherous and we followed him at a respectful distance." At times, the ice had wide crevices with water exposed, requiring jumping across and making bridges of branches. Cadieux, *Letters from the New Canada Mission*, 58.

35 Corbiere, *Gechi-Piitzijig Dbaajmowag*, 99.

36 Tanner, *Narrative of the Captivity*, 44, 84.

37 Ibid., 44–5.

38 Ibid., 77, 173, 176, 211–12, 236.

39 Kohl, *Kitchi-Gami*, 109.

40 Ibid., 109–10.

41 Hallowell, *Culture and Experience*, 120, 173.

42 Ibid., 282, 284.

43 Hallowell et al., *Contributions to Ojibwe Studies*, 542–59.

44 Rogers, *Round Lake Ojibwa*, A8.

45 Ibid., C26.

46 Ibid., D17.

47 Ibid., D26.

48 The authors caution that the index is not a complete record. Decades of missing information are apparent, particularly in the mid-twentieth century. Nevertheless, it provides a useful starting point to get a sense of historical Anishinaabek accidents on Manitoulin Island. See Manitoulin Genealogy, 2004, Manitoulin Death Index, https://sites.rootsweb.com/~onmanito/death-index.html.

49 Cadieux, *Letters from the New Canada Mission, 1843–1852*, part 2, 135–8.

50 Ibid., 149.

51 Ibid., 161.

52 The reserve was sold to settlers who agitated for the land; see Myers, "History of Obidgewong," 13.

53 Ibid., 16.

54 Indian Office Manitowaning, 20 January 1885, Indian Affairs, RG 10, vol. 2288, file 57 261, LAC.

55 Indian Office Manitowaning, 24 January 24, RG 10, vol. 2288, file 57 261, LAC.

56 Department of Indian Affairs, Ottawa, 16 February 1885, RG 10, vol. 2288, file 57 261, LAC.

57 Wikwemikong Diary, 51–3. For a history of the Wiikwemkoong Industrial School and Spanish Residential Schools, see Shanahan, *Jesuit Residential School at Spanish*. For more on Jesuit provincials in Canada, see Jesuits of Canada, 2023, "About Us," https://jesuits.ca/about-us/frequently-asked-questions/.

58 McQuarrie, *Through the Years*, 2 June 1985, 6.

59 Don Delaplante, "The Black Magic Murder Case," *Maclean's*, 1 August 1950, 41. Bearwalking is comparable to Anishnaabek stories of shapeshifting into a cannibal known as the windigo. See Manitowabi, "Gambling with the Windigo." We are unaware of windigo incidences on Manitoulin.

60 Delaplante, "Black Magic Murder Case," 41.

61 Ibid.

62 Delaplante gives the trial month of November 1951 but limited trial details. See Delaplante, "The Eden Isle of Evil Spirits," *Maclean's*, 1 December 1952, 30. Details of the trial (without a date or author) are provided in McQuarrie, *Through the Years*, 1 July 1988, 31.

63 Tanner, in *Narrative of Captivity*, 343, writes of a medicine man wearing the hide of a bear with fire coming from its mouth via gun power.

64 Cadieux, *Letters from the New Canada Mission, 1843–1852*; see both parts 1 and 2.

65 For a discussion of the "major expansion (or explosion) of local histories, historical societies, museums and genealogical groups" in Ontario from the 1950s, see Boyce, "Fifty Years in the Trenches of History," 237–43.

66 Marshall et al., "Two-Eyed Seeing in Medicine," 50–1; Roher et al., "How Is Etuaptmumk/Two-Eyed Seeing Characterized in Indigenous Health Research?"

67 Manitoulin Genealogy Club, https://manitoulinroots.ca/histories/feature2.php.

68 Manitoulin Genealogy Club, Manitoulin Obituary Index, https://sites.rootsweb. com/~onmanito/obituary/index.html); Manitoulin Death Index, https://sites. rootsweb.com/~onmanito/death-index.html; History Bites, https://sites.rootsweb. com/~onmanito/bites.html.

69 To obtain a certificate, applicants must be a direct descendant of a qualified pioneer, early settler, or centennial settler ancestor. https://sites.rootsweb.com/~onmanito/ certificate/certificateinstr.html

70 Gore Bay Museum, https://www.gorebaymuseum.com/. Other museums: Assiginack Museum, https://www.assiginack.ca/assiginack-museum-heritage-complex/; Centennial Museum in Sheguiandah, https://www.townofnemi.on.ca/p/museum; Fathom Five (Tobermory); Little Red School House (South Bay Mouth); Mississagi Lighthouse Museum (Meldrum Bay); Net Shed Museum (Meldrum Bay); Museum of the Great Lakes (Manitowaning).

71 Doctors Simpson, Thomas, 1867–1872 file, Gore Bay Museum.

72 Archie Wickett file, Gore Bay Museum.

73 For a review, see *Expositor* staff, "True Tall Tales of Manitoulin – Jack McQuarrie Spins Colourful Island Yarns for the Ages," *Manitoulin Expositor*, 3 July 2019.

74 McQuarrie, *True Tall Tales*, 127.

75 In other sections, McQuarrie makes explicit an understanding that accidents can be deemed a product of misfortune or fate. See McQuarrie, *True Tall Tales*, 27, 83, 117, 127, 165, 230, 257, 164.

76 Figlio, "What Is an Accident?," 180–206; Cooter and Luckin, "Accidents in History," 1–16, at 5.

77 For a discussion of the secularization of accident in European societies, see Cooter and Luckin, "Accidents in History," 1–16.

78 McQuarrie, *True Tall Tales*, 7.

79 Ibid., italics added. For the objective western lens, see Jeffery et al., "Two-Eyed Seeing: Current Approaches, and Discussion of Medical Applications," 321; for community engaged, qualitative, and relational, see Wright et al., "Using Two-Eyed Seeing in Research with Indigenous Peoples," 2.

80 For a discussion of settlement rules on the Island, see Derry, *Manitoulin and Region*, 83.

81 McQuarrie, *True Tall Tales*, 107. For other accident references, see ibid., 118, 230–1, 258, 308–9. For discussion of the sinking of the ss *Asia*, see Derry, *Manitoulin and Region*, 170–9; McQuarrie, *Through the Years*, June 1987 and December 1993.

82 Ishiguro, "Growing Up and Grown Up in Our Future City," 36–7.

83 Coates, "Wind, Error, and Providence," in this volume, 274.

84 Trimble, "Storying Swí:lhcha," 50.

85 Dalley, "Becoming a Settler Descendant," 356.

86 Since this section of the chapter is focused on settlers, the following discussion excludes twenty individuals listed in the Death Index who are identifiably Indigenous. No suicides are listed as accidents. Most on the list are from earlier periods: 67 of 185 died prior to 1900, 60 between 1900 and 1919, and the rest after 1920.

87 Burden, *Manitoulin*, 141–2.

88 Bertrand, *Timber Wolves*, "Men of the Bush" chapter. For an example of a fatal logging accident, see "Accidental Death of Herbert Wilson Wright," McQuarrie, *Through the Years*, February 1990.

89 McCullough, *Commercial Fishery*; see esp. "Labour and Working Conditions," chap. 69. See also Derry, "The Fishing Industry," *Manitoulin and Region*, 194–218. For an example of a fishing accident, see McQuarrie, "Wreck and Members of Ill Fated Fishing Expedition," *Through the Years*, April 1991.

90 Obituaries, *Gore Bay Recorder*, 2 May 1912. For other examples, also in Obituaries, see Robert Ednie, 30 August 1934; Daniel Campbell, 20 January 1935, Clark Wallace, 21 March 1935.

91 Carter, *Imperial Plots*.

92 *Manitoulin Expositor*, 16 August 1934, cited in Manitoulin Genealogy Club, History Bites.

93 Dalley, "Becoming a Settler Descendant."

94 Porter, "Accidents in the Eighteenth Century"; Spence, "Accidents and Violent Death in Early Modern London."

95 *Manitoulin Expositor*, 30 August 1884, 20 September 1884, 20 December 1884, 21 March 1885, 10 October 1885, 26 December 1885, 30 January 1886, 10 April 1886, 17 April 1886, cited in History Bites.

96 *Manitoulin Expositor*, 17 October 1885, 9 January 1886, 6 February 1996, 20 March 1886, 27 March 1886, cited in History Bites.

97 *Manitoulin Expositor*, 10 February 1910, cited in History Bites.

98 *Manitoulin Expositor*, 28 March 1885, cited in History Bites; for detailed discussion, see Derry, *Manitoulin and Region*, chap. 7.

99 *Manitoulin Expositor*, 12 December 1885, cited in History Bites.

100 McQuarrie, *True Tall Tales*, 175–6.

101 Carrez, *Letters from Manitoulin Island*, 221–2.

102 For discussion of the divide between the English Protestant and French Catholic settlers see Nazar, "Nineteenth Century Wikwemikong," 9–12. For recent consideration of the multicultural dimensions of settlers in the wider empire, see Dalley, "Becoming a Settler Descendant," 365.

103 Parliament of Canada, "Narrations of the Indians, 4th July, 1863."

104 For the poems on which the song drew inspiration, see McQuarrie, "Wreck of the Asia," *Through the Years*, June 1987, 23. The earliest version was from 1882.

105 Ontario Trillium Foundation, *Island of Great Spirit*.

106 Dalley, "Becoming a Settler Descendant," 356, 364.

107 Ibid., 365.

108 Discussion of "Guide for Life" in Roher et al., "How Is Etuaptmumk/Two-Eyed Seeing Characterized," 7.

109 Dalley, "Becoming a Settler Descendant."

BIBLIOGRAPHY

Archives

Algoma University Archives, Brampton
Archives of Ontario, Toronto
Assigninack Museum, Manitowaning
Gore Bay Library, Gore Bay
Gore Bay Museum, Gore Bay
Library and Archives Canada, Ottawa

Newspapers and Periodicals

Maclean's
Manitoulin Expositor
Owen Sound Times
Gore Bay Recorder

Other Sources

Angus, James T. *A Deo Victoria: The Story of the Georgian Bay Lumber Company, 1871–1942.* Thunder Bay: Severn Publications, 1990.

Assiginack Historical Society. *A Time to Remember: A History of the Municipality of Assiginack.* Assiginack, ON: Assiginack Historical Society, 1996.

Baraga, Frederic. *A Dictionary of the Otchipwe Language Explained in English.* Cincinnati: Jos. A. Hemann, 1853.

Barwin, Lynn, Marjory Shawande, Eric Crighton, and Luisa Veronis. "Methods-in-Place: 'Art Voice' as a Locally and Culturally Relevant Method to Study Traditional Medicine Programs in Manitoulin Island, Ontario, Canada." *International Journal of Qualitative Methods* 14, no. 5 (2015): 1–11.

Bertrand, J.B. *Timber Wolves: Greed and Corruption in Northwestern Ontario's Timber Industry, 1875–1960.* Thunder Bay: Thunder Bay Historical Museum Society, 1997.

Blackbird, Andrew J. *History of the Ottawa and Chippewa Indians of Michigan: A Grammar of Their Language, and Personal and Family History of the Author.* Ypsilanti, MI: Ypsilantian Job Printing House, 1887.

Bogue, Margaret Beattie. *Great Lakes: An Environmental History, 1783–1933.* Madison, WI: University of Wisconsin Press, 2000.

Boyce, Gerry. "Fifty Years in the Trenches of History." *Celebrating One Thousand Years of Ontario's History.* Willowdale: Ontario Historical Society, 2000, 237–43.

Burden, Harold Nelson. *Manitoulin; or, Five Years of Church Work among the Ojibway Indians and Lumbermen, Resident upon That Island or in Its Vicinity.* London: Simpkin, Marshall, Hamilton, Kent, 1895.

Cadieux, Lorenzo, ed. *Letters from the New Canada Mission, 1843–1852.* Translated by William Lonc and George Topp. Early Missions in Canada series no. 6. Toronto: William Lonc, 2004.

Cadieux, Lorenzo, and Robert Toupin, eds. *Letters from Manitoulin Island, 1853–1870.* Translated by Shelley J. Pearen and William Lonc. Early Jesuit Missions in Canada series no. 6. Toronto: William Lonc, 2007.

Cameron, Scott L. *The Frances Smith: Palace Steamer of the Upper Great Lakes, 1867–1896.* Toronto: Natural Heritage Books, 2005.

Canada. *A Report on the Affairs of the Indians in Canada, Laid before the Legislative Assembly, March 20, 1845, Section II, 35.* http://archive.org.

Carey, Jane, and Ben Silverstein. "Thinking with and beyond Settler Colonial Studies: New Histories after the Postcolonial." *Postcolonial Studies* 23, no. 1 (2020): 1–20.

Carter, Sarah. *Imperial Plots: Women, Land and the Spadework of British Colonialism on the Canadian Prairies.* Winnipeg: University of Manitoba Press, 2016.

Cooter, Roger, and Bill Luckin, eds. *Accidents in History: Injuries, Fatalities and Social Relations.* Amsterdam: Rodopi, 1997.

– "Accidents in History: An Introduction." In Cooter and Luckin, *Accidents in History,* 1–16.

Corbiere, Alan, ed. *Gechi-Piitzijig Dbaajmowag: The Stories of our Elders.* Translated by Kay Roy and Evelyn Roy. M'Chigeeng, ON: Ojibwe Cultural Foundation, 2011.

Cox, Alicia. "Settler Colonialism." Oxford Bibliographies. 26 July 2017. https://www.oxfordbibliographies.com/view/document/obo-9780190221911/obo-9780190221911-0029.xml.

Dalley, Cameo. "Becoming a Settler Descendant: Critical Engagements with Inherited Family Narratives of Indigeneity, Agriculture and Land in a (Post) Colonial Context." *Life Writing* 18, no. 3 (2021): 355–70.

Derry, Margaret E. *Manitoulin and Region: Voices from the Past.* Caledon, ON: Poplar Lane Press, 2010.

Figlio, Karl. "What Is an Accident?" In *The Social History of Occupational Health,* edited by Paul Weindling, 180–206. London: Croom Helm, 1985.

Greene, J.E.C. "Wikwemikong First Nation: Unceded Aboriginal Title to Manitoulin Island?" LLM thesis, University of Ottawa, 2005.

Griezic, F.J.K. "'Power to the People': The Beginning of Agrarian Revolt in Ontario, the Manitoulin By-Election, October 24, 1918." *Ontario History* 69, no. 1 (1977): 33–54.

Hallowell, A. Irving. *Culture and Experience.* Philadelphia: University of Pennsylvania Press, 1955.

Hallowell, A. Irving, Susan Elaine Gray, and Jennifer S.H. Brown. *Contributions to Ojibwe Studies: Essays, 1934–1972.* Lincoln: University of Nebraska Press, 2010.

Ishiguro, Laura. "'Growing Up and Grown Up in Our Future City': Discourses of Childhood and Settler Futurity in Colonial British Columbia." BC *Studies* 190 (Summer 2016): 15–37.

Jason, Patricia. *Wild Things: Nature, Culture and Tourism in Ontario, 1790–1914.* Toronto: University of Toronto Press, 1995.

Jeffery, Tristen, Donna L.M. Kurtz, and Charlotte Ann Jones. "Two-Eyed Seeing: Current Approaches, and Discussion of Medical Applications." BC *Medical Journal* 63, no. 8 (October 2021): 321–5.

Jones, Arthur E. "'8ENDAKE EHEN' or Old Huronia." In *Fifth Report of the Bureau of Archives for the Province of Ontario by Alexander Fraser.* Toronto: L.K. Cameron, 1908.

Jones, William. *Ojibwa Texts, Part 1.* Collected by William Jones and edited by Truman Michelson. New York: G.E. Stechert & Co., 1917.

– *Ojibwa Texts, Part 2.* Collected by William Jones and edited by Truman Michelson. New York: G.E. Stechert & Co., 1919.

Julig, Patrick. "Archaeological Conclusions from the Sheguiandah Site Research." In *The Sheguiandah Site: Archaeological, Geological and Paleobotanical Studies at a Paleoindian Site on Manitoulin Island, Ontario,* edited by Patrick Julig. Hull, QC: Canadian Museum of Civilization, 2002.

Kamckey, Jessica Grace. "Manitoulin Island in Transition: An Eco-Epidemiological Explanation of Late 19th and Early 20th Century Mortality." MSc thesis, Lakehead University, ON, 2018.

Kelm, Mary-Ellen. *Colonizing Bodies: Aboriginal Health and Healing in British Columbia, 1900–50.* Vancouver: University of British Columbia Press, 1998.

Kohl, Johann Georj. *Kitchi-Gami: Wanderings Round Lake Superior.* First published 1860. Minneapolis: Ross and Haines, Inc., 1956.

Laidlaw, Zoë, and Alan Lester, eds. *Indigenous Communities and Settler Colonialism: Land Holding, Loss and Survival in an Interconnected World.* Houndmills, UK: Palgrave Macmillan, 2015.

Leighton, Douglas. "The Manitoulin Incident of 1863: An Indian-White Confrontation in the Province of Canada." *Ontario History* 69, no. 2 (June 1977): 113–24.

Lower, Arthur. "The Wreck of the George A. Graham." *Ontario History* 78, no. 1 (March 1986): 57–62.

Major, Frederick. *Manitoulin, the Isle of the Ottawas, Being a Handbook of Historical and Other Information on the Grand Manitoulin Island.* Gore Bay, ON: Recorder Press, 1934.

Manitowabi, Darrel. "Gambling with the Windigo: Theorizing Indigenous Casinos and Gambling in Canada." *Critical Gambling Studies* 2, no. 2 (2022): 113–22.

Marshall, Murdena, Alberta Marshall, and Cheryl Bartlett. "Two-Eyed Seeing in Medicine." In *Determinants of Indigenous People's Health: Beyond the Social*, edited by Margo Greenwood, Sarah de Leeuw, and Nicole Marie Lindsay. 2nd ed. Toronto: Canadian Scholars, 2018.

McCullough, A.B. *The Commercial Fishery of the Canadian Great Lakes*. Ottawa: Ministry of the Environment, 1989.

McQuarrie, W. John. *True Tall Tales of Algoma-Manitoulin: 400 Fascinating Stories of Happenings from Communities along the North Shore, St. Jos. Island, the Manitoulin and Cockburn Islands, and Areas*. Gore Bay, ON: Mid-North Printers, 2006.

– ed. *Through the Years: Manitoulin District History and Genealogy*. Series of 151 booklets. Gore Bay, ON: Mid-North Printers, 1983–97. https://freepages. rootsweb.com/~throughtheyears1980/history/.

Murray, Florence B. "Agricultural Settlement on the Canadian Shield: Ottawa River to Georgian Bay. In *Profiles of a Province: Studies in the History of Ontario*, edited by Edith Firth, 178–86. Toronto: Ontario Historical Society, 1967.

Nazar, David. "Nineteenth Century Wikwemikong: The Foundation of a Community and an Exploration of Its People." *Ontario History* 86, no. 1 (March 1994): 9–12.

Noël, Françoise. "Childhood Accidents, Illness and Death." Chap. 7 in *Family Life and Sociability in Upper and Lower Canada, 1780–1870: A View from Diaries and Family Correspondence*. Kingston and Montreal: McGill-Queen's University Press, 2003.

Norris, Mary Jane. "The Demography of Aboriginal People in Canada." In *Ethnic Demography: Canadian Immigrant, Racial and Cultural Variations*, edited by S.S. Halli, F. Trovato, and L. Driedger. Ottawa: Carleton University Press, 1990.

Oden, Derek, S. *Harvest of Hazards: Family Farming, Accidents, and Expertise in the Corn Belt, 1940–1975*. Iowa City: University of Iowa Press, 2017.

Ontario Trillium Foundation, Lock 3 Media and Living History Multimedia Association. *Island of Great Spirit: The Legacy of Manitoulin*. Video. Ontario Visual Heritage Project Series. St Thomas, ON: Living History Multimedia Association, 2008.

Parliament of Canada. "Narrations of the Indians, 4th July, 1863, Wekwemikong." In *Sessional Papers: First Session of the Eight Parliament of the Province of Canada*, vol. 22. Quebec: Hunter Rose & Co., 1863.

Pearen, Shelley J. *Exploring Manitoulin*. 3rd ed. Toronto: University of Toronto Press, 2001.

– *Four Voices: The Great Manitoulin Island Treaty of 1862*. Ottawa: Shelly J. Pearen, 2012.

Porter, Roy. "Accidents in the Eighteenth Century." In Cooter and Luckin, *Accidents in History*, 90–106.

Rogers, Edward S. *The Round Lake Ojibwa*. Occasional paper 5, Art and Archaeology Division, Royal Ontario Museum. Toronto: Ontario Department of Lands and Forests, 1962.

Roher, Sophie, Ziwa Yu, Debbie Martin, and Anita Benoit. "How Is Etuaptmumk/Two-Eyed Seeing Characterized in Indigenous Health Research? A Scoping Review." *PLoS ONE* 16, no. 7 (2021): 1–22.

Shanahan, David F. *The Jesuit Residential School at Spanish: "More Than Mere Talent."* Toronto: Canadian Institute of Jesuit Studies, 2004.

Smith, Theresa S. *The Island of the Anishnaabeg: Thunderers and Water Monsters in the Traditional Ojibwe Life-World*. Moscow, ID: University of Idaho Press, 1995.

Spence, Craig. *Accidents and Violent Death in Early Modern London, 1650–1750*. London: Boydell Press, 2016.

Tanner, John. *A Narrative of The Captivity and Adventures of John Tanner [U.S. Interpreter at the Sault de Ste. Marie] during Thirty Years Residence among the Indians in the Interior of North America [...]*. New York: G. & C. & H. Carvill, 1830.

Travers, Karen. "Seeing with Two Eyes: Colonial Policy, The Huron Tract Treaty and Changes in the Land in Lambton County, 1780–1867." PhD diss., York University, 2015.

Trimble, Sabina. "Storying Swí:lhcha: Place Making and Power at a Stó:lō Landmark." *BC Studies* 190 (Summer 2016): 39–66.

Veracini, Lorenzo. *Settler Colonialism: A Theoretical Overview*. New York: Palgrave Macmillan, 2010.

Weaver, John C. *The Great Land Rush and the Making of the Modern World, 1650–1900*. Montreal and Kingston: McGill-Queen's University Press, 2003.

Wightman, W.R. *Forever on the Fringe: Six Studies in the Development of the Manitoulin Island*. Toronto: University of Toronto Press, 1982.

Wolfe, Patrick. *Settler Colonialism and the Transformation of Anthropology: The Politics and Poetics of an Ethnographic Event*. London and New York: Cassell, 1999.

Wright, A.L., C. Gabel, M. Ballantyne, S.M. Jack, and O. Wahoush. "Using Two-Eyed Seeing in Research with Indigenous Peoples." *International Journal of Qualitative Methods* 18 (2019): 1–19.

Young, T. Kue. *Health Care and Cultural Change: The Indian Experience in the Central Subarctic*. Toronto: University of Toronto Press, 1988.

11

An Accident's Afterlife

Childhood, Disability, Maternalism, and Rehabilitation

Megan J. Davies and Tamara Gene Myers

Othoa Scott's life was peripatetic even before her accident. Born on Hornby Island, BC, to parents Daisy (née Godkin) and Caesar Scott in 1911, Othoa was not yet five when she lost her mother to tuberculosis.[1] Taken in by her maternal grandmother in Seattle, she faced her grandmother's death a short year later. A return to Hornby to the care of her father, Caesar, and his new wife, Edith (née Card), in 1917 should have inserted the young girl into the life of an average rural child, but this was not to be the case.

In 1920, eight-year-old Othoa was playing with friends when they were chased by two older boys. In trying to escape, she climbed a fence and fell, landing on rocks. She suffered a badly injured back. Another accident story holds that she was thrown from a wagon at age two, but the tale recounted by her stepmother involving childhood play is more reliable and fits with the extant archive of Othoa's life.[2]

The accident left her bedridden, and after two weeks, Edith and Caesar sought help for her in Vancouver. According to Edith, the spine specialist they consulted put Othoa in a plaster cast and sent her home because the Vancouver General Hospital would not provide ongoing treatment to a non-resident. A hospital x-ray revealed why her accidental injury was so devastating: she had tuberculosis of the spine. For the next year or more, she languished on the island, unable to get appropriate medical attention, until one day in 1922 when her stepmother attended a meeting of the Hornby Island Women's Institute (WI). Hearing that they were raising money for disabled Russian children, Edith was incensed. What about Othoa and other injured Canadian children in desperate need of medical care? She wrote to Evangeline (Vandie) MacLachlan, secretary to the Women's Institutes in the province.[3] Three months later, MacLachlan persuaded the WIs to create a provincial fund for disabled children, Othoa had been sent for treatment to the Vancouver General Hospital, and the seeds for two pediatric healthcare facilities, the Crippled Children's Hospital in Vancouver, and the Queen Alexandra Solarium for Crippled Children on Vancouver Island, were sown.

Early local history adheres to the accident story, possibly because tuberculosis in children was difficult to detect and Othoa's bodily troubles seemed to begin after her fall.[4] Her accident, a brutal but ordinary consequence of childhood play,[5] was in fact a precipitating event in the development of services for disabled children in BC. What is more, it transformed obscure Othoa into public "Polly," the face of disability in the province in the 1920s. For more than a decade, Othoa stayed engaged with the movement that her stepmother's advocacy had initiated, becoming a figurehead in fundraising, a solarium patient and worker, and – briefly – a voice for disabled children and institutional care.

Complementing other chapters in this collection that examine industrial accidents and spectacular accidents like shipwrecks, this chapter is animated by an accident of the "banal and everyday" sort, almost imperceptible to history except that it was put to work in shaping the narrative of a settler girl and contemporary ideas of collective responsibility for her disability. As Cooter and Luckin make clear, accidents operate in a moral realm.[6] In this case, the accident's moral geometry juxtaposed an innocent child's misfortune and early twentieth-century settler womanhood's institution building. In this parable, the accident served as an ethical catalyst for a highly successful grassroots fundraising campaign and the founding of the province's first therapeutic institutions for disabled children in the 1920s. By examining the non-fatal accident and its afterlife, this chapter illuminates a trend in modern medicine that accidents could be overcome and managed – in this case, that Othoa's damaged spine could be cured – an optimism echoed in Sasha Mullally's chapter on kitchen-table surgery practice.

This is also a biography of a girl and young woman scripting the afterlife of her accident. Like the national myth of American president Franklin Delano Roosevelt, who famously triumphed over polio, Othoa's narrative centres on the series of steps that led from her accident and disability to "normal" young womanhood.[7] For an explanatory framework of this process, we look to the histories of the body and childhood, rehabilitative therapeutics and institutions, and critical disability and feminist studies. Children's hospitals, while still a small player in the field of institutionalized medicine, were growing in number in Canada, the United States, and across the British Empire, part of an increased interest in children's health and highly dependent on women's organizations for fundraising them into existence.[8] In BC, the efforts of Women's Institutes and a small group of pediatric health advocates in private and state health care were central to the emergence of youth rehabilitative medicine and services rationalized by contemporary humanitarian and economic arguments about the rights of the child and the need to turn the disabled body into a productive one.[9] Like Women's Institutes across the country, they were inspired by maternalism, eugenics, and a patriotic imperative.

Othoa was born into an era in which meanings of the child, the body, and health were rapidly changing. Campaigns to reduce infant and child death and eradicate the diseases of childhood held significant cultural valence, producing what historian Mona Gleason has termed "the public child." In 1924, the League of Nations adopted the Geneva Declaration of the Rights of the Child, recognizing the rights of youth and the obligation of adults to care for the young – an acknowledgment of society's responsibility to children like Othoa. Her accident rendered her "defective," pointing to a "compromised, if not failed, childhood" and body.[10] Through the WI and its crippled children's charity work, her body and ailment were harnessed into representing public responsibility for children and the promise of rehabilitation, cure, and ultimately youth itself.

The emergence of the public child coincided with another cultural fixation on what historian Jane Nicholas has termed the "making of the modern able body."[11] Schools in BC and elsewhere in Canada helped define that modern able body and move eugenicist thought into the mainstream by introducing health standards and monitoring, measuring, and examining children's bodies and behaviours.[12] In her study, *Canadian Carnival Freaks*, Nicholas shows that the modern exhibitionary complex "made bodies spectacles of meaning that were generative and reflective of social values."[13] Othoa became both a public child and a public spectacle as others strove to make sense and take control of her bodily difference and future. As a vehicle for WI fundraising, her disabled body was literally on display in the 1925 Exhibition Queen contest. During her time as a patient and then staff member at the new Queen Alexandra Solarium on Vancouver Island, she represented the promise of institutional therapy for children whose future was once deemed hopeless. Her innocence, her potential to outgrow her disease, and her alleged unrelentingly positive attitude – earning her the nickname Polly, derived from Pollyanna, the optimistic heroine of the 1913 children's novel of the same name – made her BC's original poster child for children with disabilities.[14]

Following the theme of the afterlife of an accident, we begin by telling the story of Othoa's early life and illness, moving on to her role as a poster child for disability and as a figurehead for WI fundraising campaigns pivotal to the founding of the Crippled Children's Hospital in Vancouver and the Queen Alexandra Solarium. The final section explicates Othoa's transformation into Polly, a patient and then staff member at the solarium, foregrounding the facility's social role in rehabilitating disabled children.

SETTLER FUTURITY, MATERNALISM, AND THE BC WOMEN'S INSTITUTES

One of the province's Northern Gulf Islands, Hornby Island is located about one-third of the way up the east side of Vancouver Island. This island is the traditional Indigenous territories of the Puntledge People, decimated by the 1862 smallpox epidemic.[15] White settlers began living on Hornby in the 1870s, with Caesar Scott's family among the first. By the early years of the twentieth century, the island had a population of about fifty settlers, including a small but active farming community.[16]

Along with his brother Alphonso, Caesar took possession of land on Hornby's north shore. He listed himself as a farmer on the census but, like most Gulf Islanders of the period, probably made his living from a combination of farming, fishing, game hunting, and logging.[17] Daisy and Caesar married in Vancouver in December 1910.[18] The newlyweds were on Hornby for the June 1911 census and for Othoa's birth in October. Daisy died on the island in May 1916, aged twenty-six.[19] A year later, Caesar, now thirty, married twenty-three-year-old Edith Card, a laundress from Victoria.[20]

The Hornby Island to which Caesar took his second bride in 1917 was very different from the community Daisy had encountered six years earlier. Roads now connected clusters of settlement and economic activity, an island school, a small store, and a Farmer's Institute that distributed literature and presented speakers from the Provincial Agricultural Department.[21] This kind of civic self-improvement underpinned the creation of a Women's Institute on Hornby in 1921, which Edith and other island women joined in its first year of operation.[22]

The afterlife of Othoa's accident hinges on this last island initiative, for by the 1920s BC Women's Institutes were a strong middle-class maternalist voice for promoting health and social care for settler families, particularly in the province's rural regions.[23] An emphasis on health and home was in the organization's DNA: the original Women's Institute was founded in Stoney Creek, Ontario, in 1897 by Adelaide Hoodless after her toddler died from tainted milk.[24] From the outset, the organization was politically activist, informed and empowered by middle-class maternalism, and concerned with the settler home, children, and community.[25] British Columbia's WIS, supported by the provincial government, petitioned the state to offer maternal and child health services in local health centres established in the interwar years and then helped fund and deliver them. This chapter thus presents a model of accident management through grassroots female settler advocacy that occupies the midway point between full philanthropy (for example, the Grenfell mission) and government response (for example, Workmen's Compensation), noted respectively by John Matchim and Ceilidh Auger-Day in this volume.

We build on early work by Seth Koven, Sonya Michel, and Anna Davin in characterizing the BC institutes as maternalist organizations.[26] Robin Teske and Mary Ann Tétreault help us appreciate how institute leaders and members took their roles as homemakers, nurturers, and moral beings into the public sphere, where the organization could be mobilized quickly and effectively to realize political and social goals.[27] The cause of BC's disabled children demonstrates how maternalism and the institutes worked in tandem with medicine, colonialism and eugenics, and how in the wake of World War I, WI members joined others in tackling disability as a patriotic duty and expression of women's recently acquired citizenship.[28] These links between the management of the accident, modern medicine, and the creation of the good citizen echo themes developed in John Matchim's chapter on the Grenfell mission in Newfoundland and Labrador in an earlier period.

The BC government launched the Women's Institute in 1909 – a time when the province was undergoing dramatic expansion in population, resource extraction, and rural settlement – beginning a tradition of hiring women to lead the organization and providing resources to each local institute (fifty cents per member annually).[29] These female leaders positioned the group as a civic and moral force in a province where men still greatly outnumbered women and concern about the racial diversity of the province, especially the presence of Asians, simmered.[30] Operating under the provincial Department of Agriculture, the group was given legal status as an independent provincial agricultural organization in 1911.[31]

Lillian Beall and Margaret Acton, the two island women who founded the Hornby chapter, were English farmers' wives, part of this national settler sisterhood. Unlike the female reformers who Margaret Jacobs considers in her work on maternal colonialism in the United States and Australia, institute women north of the forty-ninth parallel did not regard Indigenous children as part of their mandate.[32] Rather, they were engaged in a project that historians call "settler futurity," enacting colonialism through creating healthy white children – or restoring them to health – in their quest to produce future settler citizens.[33] WI members would have been aware of tuberculosis work being done by public health and school nurses.[34] As Daisy Scott and her daughter Othoa demonstrate, the disease was common in settler populations, with a fatality rate of 143 per 100,000 deaths in Vancouver during 1919, and it would be to this health challenge to which the WI turned.[35]

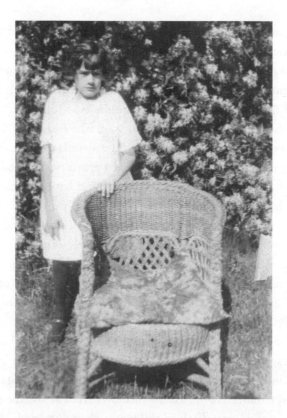

Fig. 11.1 Othoa Scott, in a family photograph likely taken in the garden of the Scott island homestead, spring 1925.

This colonial project took place at all levels of the wi. MacLachlan, who held key positions in the provincial organization from 1918 to 1946, had a history of health activism – including tuberculosis work – that was reflected in the direction of the organization under her tenure.[36] Local institute members like Beall, Acton, and Edith Scott educated themselves in health matters, pushed for medical inspection of rural schools, and staffed baby clinics.[37] They might well have agreed with accident sociologist Judith Green's statement, "Stories about accidents are vehicles for reaching a consensus about proper responsibilities and apportioning of blame."[38] Evoking the institute's commitment to child welfare, and framing her 1922 appeal for help as a mother unable to meet the health needs of her injured child,

Edith Scott employed the language of settler maternalism and the ethos of WI public responsibility.[39]

A defining feature of MacLachlan's life story was her "saviour" role in securing treatment for Othoa Scott. The WI leader drafted two highly placed BC medical men who were key to the events that followed.[40] Dr Frank McTavish, the Vancouver orthopedic surgeon who had seen the young girl following her accident, was asked to confirm details of Othoa's condition and treatment.[41] Dr Henry Esson Young, the provincial medical officer and a staunch ally of the Women's Institutes, would have seen this initiative fitting into his ambitious provincial public health program.[42] He advised MacLachlan to find a local institute willing to solicit funds and he secured money to cover transporting Othoa to Vancouver and placing her in the hospital children's ward.[43] According to Edith Scott, Othoa remained in treatment for eight months and "came out cured."[44] This success of long-term treatment in an acute-care hospital underscored the need for a pediatric rehabilitation facility.[45]

Unable to raise support from chapters in Victoria, MacLachlan took Edith Scott's request to the Central Park Women's Institute in Vancouver.[46] The group donated $25 to buy a back brace for Othoa and began the Fund for Crippled Children of BC, asking members from across the province to donate money and locate disabled children in their districts.[47] Membership response to the story of a needy white settler girl on a remote island was overwhelming, and by early 1924 organizers had $1,400.[48] Money was set aside to found a hospital for disabled children, and a year later the Women's Institute Hospital Association for Crippled Children (aka the Crippled Children's Fund) was incorporated as a "daughter organization" of the BC Women's Institutes, splitting into two committees – one to support a Vancouver institution and another to work toward a facility on Vancouver Island.[49]

PRINCESS OTHOA AND THE GLEAM O' HOPE CAMPAIGN

In the mid-1920s, "little" Othoa became a household name in the lower mainland. As the first child selected to benefit from the Crippled Children's Fund, her name was quickly associated with the fundraising efforts of the Women's Institutes to create rehabilitation services for BC's disabled youth.

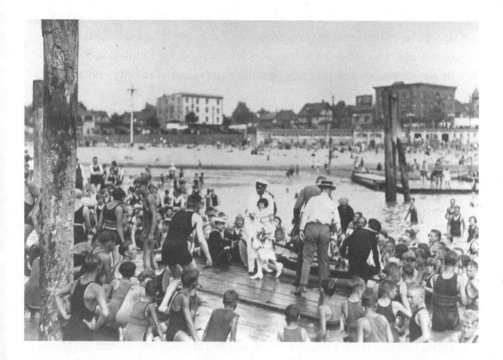

Fig. 11.2 Dressed in white and surrounded by a crowd of young people, a grinning Othoa arrives in English Bay for the Queen of the Vancouver Exhibition pageant, 1925.

Her celebrity peaked in the summer of 1925, when she ran as a contestant in the Queen of the Vancouver Exhibition pageant. The exhibition's inaugural beauty pageant generated great excitement and substantial funds for the fifteenth annual fair as well as for the wɪ's province-wide Hospital Association for Crippled Children campaign. The pomp of the pageant was very much of its era and in line with the wɪ's British connection, although the inclusion of a "crippled" girl heralded a shift in exhibitionary culture.

As a pageant contestant, fourteen-year-old Othoa joined a long tradition of bodily spectacle involving children. Agricultural and industrial fairs of the nineteenth century emphasized the gendered labour of rural life. But as fairs transitioned away from spectacles of production toward consumption and entertainment, beauty contests and baby shows were added – the latter an example of the sentimentalization and public commodification of childhood.[50] Modern Canada's exhibitionary culture comprised "visual spectacles available for easy consumption"[51] that reinforced racial, class, national, age, and gendered hierarchies. The Vancouver Exhibition pageant in 1925 carried on this tradition, instilling the values of the city's dominant and aspirational classes.

This local exhibition, later known as the Pacific National Exhibition, had begun in 1910 as an industrial and agricultural fair to promote animal husbandry and "the improvement of the breed of horses, cattle, sheep, pigs, dogs" and to develop the province's natural resources.[52] By 1925, children and youth were well integrated into the exhibition: that year, the Elks sponsored a flag day for youngsters, providing free ice cream and Union Jacks to 25,000 visitors.[53] The pageantry of thousands of children waving the Union Jack reminded exhibition attendees of the superiority of British culture and white settler society and their deep connection to it.

The 1925 Queen of the Exhibition pageant was part fundraiser for the fair, local businesses and causes, and part beauty contest. As Patrizia Gentile shows in her history of Canadian beauty contests, such public spectacles helped create a visual norm about beauty, bodies, and nation that asserted racial hierarchy and promoted white settler femininity as foundational for a strong, prosperous, and healthy nation.[54] Spectacles where bodies were displayed – from beauty contests to freak shows – abounded in this era, reinforcing standards of beauty and ugliness that defined each other, as Nicholas reminds us.[55] Othoa, however, did not fit neatly into this binary. Her disability should have exempted her from a place in the pageant, yet it did not: her place depended on the flexibility of the social category "disabled," her cuteness and innocence, and her ability to represent hope and recovery for a white settler child.

The BC Women's Institute collaborated with a Vancouver businessman, W.C. Shelly of Shelly Brothers Bakery, to enter Othoa in the competition and name her "Gleam O' Hope Princess." Beginning in the early 1920s, the Crippled Children's Fund sought financial donations using stories such as Othoa's in which medical interventions into the lives of disabled children allowed for "complete recovery" and therefore hope. In 1926, the *Vancouver Province* pictured three smiling girls, the text proclaiming, "Where once their future held nothing but gloom, it now holds hope for complete recovery."[56] Othoa was eminently marketable as a "gleam of hope" because her spinal injury was largely hidden, detectable only in her stiff posture; unlike the three girls pictured in the newspaper, she did not need crutches or remedial footwear. Perhaps most important-ly, her diminutive size, whiteness, and smile made her "cute," a commod-ity aesthetic that was part and parcel of save-the-children campaigns by 1925.[57] Othoa fit the interwar era look of "cute," exuding joy and determi-nation despite her accident and disease, and a pixie quality that played on the feminine maternal empathy displayed by the women behind the Crippled Children's Fund.[58]

As a contestant, Othoa was fêted in the weeks leading up to the com-petition at functions designed to stimulate donations to the exhibition in the form of VanEx bonds, a portion of which would go to the WI's Crippled Children's Fund. Her sponsors ran advertisements describing her as the "first cripple cured under the Crippled Children's Fund." A $1 bond was good for admission to the fair and counted as a thousand votes for Othoa. Her picture accompanied the advertisements of the VanEx bonds. Her story included her life on remote Hornby Island, where "the steamer calls but once a week."[59] To launch her campaign, the WI organized a spectacu-lar trip to Vancouver for her by seaplane. "Out of a Clear Sky – a Gleam of Hope," the newspapers reported.[60] Dressed for the occasion in a white dress with matching shoes, she was met by thousands of children at English Bay where she was scooped up in a "pure white car" and taken to the Hotel Vancouver for a tea in her honour. The white imagery abounded in her campaign reinforcing her innocence, youth, and white settler background. Audiences were reassured that this girl who had suffered tragedy as a child had talents in the form of piano, singing, and reciting, as well as ambition – she intended to leave her rural roots to pursue a business course.[61] Role-modelling determination to lead a "useful" rather than parasitic life was key to her designation as princess of the pageant.

The contest was held on the first night of the exhibition with the pag-eant/crowning to follow. The latter mimicked the 1837 coronation of Queen Victoria. Photographs of Othoa show her decked in white with a crown on her head, looking much younger than the other contestants. She appears small and her body stiff, as if in a brace. She was not crowned queen, but she was runner-up, her prize a course in stenography.

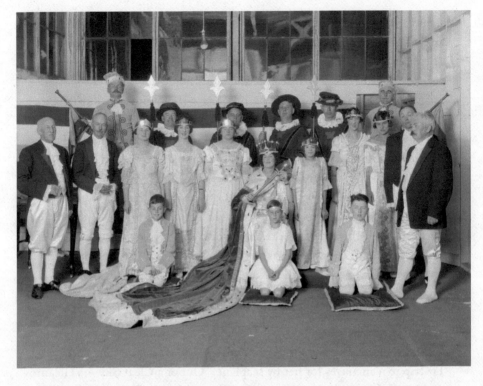

Fig. 11.3 Princess Gleam O' Hope, the smallest contestant in the Queen of the Vancouver Exhibition pageant, to the right of the crowned queen. Othoa's rigid posture indicates the use of a back brace.

Although Othoa would later be a patient at the newly founded Queen Alexandra Solarium on Vancouver Island, the pageant turned her into a "cured cripple," a label that was reproduced frequently in the coverage of the pageant. This can be read as her first decisive step away from her accident; receipt of Crippled Children's funds and medical attention launched her on a path toward recovery and a return to "normal." Rather than remind children and parents of the dangers of childhood accidents and disease, the discursive Othoa represented "hope" for a new generation of disabled children who could aspire to bodily normalcy. By the time of the pageant, the wi's Crippled Children's Fund boasted more than forty cured children. Othoa's campaign and participation in the pageant was part of a larger movement to educate the public about disability, and the rise of the disabled poster child would become a feature of fundraising campaigns across the twentieth century. Othoa was impish, not helpless, and was easily turned into a beloved icon of hope for childhood.[62]

INSTITUTIONALIZING CHILD REHABILITATION IN BC

Rehabilitative medicine was in its infancy in Canada when Othoa fell from the fence, but hospitals for children had been founded in most Canadian cities by the 1920s and sanatoriums dotted the nation's rural landscape.[63] An institutional and civic response – often initiated by women's organizations – to long-standing concerns about childhood disease, these facilities offered hope for the future to a society ravaged by war-related death and disability.[64] Medical and rehabilitative staff in pediatric hospitals and sanitoriums undertook the painstaking process of correcting the defective bodies of disabled children and bolstering the health of "delicate" children, invoking a humanitarian and economic rationale infused with eugenics.[65]

wi fundraising efforts like the Gleam O' Hope Princess and contributions from local chapters provided operational funds for bc's first pediatric rehabilitation facilities.[66] Frank McTavish, Othoa's physician, was pivotal to the 1928 establishment of the Vancouver Crippled Children's Hospital.[67] wi funding underwrote a Vancouver clinic from 1923 to 1926, where seventy-six children from across the province were treated under McTavish's direction.[68] In 1928 the Crippled Children's Hospital (ccH) opened in the city's Marpole district, demonstrating the prestige of orthopaedic surgery.[69] In its first five years, the hospital cared for 354 patients, holding a Saturday-morning outdoor clinic. Eighty per cent of its patients were unable to pay for the treatment.[70]

Touting the facility as a "Repair Shop for Broken Children" in a 1929 article, a journalist described how the "twisted limbs" of children like Albert, a "little Japanese boy from Prince Rupert," were "repaired" through a combination of Dr McTavish's surgical skills, corrective exercise, massage and physiotherapy, and daily sunbaths using an Alpine lamp with "healing violet rays."[71] More boot camp than hospital, the ccH expected its young patients to work hard, overcome their disability, and become productive citizens – regarded by critical disability scholars as the standard prescription for crip-success in the early twentieth-century.[72] The WI had stepped back from funding the hospital by the time it opened a large new facility in 1933.[73]

The Queen Alexandra Solarium (QAS), which opened its doors on Vancouver Island in March 1927, with Othoa Scott as one of its first patients, had a different orientation but a continued connection with the Women's Institutes.[74] Its founding physician Cyril Wace had conducted a provincial survey on children in need of orthopaedic treatment and was keen to use ideas and practices of Swiss physician Auguste Rollier and the British practitioner Sir Henry Gauvain to treat the patients he had identified.[75] Rollier employed a combination of simple splints, heliotherapy (sun bathing), craft activity, and light manual work for patients who came to his clinics in Leysin, Switzerland with tuberculosis, Pott's disease, and ailments of the hips, knees, and ankles.[76] Gauvain was medical superintendent at Lord Mayor Treloar Cripples Hospital in Alton, England, where treatment was based on the idea that healthy outdoor living and meaningful activity could rectify psychological damage caused by extended illness and long separation from home and kin. "Sunlight," Gauvain wrote, "exhilarates and enlivens ... like a draught of good champagne" but was also "the world's greatest antiseptic" and was believed to act on deep-seated lesions like those created by tuberculosis.[77]

Wace became an avid promoter of a similar facility for children on Vancouver Island and quickly raised $25,000 from Victoria businesses and community organizations. Hearing of the plan, MacLachlan committed the Women's Institutes to immediate action. In April 1926 the Queen Alexandra Society for Crippled Children was incorporated as a separate society, independent from the Vancouver-based Women's Institute Hospital Association for Crippled Children. Wace's daughter, nurse Elizabeth Wace, learned how to manufacture celluloid splints for children from Gauvain, and Alton nurse Miss H.I. Willis was hired.[78] Wace was careful to differentiate between the preventative and curative solarium and the surgical acute-care hospital.[79] In addition, he built on the practices of Gauvain and Rollier by stressing that a system of education and occupational training would be undertaken alongside treatment.[80]

A rural site north of Victoria on the scenic west side of Saanich Inlet was selected because it provided the pure air, record hours of sunshine, and access to safe sea bathing that were considered ideal for healing chronic conditions and disability.[81] For Othoa, coming from Hornby Island, the natural elements of the site would have been familiar, but these were now paired with "scientific" physiotherapy employing splints for "patient re-education of the injured and wasted muscles," helio-sun-therapy, and daily school lessons.[82] First-person descriptions, government and media images, and other contemporary accounts of the solarium noted the homelike ambiance and extolled the outdoor veranda that ran the entire length of the building, accessed directly from the three wards by large patio windows – a feature that borrowed heavily from Leysin and Alton.[83] Plans included gently sloping walkways at either end of the building leading to the garden and a tidal saltwater swimming pool.[84]

Wace had a genius for engaging the well-connected and well-qualified with his project. The English educator and eugenicist Alice Ravenhill joined the solarium committee at its inception in 1925 and took responsibility for convening its women's auxiliary and selecting hospital equipment.[85] Ravenhill published a 1927 article in the American journal *Modern Hospital* lauding the many merits of the new rehabilitative institution and recounting Othoa's story.[86] In September of that year, Gauvain himself twice toured the site, the second time with the lieutenant governor, the premier of Northern Ireland, and the bishop of Columbia, who led a short inaugural religious service.[87] Letters of endorsement flooded in from medical societies and the National Federation of Women's Institutes in Great Britain; donations for the new facility included an ambulance, thirty beds and cots, two invalid chairs, and a pair of hand-propelled ambulances of "excellent design."[88]

With his professional commitment to health innovation, child welfare, and the Women's Institutes, provincial health officer Henry Esson Young was another obvious ally for this project. This hybrid scheme that secured grassroots support, high-level patronage, and professional involvement would have attracted his interest. Esson Young's presence on the solarium committee and his 1928 article about the project in the Canadian Public Health Association's professional journal were clear demonstrations of his – and hence the provincial health state's – support for a therapeutic program that was new to Canada. The influential provincial bureaucrat wrote that the solarium's care regime for its young patients aimed to tap the power inherent within the "living tissues" of the ailing child body, following a careful regime of "sunshine, fresh air, sea bathing, simple food and suitable exercise."[89] The solarium was to be Othoa's home and community in her young adult years.

WHEN OTHOA BECAME POLLY

Sanatorium facilities like the QAS would give disabled youth what child savers had long been arguing for on behalf of the nation's children: a childhood spent in school, time in a safe and clean environment, fresh air, sunshine, good food, appropriate exercise, and rest. The institution facilitated the removal of disabled and unhealthy children from impoverished families and replaced homes deemed inadequate with rehabilitative medicine and middle-class values and practices to remake the imperfect child into the productive citizen. Despite the fragmenting of family, these institutions were conceived as positive substitutes for home, in the same way that compulsory schooling had replaced what was seen as substandard home education decades earlier.

In 1927, two years after Othoa stood as the Gleam O' Hope princess and helped raise funds for the cause of crippled children's facilities, she became a patient at the QAS, her treatment paid for in small amounts sent by local WI chapters from Lynn Valley (North Vancouver), Peachland (Okanagan), and the Valdez Island (Salish Sea) groups.[90] It was during her time at the QAS that Othoa became known as Polly, the ever-optimistic girl who overcame her physical disability. Othoa/Polly's central place in the origin story of the institution persisted and was embellished in the press. In this retelling she is "a lonely little girl with a crippled spine keeping her from enjoying life as did others on Hornby Island and who knew nothing of the outside world."[91] She was just one of the children who were "fortunate enough to be received there, as compared with their former existence under trying and oftentimes hopeless conditions." Likely using her time as a patient to gain further education, Polly then took up her Gleam O' Hope award for a secretarial course in Victoria, returning afterwards to QAS to work in the office and with the younger children. In this way, the institution fulfilled its promise to her for "a normal life" upon release and facilitated her second step away from accident victim and crippled child to young professional woman and (briefly) experiential expert on disability.

Polly's public persona was further enhanced when she was invited in 1928 to write a series of letters about life at the QAS for Victoria's *Daily Times*, putting a face on the experience of children in this new institution, and creating awareness about treatment for disabled youth. Another resident, Audrey Alexandra Brown, also wrote about her stay at QAS in her memoir, *The Log of a Lame Duck*. The lame ducker recounts her long road to recovery, painful treatments for arthritis in 1934, and the ultimate ability to walk away from the institution after a year. Both Polly and Audrey present narratives of overcoming adversity and hopelessness, and with the help of the QAS, achieving the promise of a near-"normal" life.

Polly and Audrey were not typical QAS residents. The facility accepted boys to the age of twelve years and girls to the age of fourteen, and the two young women, aged sixteen and thirty when they entered QAS, must have stood out among the patient population. Polly was a charity case but a local celebrity, and Audrey was already a published poet recognized in Canada's literary community.[92] In contrast, many QAS patients were young charity cases from remote regions of the province. Polly divided residents into "up-children" and those who were bedridden, a functional categorization likely used by staff as well.[93] In her memoir, Audrey relied on racist tropes common in 1930s BC to describe patients: an Indigenous girl lay reserved and quiet, while two Chinese-Canadian girls – believed to be undervalued because of their sex – required rescue from a cruel father who had kept them in a basement.[94] Both writers were captivated by the QAS's luxurious surroundings, delighting in its routines, ambiance, and large windows and wide verandah offering scenic views.

Polly's solarium vignettes underscore a particular affective experience for disabled children in treatment. The strongest emotion was gratitude: we "don't talk about being crippled," Polly wrote, knowing things "could be worse."[95] The loneliness and isolation of a disabled childhood, she suggested, were cured by this collective living. This focus on the social benefits of solarium life rather than home sickness reassured the public that the QAS and institutionalization of disabled children was far better than a hopeless, isolated childhood spent in a family home without constructive training or treatment.

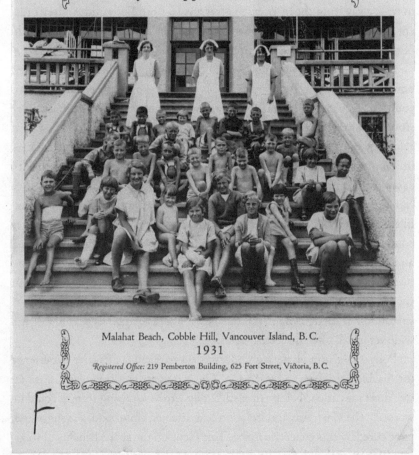

Sixth *Annual Report*

Queen Alexandra Solarium
for Crippled Children

Malahat Beach, Cobble Hill, Vancouver Island, B.C.
1931
Registered Office: 219 Pemberton Building, 625 Fort Street, Victoria, B.C.

Fig. 11.4 "Up-children" and staff pose for the cover of *Sixth Annual Report: Queen Alexandra Solarium for Crippled Children, 1931.*

Indeed, Polly's newspaper columns conform to a genre of children's letter writing exemplified in summer camp correspondence, with details of place and space animated by accounts of daily routine and special events. She describes delicious roasts and fish (sometimes caught by residents), ice cream for dessert, games, story-time, prayers, and small chores.[96] Weather permitting, the day started with an adventure in the pool at the sea's edge, she wrote. The up-children made their way down to the pool alongside those in wheelchairs or on the trolley. Lessons occupied the main part of the day, with handiwork and crafting punctuating the QAS curriculum.[97]

In an era when occupational therapy was becoming mainstream, QAS offered embroidery, knitting, and sewing to both girls and boys.[98] Discussing crafting at QAS gave Polly an opportunity to address gender and anxieties about the feminine setting of the institution. Teaching both girls and boys handiwork, she maintained, did not interfere with boys becoming "He-Men." In an era of concern over boys' "sissy" tendencies, when the very definition of masculinity centred on able-bodiedness, it's not surprising that Polly commented multiple times about male patients' potential to become men despite their disability – a touchstone in veteran rehabilitation programs of the era.[99] She helped her public to imagine that QAS boys defined themselves in contrast to girls – eschewing "girls'" literature and playing games and roughhousing like "ordinary" boys, and of course overcoming physical challenges.[100]

Polly repeatedly makes the point that disabled children are capable and "normal." She chides the reader for thinking that a "paralyzed leg or a stiff knee" would keep children from swimming – they held swimming races and elaborate water games and "all enjoy it very much."[101] Despite the absence of a schoolroom, lessons were held daily in the mornings and afternoons, in the wards or on the verandah. Like Cyril Wace, her former physician and now her supervisor, Polly emphasized that the QAS followed the same curriculum as any "ordinary" school, reassuring her readers that they had schoolbooks and were learning reading, writing and arithmetic, doing physical drills, and taking singing lessons.[102] Her focus on education at the QAS relates to the perception that disabled children left at home were often deprived of schooling, reinforcing their poor chances for a productive future.[103]

In 1932, Polly returned to the QAS to celebrate her twenty-first birthday. Fêted as the institution's first patient, one with extraordinary "pluck," she literally stood as proof of the power of remedial treatment as she now walked without effort.[104] She became a staff member, Dr Wace's stenographer and assistant, a "living testimonial to the excellent work it is accomplishing on behalf of crippled children."[105] Polly and Audrey confirmed to their reading publics that disabled children could become "useful" and happy members of society.[106] Polly continued to work at QAS before launching herself into adulthood, meaning marriage to local schoolteacher Malcolm Dunnett and motherhood; her former name, Othoa Scott, lived on as the title of the WI's fundraising efforts on behalf of "crippled children."

CONCLUSION

In 1920 Othoa Scott experienced a devastating accident while playing. Like many other children who suffered from serious injury or disease, she was left to languish in a remote island community. Othoa lying abed, tormented by pain that her parents could not alleviate, encapsulates the element of disorder that is the essence of the accident, a state that appears "to challenge the logic of linear positivist explanations of progress and to mock the metanarratives of philosophy and sociology."[107] Reading Sasha Mullally's chapter in this volume, it is easy to image a similar scene in the MacCormack farmhouse in rural Prince Edward Island as a distraught mother strove to help her child through a long process of healing and rehabilitation. Yet in this post–World War I moment in BC, a convergence of professional and state development, female agency, and settler futurity, along with Othoa's personal attributes, gave her particular accident a prodigious afterlife.

Othoa's fall from the fence became a public accident, affecting professional and community groups and offering hope to disabled children across the province. Inspired by the power of her story, BC's Women's Institutes partnered with provincial pediatric and rehabilitation specialists to found two path-breaking institutions for disabled and delicate children. At the Vancouver Crippled Children's Hospital and the Queen Alexandra Solarium, damaged and diseased young bodies could be reclaimed through a combination of science and nature, neglected minds educated, and idle hands trained in useful skills. Removed from what were considered deficient, ignorant, and neglectful families, these broken children could be recreated as useful citizens. The first-person accounts by two young settler women, Othoa Scott and Audrey Brown, along with contemporary commentaries, suggest that the Queen Alexandra Solarium improved the lives of its young patients; yet it is important to remember that the majority of them were very young and vulnerable, and the history of children's institutions is riddled with abuse and suffering.[108] More biographical and institutional studies need to be done on the boundary of disability studies and the history of the accident.

Othoa remained central to these developments until the mid-1930s. As Princess Gleam O' Hope, her cuteness, diminutive size, and white settler background afforded her the powerful cultural designation that could be deployed to maximum fundraising effect. As Polly, first a patient and then a staff member at the QAS, her pluck, Pollyanna disposition, and determination to succeed in the "normal" adult world were harnessed to sell a new future for modern children with disabilities. With her marriage and subsequent life as wife and mother of three children, Othoa took her final steps beyond the social and physical barriers created by her youthful accident, fulfilling the Women's Institute's normative expectations of her gender in the able world. Perhaps as a reminder of this long transition, she kept the name Polly for the rest of her life.[109]

ACKNOWLEDGMENTS

We acknowledge funding from the UBC History Department, the exceptional research of Georgia Twiss, the efforts of UBC Okanagan archivist Paige Hohmann, and the generosity of Regan Fahey and the Hornby Island Archives.

NOTES

1 Edith Wilcox née Scott, notebook (ca. 1978), file 6, box 1, Early Settlers Collection, Scott Family: Othoa Scott and the BC Children's Hospital, Hornby Island Archives (hereafter HIA); Edith Wilcox née Scott, typed document (ca. 1981), Early Settlers Collection, HIA.

2 Corrigall, *History of Hornby Island*, 22.

3 Wilcox, notebook, Early Settlers Collection, HIA; Wilcox, typed document, Early Settlers Collection, HIA; Forbes, *Wild Roses at Their Feet*, 82–3; British Columbia Women's Institutes, *100 Years of BC Women's Institutes, 1909–2009*, 17.

4 McCuaig, *Weariness, the Fever, and the Fret*, 158.

5 Gleason, "From "Disgraceful Carelessness" to "Intelligent Precaution"; Myers, "Didactic Sudden Death."

6 Cooter and Luckins, "Accidents in History: An Introduction," 3.

7 Fairchild, "Polio Narrative."

8 Wright, *Sick Kids*, 21.

9 "Solarium Planned for Vancouver Island," *Victoria Daily Times* (7 March 1928), 7.

10 Gleason, *Small Matters*, 135.

11 Nicholas, *Canadian Carnival Freaks*, 7.

12 Gleason, *Small Matters*, 9–10; Ellis, *Class by Themselves?*, 11–51; Clarke, "Sacred Daemons."

13 Nicholas, *Canadian Carnival Freaks*, 3.

14 Longmore, "Heaven's Special Child," 34–41.

15 John Millan, "The Pentlatch People of Denman Island," unpublished paper presented at Islands of British Columbia 2004: An Interdisciplinary Exploration Conference, Denman Island, BC, August 2004.

16 Corrigall, *History of Hornby Island*, 29–31.

17 Sandwell, *Contesting Rural Space*, 21–2.

18 Marriage Registration 023165 to 023677, 1910, BC, Division of Vital Statistics, GR 2962, vol. 062, BC Archives (hereafter BCA).

19 Denman Island, District 8, 5,1911, Canada Census, 1911; Daisy Scott, BC Death Registrations, 1872–1986, BC Division of Vital Statistics, GR 2951, BCA.

20 Marriage Registration 040879 to 040991, 1917, BC, Vital Statistics, BCA.

21 Corrigall, *History of Hornby Island*, 35–39.

22 Ibid., 31; British Columbia Women's Institute, *Modern Pioneers*, 36, 82.

23 Zacharias, "British Columbia Women's Institute in the Early Years"; Green, "Rise of Motherhood."

24 For the founding story of the Ontario organization, see Ambrose, *For Home and Country*.

25 See Andrews, *Acceptable Face of Feminism*, 1–16, 79–99; Halpern, *And on That Farm He Had a Wife*, 3–18; Ambrose, *Great Rural Sisterhood*, 69–96.

26 See Koven and Michel, "Introduction: Mother Worlds"; Davin, "Imperialism and Motherhood."

27 Teske and Tétreault, introduction to *Conscious Acts and the Politics of Social Change*, 1–25.

28 Devereux, *Growing a Race*; Wright, *Sick Kids*, 175. On BC suffrage, see Campbell, *Great Revolutionary Wave*.

29 Zacharias, "British Columbia Women's Institute in the Early Years," 55–61; Jean Barman, *West beyond the West*, 129–50; Notes re Women's Institutes in B.C., 5 January 1915, Advisory Board of Women's Institutes of British Columbia, 1911–27, PR-1031, MS-0178, Minutes and Scrapbook, BCA.

30 Davies, *Into the House of Old*, 17; Barman, 129–50.

31 Zacharias, "British Columbia Women's Institute in the Early Years," 58–9.

32 Jacobs, *White Mother to a Dark Race*.

33 Ishiguro, "Histories of Settler Colonialism," 5–14; Megan Davies, extracts from the Report of the Women's Institutes of British Columbia, 1909–1914, PR-1031, MS-0178, BCA.

34 Davies, "Competent Professionals and Modern Methods;" Forbes, *Wild Roses at Their Feet*, 82–3; Zilm and Warbinek, TB *Nurses in B.C.*, 10.

35 Zilm and Warbinek, TB *Nurses in B.C.*, 15. In 1921 the provincial government took over Tranquille Sanitorium, a private tuberculosis facility near Kamloops. Norton, *Whole Little City by Itself*, 102–6.

36 Forbes, *Wild Roses at Their Feet*, 17. MacLachlan's commitment to health care also appears to have been personal, linked to a serious prolonged family illness that could have been averted by prompt hospital treatment. H.L. Baley, "Fund for Crippled Children," *Country Life in British Columbia*, ca. 1923.

37 Zacharias, "British Columbia Women's Institute in the Early Years," 8–32; Davies, "Mother's Medicine."

38 Green, *Risk and Misfortune*.

39 V.S. MacLachlan, "History to Date of Women's Institute Crippled Children's Hospital Fund," Women's Institute Hospital Association Minutes and Reports, 1925–1926, box 18, file 002, Queen Alexandra Solarium Archives (hereafter QASA).

40 Forbes, *Wild Roses at Their Feet*, 82–3; British Columbia Women's Institutes, *100 Women*, 17.

41 MacLachlan, "History to Date"; British Columbia Women's Institutes, *Modern Pioneers*, 17.

42 Davies, "Young, Henry Esson."

43 MacLachlan, "History to Date."

44 Wilcox notebook, Early Settlers Collection, HIA; Wilcox, typed document, Early Settlers Collection, HIA.

45 Marcellus, "'Tiny Cripples and the Sunshine of Life.'"

46 Mira A. Barber, Early History of the Crippled Children's Hospital of Vancouver, undated, BC, PR-1129, MS-1592, BCA.

47 Mina Barber to Secretaries of the Women's Institutes, 3 April 1923, folder 6, box 09, British Columbia Women's Institute fonds, OSC ARC 08, University of British

Columbia – Okanagan, Okanagan Archives and Special Collections (OASC); Log Book of the Crippled Children's Hospital, ca. March 1923, folder 45, box 05, OSC ARC 08, OASC.

48 MacLachlan, "History to Date"; British Columbia Women's Institute, *Modern Pioneers*, 16–17; British Columbia Women's Institute, *100 Years*, 35–7.

49 British Columbia Women's Institute, *Modern Pioneers*, 17; H.L. Bayley to Cloverdale Women's Institute, 6 January 1925, folder 6, box 09, OSC ARC 08, UBCOA; undated document, ca. 1925, 018-002, QASA.

50 Pearson, "Infantile Specimens," 361.

51 Nicholas, *Canadian Carnival Freaks*, 23.

52 *Official Catalogue and Programme of Vancouver's First Exhibition* (Vancouver: Sunday Sunset Presses, 1910).

53 "Record Crowd at Gates of Big Fair," *Vancouver Province*, 10 August 1925, 1.

54 Gentile, *Queen of the Maple Leaf*, 5.

55 Nicholas, *Canadian Carnival Freaks*, 17.

56 "These Are Happy Wards of the Crippled Children's Fund," *Vancouver Province*. 13 May 1926, 30.

57 Nicholas, *Canadian Carnival Freaks*, 174.

58 Ibid., 176–7.

59 "Shelly Bros' Candidate for Queen of the Fair Enters the Contest," *Vancouver Province*, 18 June 1925, 13.

60 "Out of a Clear Sky – a Gleam of Hope," *Vancouver Sun*, 9 July 1925, 7; "Princess Coming Here by Seaplane," *Province*, 6 July 1925, 2.

61 "Shelly Bros' Candidate for Queen of the Fair Enters the Contest."

62 For iconic disabled children, see Longmore, "Heaven's Special Child."

63 Friedland, *Restoring the Spirit*; Boyd-Scriver, *Montreal Children's Hospital*; Medovy, *Vision Fulfilled*; Wright, *Sick Kids*; Burke, *Building Resistance*.

64 Wright, *Sick Kids*, 34; Burke, *Building Resistance*.

65 Friedland, *Restoring the Spirit*; Marcellus, "Tiny Cripples," 412; Wright, *Sick Kids*, 86

66 MacLachlan, "History to Date," QASA; British Columbia Women's Institute, *Modern Pioneers*, 17.

67 "Death Claims Dr. F. McTavish." *Vancouver Daily Province* (9 November 1936), 6.

68 President's Address, February 1926, Women's Institute's Hospital Association for Crippled Children, Third Annual Report, 018-002, QASA.

69 Mrs. W.H. Carswell, Secretary-Treasurer, 30 December 1927, Women's Institute/ Canadian Red Cross Society, Crippled Children's Hospital Branch, folder 07, box 07, OSC ARC 08, UBCOA; Wright, *Sick Kids*, 71–95.

70 Key sources of information about the early CCH were the BC Women's Institute Honor Roll, PR-1129, MS-1592, BCA; Barber, Early History of the Crippled Children's Hospital, PR-1129, MS-1592, BCA; A Decade of Successful Achievement in the History of the Crippled Children's Hospital, ca. 1935, folder 07, box 09, OSC ARC 08, UBCOA.

71 Cecilia McReavy, "Repair Shop for Broken Children," *Sunday Sun*, magazine supplement, 30 November 1929.
72 McReavy, "Repair Shop"; Wright, *Sick Kids*, 85–6; Reaume, *Lyndhurst*.
73 A Decade of Successful Achievement, file 07, box 09, BCWI collection, UBCOA.
74 The solarium was named after Britain's Queen Alexandra, a champion of the disabled and herself disabled. Barbara McDonell, "Hope for the Handicapped: Queen Alexandra Hospital for Children," *The Islander*, November 1984, 4.
75 McDonell, "Hope for the Handicapped," 4.
76 Rollier, "'Sun Cure.'" For a full explanation of Rollier's techniques, see Hobday, "Sunlight Therapy and Solar Architecture."
77 Gauvain, "Effect of Sun, Sea and Open-Air in the Treatment of Disease."
78 First Annual Report of the Queen Alexandra Solarium for Crippled Children, ca. 1927, folder 14, box 05, OSC ARC 08, UBCOA.
79 Wace, "Queen Alexandra Solarium for Crippled Children," 702–6.
80 Ibid.
81 Vancouver Island Committee, Women's Institute Hospital Association for Crippled Children, ca. 1925–26, folder 06, box 09, OSC ARC 08, UBCOA; Wright, *Sick Kids*, 180, details work done at the Toronto Children's Hospital's Thistletown location to create a pastoral setting, but this was not necessary at Mill Bay.
82 Vancouver Island Committee, ca. 1925–26, folder 06, box 09, OSC ARC 08, UBCOA.
83 First Annual Report, file 14, box 05, OSC ARC 08, UBCOA; Hobday, "Sunlight Therapy."
84 The pool is mentioned in First Annual Report, folder 14, box 05, OSC ARC 08, UBCOA.
85 Ibid.
86 Ravenhill, "Where Health Is Found in Sunbathing," 118, 120, 122; de Zwart, "Alice Ravenhill."
87 First Annual Report, folder 14, box 05, OSC ARC 08, UBCOA.
88 Ibid.
89 Young, "Queen Alexandra Solarium," 374–7.
90 C. Wace to Mrs. M.L. Murrey, 11 February 1928, folder 45, box 05, OSC ARC 08, UBCOA; Accounts, Othoa Scott Fund, 30 April 1928, folder 45, box 05, OSC ARC 08, UBCOA; 11 C. Wace to Mrs. H.H. Pitts, September 1928, folder 45, box 05, OSC ARC 08, UBCOA.
91 A. Winnifred Lee, "Formal Opening Takes Place Tomorrow," *Daily Province*, 24 March 1928, 19.
92 Canada's Early Women Writers, SFU Library Digital Collections, Simon Fraser University, Burnaby, BC, 1980–2014, https://digital.lib.sfu.ca/islandora/object/ceww:830.
93 "Letters of Polly of the Sanitorium," *Victoria Daily Times*, 15 September 1928.
94 Brown, *Log of the Lame Duck*, 7.
95 "Letters of Polly," *Victoria Daily Times*, 1 September 1928.
96 "Letters of Polly," *Victoria Daily Times*, 8 August 1928, 25 August 1928, 15 September 1928.
97 Friedland, *Restoring the Spirit*.
98 Ibid.

99   Morton, *Winning the Second Battle.*
100   "Letters of Polly," *Victoria Daily Times,* 8 and 28 September 1928.
101   "Letters of Polly," *Victoria Daily Times,* 28 July 1928.
102   "Letters of Polly," *Victoria Daily Times,* 4 August 1928.
103   Wace, "Queen Alexandra Solarium."
104   "The Solarium Honours 'Polly,'" *Victoria Daily Times,* 4 November 1932.
105   Ibid.
106   Kinnaird, "Facilities for the Care of Crippled Children."
107   Cooter and Luckin, "Introduction: Accidents in History," 4.
108   Rossiter and Rinaldi, *Institutional Violence and Disability.*
109   Polly Dunnett died suddenly on 18 June 1981, aged seventy. Her son, Malcolm, and daughters, Diana and Robyn, survived her. Her understated obituary asked for donations to the Queen Alexandra Solarium; folder 01, box 03, OSC ARC 08, UBCOA.

BIBLIOGRAPHY

Archives

British Columbia Archives, Victoria, BC
Hornby Island Archives, Hornby Island, BC
Queen Alexandra Solarium Archives, Victoria, BC
University of British Columbia Okanagan, Archives and Special Collections, Kelowna, BC

Newspapers and Periodicals

The Islander (Victoria)
Vancouver Daily Province
Vancouver Province
Vancouver Sun
Victoria Daily Times

Other Sources

Ambrose, Linda M. *A Great Rural Sisterhood: Madge Robertson Watt and the ACWW.* Toronto: University of Toronto Press, 2015.
– *For Home and Country: The Centennial History of the Women's Institutes in Ontario, 1897–1997.* Erin, ON: Boston Mills Press, 1996.
Andrews, Maggie. *The Acceptable Face of Feminism: The Women's Institute as a Social Movement.* London: Lawrence & Wishart, 1997.

Barman, Jean. *The West beyond the West: A History of British Columbia*. Vancouver: University of British Columbia Press, 1991.

Boyd-Scriver, Jessie. *The Montreal Children's Hospital: Years of Growth*. Montreal: McGill-Queen's University Press, 1979.

British Columbia Women's Institutes. *100 Years of BC Women's Institutes, 1909–2009*. Kamloops: British Columbia Women's Institutes, 2008.

– *Modern Pioneers, 1909–1959*. Vancouver: Evergreen Press, 1959.

Brown, Audrey Alexandra. *The Log of the Lame Duck*. Toronto: MacMillan, 1934.

Burke, Stacie. *Building Resistance: Children, Tuberculosis, and the Toronto Sanatorium*. Montreal: McGill-Queen's University Press, 2018.

Campbell, Lara. *A Great Revolutionary Wave*. Vancouver: University of British Columbia Press, 2020.

Clarke, Nic. "Sacred Daemons: Exploring British Columbian Society's Perceptions of 'Mentally Deficient' Children, 1870–1930." *BC Studies* 144 (2004): 61–89.

Cooter, Roger, and Bill Luckin, eds. "Accidents in History: An Introduction." In *Accidents in History: Injuries, Fatalities, and Social Relations*, edited by Roger Cooter and Bill Luckin, 1–16. Amsterdam and Atlanta: Rodopi, 1997.

Corrigall, Margery. *The History of Hornby Island*. Comox, BC: Comox District Free Press, 1978.

Davies, Megan J. "Competent Professionals and Modern Methods: State Medicine in British Columbia during the 1930s." *Bulletin of the History of Medicine* 76, no. 1 (2002): 56–83.

– *Into the House of Old: A History of Residential Care in BC*. Montreal: McGill-Queen's University Press, 2003.

– "Mother's Medicine: Women, Home and Health in BC's Peace River Region, 1920–1940." In *Social Medicine and Rural Health in the North in the 19th and 20th Centuries*, edited by J.T.H. Conner and S. Curtis, 199–214. London: Pickering & Chatto, 2011.

– "Young, Henry Esson." In *Dictionary of Canadian Biography*. Vol. 16. University of Toronto/Université Laval, 2003–. http://www.biographi.ca/en/bio/young_henry_esson_16E.html.

Davin, Anna. "Imperialism and Motherhood." *History Workshop Journal* 5, no. 1 (Spring 1978): 9–66.

Devereux, Cecily Margaret. *Growing a Race: Nellie L. McClung and the Fiction of Eugenic Feminism*. Montreal: McGill-Queen's University Press, 2005.

De Zwart, Mary Leah. "Alice Ravenhill: Making Friends with the Powers That Be." *BC Studies* 191 (2016): 35–45.

Ellis, Jason. *A Class by Themselves? The Origins of Special Education in Toronto and Beyond*. Toronto: University of Toronto Press, 2019.

Fairchild, Amy L. "The Polio Narratives: Dialogues with FDR." *Bulletin of the History of Medicine* 75, no. 3 (2001): 488–574.

Forbes, Elizabeth. *Wild Roses at Their Feet: Pioneer Women of Vancouver Island.* Vancouver: Evergreen Press, 1971.

Friedland, Judith. *Restoring the Spirit: The Beginnings of Occupational Therapy in Canada, 1890–1930.* Montreal: McGill-Queen's University Press, 2009.

Gauvain, Henry. "The Effect of Sun, Sea and Open-Air in the Treatment of Disease." *Journal of the Royal Society of Arts* 72, no. 3709 (1923): 74–84.

Gentile, Patrizia. *Queen of the Maple Leaf: Beauty Contests and Settler Femininity.* Vancouver: UBC Press, 2020.

Gleason, Mona. "From 'Disgraceful Carelessness' to 'Intelligent Precaution': Accidents and the Public Child in English Canada, 1900–1950." *Journal of Family History* 30, no. 2 (April 2005): 230–41.

– *Small Matters: Canadian Children in Sickness and Health, 1900–1940.* Montreal: McGill-Queen's University Press, 2013.

Green, Heather. "The Rise of Motherhood: Maternal Feminism and Health in the Rural Prairie Provinces, 1900–1930." *Past Imperfect* 20, no. 1 (2017): 48–70.

Green, Judith. *Risk and Misfortune: The Social Construction of Accidents.* London: UCL Press, 1997.

Halpern, Monda. *And on That Farm He Had a Wife: Ontario Farm Women and Feminism, 1900–1970.* Montreal and Kingston: McGill-Queen's University Press, 2001.

Hobday, R.A. "Sunlight Therapy and Solar Architecture." *Medical History* 41, no. 4 (1997): 455–72.

Ishiguro, Laura. "Histories of Settler Colonialism: Considering New Currents." *BC Studies* 190 (2016): 5–14.

Jacobs, Margaret D. *White Mother to a Dark Race: Settler Colonialism, Maternalism, and the Removal of Indigenous Children in the American West and Australia, 1880–1940.* Lincoln: University of Nebraska Press, 2009.

Kinnaird, Ellen. "Facilities for the Care of Crippled Children in British Columbia." MSW thesis, University of British Columbia, 1950.

Koven, Seth, and Sonya Michel, eds. "Introduction: Mother Worlds." In *Mothers of a New World: Maternalist Politics and the Origins of Welfare State*, edited by Seth Koven and Sonya Michel, 1–43. New York: Routledge, 1993.

Longmore, Paul K. "'Heaven's Special Child': The Making of Poster Children." In *The Disability Studies Reader*, edited by Lennard J. Davis, 34–41. New York: Taylor & Francis, 2013.

Marcellus, Lenora. "'Tiny Cripples and the Sunshine of Life': 15 Years of Children's Nursing at Vancouver Island's Queen Alexandra Solarium, 1927–1942." *Journal of Pediatric Nursing* 19, no. 6 (December 2004): 411–20.

McCuaig, Katherine. *The Weariness, the Fever, and the Fret: The Campaign against Tuberculosis in Canada, 1900–1950.* Montreal: McGill-Queen's University Press, 1999.

Medovy, H. *A Vision Fulfilled: The Story of the Children's Hospital of Winnipeg, 1909–1973*. Winnipeg: Peguis, 1984.

Morton, Desmond. *Winning the Second Battle: Canadian Veterans and the Return to Civilian Life, 1915–1930*. Toronto: University of Toronto Press, 1987.

Myers, Tamara. "Didactic Sudden Death: Children, Police, and Teaching Citizenship in the Age of Automobility." *Journal of the History of Childhood and Youth* 8, no. 3 (Fall 2015): 451–75.

Nicholas, Jane. *Canadian Carnival Freaks and the Extraordinary Body, 1900–1970*. Toronto: University of Toronto Press, 2018.

Norton, Wayne. *A Whole Little City by Itself: Tranquille and Tuberculosis*. Kamloops, BC: Plateau Press, 1999.

Pearson, Susan J. "Infantile Specimens: Showing Babies in Nineteenth Century America." *Journal of Social History* 42, no. 2 (Winter 2008): 341–70.

Ravenhill, Alice. "Where Health Is Found in Sunbathing." *Modern Hospital* 29, no. 6 (December 1927): 118–22.

Reaume, Geoffrey. *Lyndhurst: Canada's First Rehabilitation Centre for People with Spinal Cord Injuries, 1945–1998*. Montreal and Kingston: McGill-Queen's University Press, 2007.

Rollier, Auguste. "'The Sun Cure,' and the Work Cure in Surgical Tuberculosis." *British Medical Journal* 2, no. 3599 (December 1929): 1206–7.

Rossiter, Kate, and Jen Rinaldi. *Institutional Violence and Disability: Punishing Conditions*: London: Routledge, 2019.

Sandwell, R.W. *Contesting Rural Space: Land Policy and the Practices of Settlement, Saltspring Island, British Columbia, 1859–91*. Montreal: McGill-Queen's University Press, 2005.

Teske, Robin L., and Mary Ann Tétreault. Introduction to *Conscious Acts and the Politics of Social Change*, edited by Robin L. Teske and Mary Ann Tétreault, 1–25. Columbia, SC: University of South Carolina Press, 2000.

Wace, C. "The Queen Alexandra Solarium for Crippled Children." *Canadian Medical Association Journal* 21, no. 6 (December 1929): 702–6.

Wright, David. *Sick Kids: The History of the Hospital for Sick Children*. Toronto: University of Toronto Press, 2016.

Young, H.E. "Queen Alexandra Solarium." *Public Health Journal* 19, no. 8 (1928): 374–7.

Zacharias, Alexandra. "British Columbia Women's Institute in the Early Years: A Time to Remember." In *In Her Own Right: Selected Essays on Women's History in BC*, edited by Barbara Latham and Cathy Kess, 55–78. Victoria: Camosun College, 1980.

Zilm, Glennis, and Ethel Warbinek. TB *Nurses in B.C., 1895–1960: A Biographical Dictionary*. White Rock, BC: n.p., 2006.

12

Kitchen-Table Surgery

Rural Risk and Accidental Care in Early Twentieth-Century General Practice

Sasha Mullally

In the summer of 1910, Dr Augustine MacDonald of Souris, Prince Edward Island, undertook a fabled bit of kitchen-table surgery. Called to the MacCormack farmhouse in St Margarets, twelve kilometres from his office in town, he was greeted by a gruesome accident: a young boy had gone out to the fields in search of his father, encountered a hay mower, and all but lost both of his feet. Arriving at the farmhouse half a day after the event, the doctor spent the next several hours hovering over the kitchen table, working on the four-year-old attempting to reattach the severed limbs. At least one account describes his return days later expecting to find that his efforts were in vain and prepared to amputate. But, as the story goes, he found good circulation in both appendages. Over the intervening months, the country doctor monitored the child's recovery back to limited mobility, his feet saved.

Farm families at the turn of the last century often lived precariously and faced risk of accidental injury, dismemberment, and even death in everyday life and work. The settler economy on Prince Edward Island, a tiny jurisdiction on Canada's Atlantic coast best known for being the fictional setting of *Anne of Green Gables*, relied on primary resources – farming and fishing – for most of its colonial and provincial history. In agriculture, mixed farms were the early twentieth-century norm, but occupational pluralism was often a necessity.[1] While farm life could be as pleasant as that depicted by L.M. Montgomery in her fictional Avonlea, life in the province and the wider region was far from idyllic. In reality, farming involved long hours of gruelling work in fields, barns, and kitchens as families attempted to make a living raising animals and bringing forth crops from the iconic red soil.

In the early twentieth century, new technologies were making the work easier, especially at planting and harvest. Families like the MacCormacks planted a range of mixed vegetables and cereals and engaged in livestock farming. They cut summer hay to feed their animals over the winter. While new farm machinery allowed for a quicker harvest of crops like hay, these machines with whirring blades and grinding gears required constant maintenance and attention. As Derek Oden observes, the farm safety movement only gained traction in the 1940s; before then, risk was assessed and managed in the individual private family farm economy.[2] Labouring bodies, now spared some of the backbreaking manual work of scythe hand-mowing and hand-threshing, were nonetheless subject to new bodily risks through encounters with mowers and combines. As the MacCormack boy, known as A.J., experienced in 1910, malfunction and mishap when interacting with machines posed a new threat. Unlike Othoa Scott's spinal injury that was the ordinary consequence of childhood play, the trauma suffered by A.J. MacCormack was the brutal by-product of new human-technology interactions. The resulting accidental injuries could be severe and often required new skills of their health providers, especially the doctors who might be called to provide surgical repair.

This chapter situates this single story of a country operation in a longer history and wider genre of "kitchen-table surgery," undertaken with increased frequency at the turn of the nineteenth century to manage the impact of accidental injury. The incident followed on the heels of a period in North American health history characterized by Christopher Lawrence and others as one of "surgical optimism."[3] Following and benefiting from the precepts of Listerism, increasingly successful surgical interventions were becoming commonplace within modern practices.[4] They were written about in medical journals and retrospectively in medical memoirs as an increasingly common component of "country practice."[5] Eventually, "modern" operations would require the controlled spaces of hospital surgical care,[6] but, as Crowther and Dupree have shown, surgery a century ago was not yet confined to specialists, and Lister's methods were adapted to suit hospitals and households, in peace and war.[7] Robust rural bodies were in some ways thought to be well-suited to withstand difficulties with both procedures and recovery.[8] But despite new understandings of the germ theory and advancements in orthopedic surgical practice, undertaking this kind of foot surgery a century ago risked the death of the child from infection. Limb reattachment was decades away, and the chances of success in a remote PEI farmhouse were slim. As techniques for paediatric surgery were undeveloped,[9] attempted reattachment might also result in greater pain and disability than a clean amputation.[10]

Why did the doctor proceed? Did surgical optimism encourage kitchen-table surgical interventions? Some have argued that doctors took on such risks to learn through practice.[11] In pursuing home-based surgery, Augustine MacDonald, a physician of long-standing tenure who eventually became known simply as Dr Gus, managed a new set of risk-reward calculations in general practice. Thomas Schlich has observed that a century ago the singular risky case might prove valuable to advance surgical knowledge, but that was not the trade of a country doctor, who was establishing and maintaining relationships of trust in a rural area with long-term practice in mind.[12] Amputation, on the other hand, compromised the future productivity of a young body; patients might retain valuable physical capacity if they retained the ability to walk. After amputation, the clinical risks from infection still loomed large. Additionally, rural workers and farmers did not always have access to prosthetic devices, such as those available to injured veterans and industrial workers, which might allow them to reconstruct themselves as productive members of society.[13] And so, what were the practical considerations for a clinician undertaking a rural operation in the early twentieth century? How might a general practitioner approach such a traumatic case in 1910? What potential reward encouraged Dr Gus to proceed, and what were the risks and rewards for the patient and his family? What was A.J.'s life like after the doctor left and the surgery was declared a "success"? I explore this extreme example of accidental harm and reconstructive surgery to see what it tells us about the structures of surgical authority and medical decision-making in farm homes a century ago.

To undertake this task, I assembled and performed a deep reading of historical narratives generated about the MacCormack foot surgery. If the event caught the attention of local residents, this is not reflected in newspapers or other print media of the day. When the incident resurfaced in media outlets in 1962, however, it turned the doctor into a minor celebrity. Still living in Souris, the avuncular and now elderly doctor became the subject of admiring attention. Eventually described as a "medical miracle," the story was celebrated in major newspapers, regional magazines, local histories, and high-school theatre.

It is also captured in an oral interview I conducted years ago. I grew up in the Souris area at the end of the twentieth century and was very familiar with the story of "the day Dr Gus sewed the feet back on." Reviewing the evolution of the surgery's narrative arc allows for an unpacking of the story, including my own unwitting role in perpetuating one particular version as I pursued my master's degree.[14] By drawing on recent work that evaluates the social negotiations of clinical decision-making in rural homes and considers gender and power within a family unit as well as the rural community context, it is possible to put old stories in new light. Exploring the narrative accounts reveals elisions and emphases that suited different purposes at different times and factored into the risk-and-reward calculus of kitchen-table surgery in 1910 as layers of storytelling emerge and recede.

REVISING THE "STORY EVERYBODY KNEW"

To begin this task, I revisited a 1994 interview I conducted with retired schoolteacher and local historian Adele Townshend. A highly regarded teacher, writer, and author, Townshend reviewed Dr Gus's career with me over tea in her Souris West living room almost thirty years ago. In the preamble to our conversation, she highlighted that "it was a story that everybody knew, that everybody grew up with."[15] Coming into her house with my own version of events as told to me by various older friends and family members over the years, I did not at the time disagree.

Though I was interested in medical work, Townshend had few surgical details to offer, simply telling me, "So, he sewed the feet back on at the kitchen table, as I heard it." She qualified some details, saying, "Some would say a bed or otherwise, wherever he did it – on the kitchen table, we'll say – and he sewed them back on." Instead, she focused on making meaning of the unexpected recovery. The doctor reattached the feet, she said, "fully expecting that he would have to come out and do what he was going to have to do first [amputate]. But anyway, he went home, and when he came home the next day, he found the toes and the feet were warm."[16] Against Dr Gus's expectations, his attempted limb reattachment proceeded without amputation, the patient survived, and the event became part of public memory and then public history.

Townshend was an accomplished local historian when I interviewed her in 1994, and this particular surgery featured at least four times in her published work. For instance, in a 1980 centennial brochure with historical highlights from the area, she celebrated the doctor who "made medical history when he sewed the feet back on a boy who had lost them in a farm accident. The operation was performed on a kitchen table in the boy's home at St. Margaret's."[17] Her book *Ten Farms Become a Town* (1986) goes into more detail. An ambitious work spanning 1700 to 1920, it features Dr Gus in two chapters. His first mention is alongside details of the foot surgery, and though it barely comprises a paragraph, this provides a backdrop for a larger discussion of the doctor's career, and an illustration of the truism that when a doctor answered a call to the country "he never knew what lay ahead of him."[18] Townshend then provides more details about the nature and extent of the injury. Dr Gus found the "four-year-old boy ... both legs severed just above the ankles. Only the Achilles tendons were still attached. He had been standing unseen in the hay field as his father passed with the mower." There is also a brief suggestion that the clinician was not the one who suggested the surgery but that he was swayed by the parents, both "very upset." The mother, in particular, "would not allow the Doctor to sever the ankles completely. And so, on the table in the farm kitchen, Dr Gus sewed the ankles ... [and] bound the legs using barrel staves as splints."[19]

Townshend stresses the rustic circumstances, the physician's ingenuity, and his responsiveness to the family's wishes. These points feed into details offered in a later chapter when she positions the doctor within the broader history of the community. Dr Gus, we then learn, practised in the area for more than sixty years from 1904 to 1968.[20] She describes personal attributes that made him a successful caregiver of long tenure who enjoyed "warm affection" from local people and was seen as a "devoted physician and friend."[21] Emphasizing the unending labours of rural medical practice of the period, she quotes other glowing accounts of the doctor, who "travelled in winter by horse and sleigh to homes from East Point to Annandale." These sources remembered that "older residents relate the feeling of peace and trust he brought to the sick and talk of his uncanny ability to diagnose an illness correctly."[22]

Townshend's interest in Dr Gus was well established by the time she wrote about him in the late 1970s and '80s because he was a close family friend. Her father, Roy MacLean, had lost a thumb to a mechanical saw in the interwar period, and Dr Gus had successfully reattached the digit.[23] While she had reason to believe in the doctor's general surgical skills, the difference between reattaching a thumb and reattaching two feet was not lost on her. The improbability of the foot surgery's success was something she grappled with in our interview: "It seems a miracle that they could get word to Dr Gus and that he would come out in time to save him because I would imagine [the boy] would be bleeding very badly."[24] Recognizing the odds against surgical success, she observed, "The idea that it could be done was almost unbelievable."[25] A careful reading of the surgical narratives reveals that she is among the first to reference a higher power in the story; the "miraculous" event and its outcome inspired further creative writing. In another article on the surgery published in the *Atlantic Advocate* in 1979, Townshend takes more narrative space to describe the physician as a devout Catholic. The settler population in Souris area comprised a Catholic majority, descended from Acadian, Irish, and Highland Scottish settlers, the latter describing most branches of Gus MacDonald's family tree.[26] Perhaps thinking of this faith community, Townshend quotes Dr Gus as saying that during the operation, "his hands were guided by a higher power."[27] This formulation recurs in other iterations. Most importantly, it is a line used in a local high-school play about the event that Townshend wrote in the early 1980s and supervised as English teacher, in between her first article and the publication of her book, working to place the surgical success outside the powers of the clinician. Townshend also recalled inserting a particular dramatic moment into the script of her play: in between the operation and the doctor's return days later, an anguished Dr Gus stops at the Catholic Church to pray for the MacCormack boy. Light streaming down on him through a stained glass, the scene portrays the doctor as an actor who puts himself at the mercy of Providence, his hands the conduit of divine intervention. In a subsequent scene, he returns to the farmhouse and expresses disbelief at finding the feet warm. At this high point of the play, he proclaims with surprise and joy, "This boy will walk again!" To what degree that outcome was the result of surgical skill or the power of prayer is left to the audience to decide.

Scholars such as Roy Porter see references to and belief in miracles as a distinctly pre-modern sensibility; indeed, this seems to have been Townshend's dramatic formulation rather than a reflection on fatalistic reliance on a higher power on the part of the doctor or the local population.[28] Like the shipwrecks in Colin Coates's chapter, the boy's recovery is interpreted through a lens of culture and religion, but Townshend's narrative also contained empirical analysis, emphasizing technical details of the surgery and the skills available to the community because of the doctor's presence and his willingness to undertake such work.[29] As writer and community historian, Townshend made several important choices when placing Dr Gus in the broader history of Souris and eastern Kings County. As she sketched out in the introduction to her book, the longer history of Souris is one in which the settler communities encountered their share of challenges as primary resource producers. In 1900, rural Prince Edward Island farms were still recovering from a century and a half of absentee landlords.[30] Though the twentieth century looked promising at the outset, inhabitants still found themselves at the mercy of the elements and many external political and economic factors as they attempted to develop successful domestic economies.[31] Farm incomes, essential to provincial household income,[32] did not keep pace with industrial wages and agricultural endeavours in other parts of the country, and youth outmigration was an ongoing problem.[33]

Notwithstanding these realities, *Ten Farms Become a Town* is a typical community history, a liberal and progressive account with industry and

shared purpose winning out against hardships, and civic enterprises co-
alescing to create a modestly thriving population centre on the eastern end
of late twentieth-century Prince Edward Island. The precarity of farm life
and work can be alleviated by belief in a higher power guiding events but
can also be borne by faith in community solidarity. Townshend mindfully
deploys elements that emphasize the physician's communitarian spirit and
the moral economy of rural practice. Dr Gus neither charged nor received
a fee for the foot surgery. In her *Atlantic Advocate* article, Townshend details how the boy "recovered and learned to walk again, with some difficulty
at first. But the day arrives when he was able to accompany his parents to
Souris, walk into the Doctor's Office and present him with a brown lustre
jug." She adds, "Dr Gus never received payment he treasured more."[34] In *Ten
Farms*, she updates the story to reveal that "shortly before [Dr Gus] died in
1970, he returned the jug to the McCormack family.[35] In her telling, a miraculous recovery underscores the procedure's risk, while mitigating possible
human frailty in either the decision-making behind or execution of the surgery. Additionally, this exchange of valuables also acts as a metaphor for a
communitarianism that offers a doctor both material and ineffable rewards.

These themes are reflected in broader media representations of iconic
"country doctors." Charlotte Borst has recently argued that "the country
doctor was a contested figure whose image embodied competing ideals of a
racialized professional and masculine identity in the early twentieth century."[36] Borst sees a divergence between the professional and public narratives
about practitioners like Dr Gus. The public's idealization of communitarian altruism contests an emerging professional emphasis on scientific practice in postwar American print media. In the case of Dr Gus and the 1910
foot surgery, we see, in fact, the marriage of both. In my previous work, I
note a high degree of complementarity and ample room for narrative cohesion in such texts, mainly because I examine source materials that Borst's
analysis did not consider: the autobiographical and biographical works by
and about such physicians.[37] Life stories bring narrative cohesion and add
attention to place. Looking at the creation of source narratives reveals the
dynamism of the media renderings and how they served many different
purposes at different points in time. This cohesion is evidenced most clearly
in the co-production of memories and memorialization of Dr Gus as a

country doctor. These must be read as flexible cultural artifacts, which nonetheless offer important insight into historical general practice.

Adele Townshend was, after all, building upon the local knowledge already in circulation, some of it put to the printed page before her own efforts. "Everybody grew up with" these stories because they transitioned from oral history and informal local knowledge into print in the 1960s. Later twentieth-century writers like Townshend did not directly engage with the clinician as they crafted new iterations of the foot surgery – Dr Gus had years since passed away when he became the subject of magazine articles, community histories, and local plays. But these dramatized events were based on printed news and retrospectives formed in conversation with him. They constitute biographical – even quasi-autobiographical – accounts. The earliest print reports of the foot surgery reflect a consideration of the domestic environments of rural practices, common and well-established influence on medical decision-making in rural general practice of the period.[38] Community memories of the incident changed in ways that allowed those removed from the place and time to nonetheless connect and relate to the story and take meaning from the injury and trauma. These renderings point to modes of social interaction at the bedside and structures of medical decision-making that catered to a local and persistent "country mode" of care.[39] Earlier accounts discuss neither payment nor the presence of any "higher power" but instead put greater emphasis on the doctor's point of view, through which we learn more about the family encounter and the surgical process. In so doing, they provide more details about the decision to operate, the risks involved, and the real rewards sought.

"I SUBMIT IT WAS A MIRACLE": MEDICAL AND COMMUNITY MEMORY

It is a Prince Edward Island truism that you have to become famous and admired outside the province before you will be appreciated in the province. Perhaps this is true of most small places, but this was the case for Dr Gus. In 1962, Neil A. Matheson, a local newspaperman, was contacted by editors at the *Boston Globe*, who had gotten wind of an unusual story of kitchen-table surgery and sought out the reporter to investigate. Many

Globe readers of the day had direct ties to or roots in Atlantic Canada, and stories from Prince Edward Island often featured in its pages. Matheson was a well-established provincial farm editor for the principal island daily, the *Charlottetown Guardian*. In addition to reporting on agricultural events and affairs, a position of some importance in the jurisdiction, by the 1960s Matheson had a weekly Across the Island column where he reported human interest stories related to rural living. These often had the historical aim of "capturing" elements of island life that were fast disappearing with the modernization of the province.

Matheson knew Dr Gus, so it was an easy task to set up an interview, go out to Souris, and collect the requisite details. Matheson's report, with provocative detail of both the accident and the kitchen-table surgery that followed, so captured the editors' interest that they ran it as a feature in the *Sunday Globe* at the end of September 1962. In his report, Matheson largely deferred to the doctor, whom he quoted extensively and whose version framed the narrative. Matheson was a quintessential "pastkeeper" of his time, to use Batinski's term.[40] He did not interpret the details or the meaning of events brought to light in 1962 in any overt way but acted as a community interlocutor and faithful scribe for the stories he was told. Dr Gus's version emphasized both the clinical details and the social elements of the encounter. And it was immediately clear that, while kitchen-table surgeries were not uncommon in his early years of practice, it was no longer something that he took on.

The country doctor stressed that the contexts – the accidental and emergency nature of the injury and pressure from the family – were the main reasons he had pursued limb reattachment. The family role was foregrounded in his recollection fifty years on. He remembered the long journey to the farm, arriving fatigued to be met by the mother in the yard: "Before I'd set foot inside the house, she'd made me promise I would do everything I could to preserve [her son's] ability to walk." Matheson adds, "Having made the promise, he just had to try."[41]

Arriving at the patient's side, Dr Gus was shocked by the extent of the injury. As Adele Townshend accurately reported years later, he told Matheson that he encountered two almost entirely severed ankles, attached by some sinew and, on one side, the Achilles tendon. He went to work, however. We learn that he sterilized the surgical field with bichloride of mercury, used catgut to reattach the tendons, while the rest – arteries, blood vessels, muscle tissue, and skin – were sutured with "silk thread that he bought in a store in Souris."[42] He then bound up the boy's lower legs and ankles with gauze bandages and household cloth sterilized on the stove. As others remembered and relayed, he used barrel staves as splints. Matheson colourfully commented about the manufacture, "He smashed a barrel that was under the eave of the roof to catch the rain water – the soft water was used on wash days as there were no fancy detergents or soap powders then – sawed several stakes in two, and used them for splints to hold the bones straight, after he had completed a surgery job that required several hours."[43] Although the doctor left the scene without a good feeling, Matheson relates how "he came back two days later, thinking he would have to take them off. But there was heat in them, the blood was [in] circulation."[44]

The article reflects that Matheson was clearly enamoured by the doctor, but probative. In this first published capture of the event, Dr Gus deflects praise and acknowledges that "the job wasn't perfect." Matheson concurs, noting that "Mr MacCormack was always lame," then defends the doctor: "I submit it was a miracle of surgery in those far-off days, considering the job was performed alone. Modern surgical experts talk in glowing terms of limbs that are attached – it has been done several times, I believe – with teams of surgeons, nurses and many specialists in the most completely equipped hospitals."[45]

Two years later, Matheson returned to Dr Gus's office to ask more questions about the 1910 surgery but also expanded his enquiries to include the physician's medical work over six decades of a long career. Two events may have contributed to this renewed interest. Charlottetown doctor William Lea was publishing a new book on the *History of Medicine on Prince Edward Island*, and excerpts were being featured in the Island newspaper, while a community effort was emerging to nominate Dr Gus MacDonald for an Order of Canada, an honour he would receive from Governor General Michener in 1968. Both efforts likely turned Matheson's attention back to the history of health care and influenced his decision to write a new feature on Dr Gus, this time for his Across the Island column. He also took the opportunity to review elements of the doctor's career – including the foot surgery – in a separate article published in the Canadian medical circular *Medical Post*.[46]

These subsequent articles offer few new details about the 1910 accident and foot surgery. Matheson's second visit to Dr Gus in Souris provided an opportunity to recount the high points of his career, including the celebration of his diamond jubilee in practice held earlier that year.[47] Apparently Dr Gus extracted a promise from Matheson not to "say too much about his work, if I ever wrote about him again."[48] Instead, the reporter toured the doctor's collection of artifacts, some from former patients, and others acquired through family connections. And as Dr Gus grew comfortable, he offered details of other cases attached to the items. The conversation drifted back to accidents encountered in his career, cases he increasingly chose to send on to Charlottetown. Building modern hospital facilities in the capital effectively centralized surgical services even for rural-based doctors eighty kilometres away.[49]

"In the early days of cars," for instance, Dr Gus treated an automobile accident victim at nearby Rollo Bay, who suffered a broken arm. Matheson writes, "The doctor pulled several boards from a paling fence for splints, pulled 'soft natural grass' to cushion the bones, tied it with string and sent the man to a Charlottetown hospital for complete examination."[50] Other surgical challenges he continued to take on himself. Severed appendages were not entirely uncommon, and Roy MacLean's thumb was not the only one the doctor reattached. "My friend was at an afternoon wedding reception," Matheson reported, and "a lady there remembered the time he had put her thumb back on. I'm not sure, but I think she was the one whose thumb had been bitten off by a horse, for there were several of those replaced thumbs." Other clinical elements of the interview focused on childbirth, some of which involved a degree of surgical care. Matheson informed his readers, "Dr Gus was almost equally famous for his skill in confinement cases" and "never lost a mother." Generally, the province witnessed high maternal mortality rates in the early decades of the twentieth century.[51] These stories aside, the doctor's embargo on the history of his practice ultimately remained in place in Matheson's writing: "There are many other stories about his career ... but they are for his memoirs which he is writing. They should make most interesting reading."[52] Those memoirs have not yet surfaced.

There was certainly more to say about Dr Gus than what was offered in these occasional features. He graduated from McGill medical school in 1902 at the age of twenty-eight after having taught school for several years. He spent his life connected to Catholic institutions and organizations and was a long-standing member of the Lions Club and the Knights of Columbus. Church connections, in fact, brought him to Souris. The 1980 community history observes, "Dr Gus ... owed his education to his uncle, the Reverend Donald MacDonald, the builder of St. Mary's Church; in gratitude the young doctor chose to practice in Souris."[53] He married twice but had no children and survived both spouses, living out his life in a charming if unusual triangular house in downtown Souris.[54] Most public history emphasizes the community regard for him at the end of his six-decade career in Souris, "where he was greatly beloved and still remembered with affection."[55] He ran for public office several times, winning the seat of First Kings more often than not and serving off and on as a member of the Legislative Assembly from 1915 to 1947. There is evidence that he was an effective public advocate, especially in organizing the community behind the project to build a hospital, arguing, somewhat ironically, that such a facility would be "the incentive ... for a young surgeon to settle in our midst."[56] He apparently never hurried, was a great wit, and had a lovely singing voice. While these are engaging details of his public profile, other accounts emerge of him as an effective but also somewhat fearsome character who expected stoicism from patients, young and old. Remembering a clinical encounter with Dr Gus, Mary Malone wrote how he lanced a boil on her when she was a child. By then an old doctor, he opened his black bag and removed a surgical knife. "To a six-year-old," she recalled, "it looked like a bayonet. I sat there shivering in my shoes ... I thought I was going to die." She admitted she felt better after the procedure but could not resist a terse observation: "Doctor Gus did not believe in wasting medication to relieve pain."[57]

"THIS BOY WILL WALK AGAIN": GRIEF, GUILT, AND THE SEARCH FOR A GOOD ENDING

The theme of pain and fear management prompt a return to the patient's perspective and to the family role in shaping the surgical encounter of 1910. The story that ran in the *Boston Globe* featured a large photo of the doctor, an older man sitting at a desk holding an heirloom lancet, one of his prized medical artifacts and possessions. The original print story included a headshot of A.J. MacCormack, both living proof of and witness to the clinician's handiwork. The boy had not only lived but grew up to become a productive member of society. Townshend remembered that A.J. "walked with difficulty, but he taught school and farmed a bit and he spent his last days at Colville Manor."[58] Matheson also recalled A.J.'s years of active study followed by professional service. In fact, the two men attended Prince of Wales College together, during which time A.J. earned his teaching credentials. Although he was lame, as Matheson noted in 1962, that had not stopped his education; "he walked one and one half miles to school each day through the ten grades." Matheson went on to describe how "he taught for more than 20 years, 1926–1949 ... before a cold in the legs added so much to the discomfort that he had been developing, that he finally decided he could no longer be on his feet as much as the teaching job demanded." We learn that he then returned to the family home in St Margarets to "farm a bit" before retirement. His productivity was foregrounded as a comfort for readers, emphasizing that his story had a happy ending.

A.J.'s mind was sharp on the 1910 events, and he also provided elements to shape the incident from the family's perspective. These memories add missing but critical context to the doctor's version of events. Some of these are also corrective to community memory about events right before the accident happened. "The story goes," Townshend related in our 1994 interview, "the boy's father was out cutting hay in the field. And the little four-year old boy, his mother was busy, and he slipped away from her." Apparently "the little fellow [then] went looking for his father and he heard the hay mower in the field and he saw the horse, and he thought he'd run and get a drive with his father. I suppose farm boys often did. But, as he approached the horse and mower, the long cutting bar caught his ankles and cut his feet and severed the feet almost totally except for the tendon at the back of his feet."[59] In 1964, however, Matheson extracted a different version from the patient: "He was just four years old on that summer day in 1910 when he locked his sister in the house, and went out to stroll in the field where his father was cutting hay with a horse-drawn mower" – a slight difference, but one that absolves family members from any lack of attention or oversight. This is important because all accounts centre the decision to operate on the wishes of the mother, who strongly expresses her thoughts and feelings in many extant versions. The family response is otherwise almost entirely lost to history. Fifty-two years later, A.J. remembered being conscious after the accident, though not apparently in pain. But as Matheson explains, "The child couldn't understand the extent of the disaster." As a four-year-old, he looked up and asked his mother, "Why is everyone crying?"

For others in the family, the implications of the disastrous event were clear and lived on beyond the 1910 event itself. Townshend remembered the play she staged at the high school in the 1980s. "At the end of the performance," she recalled, "I looked down and Cathy MacIntyre the leading lady in the play was with this older woman. Cathy had her arms around her and the woman was sobbing." When Townshend questioned the student later on, she learned that the sobbing woman was A.J. MacCormack's older sister and "she was there in the kitchen when it happened … It was a sad little play anyway, but apparently it was very real to her."[60] And more than Townshend might have articulated at the time, A.J. MacCormack's version of events, especially where he "locked his sister in the kitchen" before going outside, absolved his sister, too.

Ultimately, the story of this foot surgery came to "belong" to Dr Gus in that it evolved and adapted to foreground the physician's activities and situate him at the centre of a dramatic and heroic surgical feat. Spilling from the pen of pastkeepers like Neil Matheson in the 1960s and honed by the creative expressions of local writers like Adele Townshend, stories emerge and converge on depictions of Dr Gus as a beloved and unusually skilled community clinician who expressed a great deal of community sensitivity. The first stories were co-produced by him and the friends and acquaintances who became chroniclers of his life and career. With them, he actively participated in framing the story to underscore the need for hospital facilities in Eastern Kings County, a project he supported since the interwar period. Over time, new writers emphasized the "miraculous" recovery of A.J. MacCormack after the "fuss" made by his mother when the doctor arrived on the scene. Mid-century revisions used the mother's insistence to deflect the questionable undertaking of the procedure, mediating any possible criticism of the doctor's decision to step outside the typical mid-century scope of practice of an average rural general practitioner. Later twentieth-century writers, including myself, continued to centre the heroic risk-taking doctor in the telling and retelling of such tales.

Stories can be a rich source for historians but must be understood in cultural context. Unlike those Indigenous stories examined in Hudson and Manitowabi's chapter, these are not "mythic" accounts with their own consciousness, as that concept is understood by the Anishnaabek.[61] Yet settler stories of accidents can be seen as deep and important expressions of individual and community values. There is a lot to learn, for instance, in the family's response to the event, particularly their efforts in the immediate aftermath to save the child pain and disability. Equally important are A.J.'s efforts years later to craft a version of events that attempted to spare his family blame and sorrow.

One unnamed character deserves greater attention. Most accounts depict A.J.'s mother as an emotional woman whose reaction overwhelms the otherwise good judgment of a local medical professional. Then, despite the odds, a divinely guided surgical intervention saves the boy's ability to walk in a "miraculous" recovery. Putting miracles aside, one might consider a more mundane reality: the mother might well have been the reason there was a successful outcome, not only because she was determined that the doctor try to save her son's severed feet.

The first print account in 1962 says she met Dr Gus in the yard and extracted a promise from him to take a medical risk with her son's life, and with his own reputation, banking on the prospect of A.J. walking again. That encounter reflects Claire Brock's findings in research that explores how surgeons, patients, and the lay public conceptualized risk and responsibility in the late nineteenth and early twentieth centuries. By 1910, surgery could be simultaneously seen as safe (owing to developments in surgical science) and increasingly risky (because such progress allowed for greater experimentation). Paradoxically, Bock argues, the age of surgical optimism for doctors could be experienced as the age of surgical anxiety for patients.[62] Moreover, while the *Boston Globe* featured photos only of the doctor and his patient, the analysis here supports Nancy Theriot's observation that the triad of doctor-patient-family interaction is critically important to understanding clinical decisions and negotiations at the early twentieth-century bedside.[63] The mother made the decision, extracted the promise, and determined the course of treatment. This largely forgotten layer of the narrative history reveals what Sally Wilde, studying the context of rural Australia, has characterized as a high degree of patient autonomy with surgical interventions. Clinicians deferred to family to cultivate trust over a long relationship of care.[64] This deference ultimately empowered patients and engaged whole families in decision-making. In 1962 or 1986, one might comfortably assume that the doctor would assess and determine procedural risk; the 1910 reality was that this power often rested with the mother.[65]

Authority is often accompanied by responsibility, and A.J.'s mother's role did not end in the yard in negotiation with a country doctor. Apart from the question of blame and guilt over who or what might have led to or prevented the mowing accident, it was almost certainly she who took on the task of managing recovery, a process at least as important as the surgical work. Dr Gus might have found the feet "warm," but they could still have easily developed an infection, possibly advancing to gangrene, in the absence of constant surveillance and innumerable dressing changes. Once surgery is over, the only bulwark against life-threatening infection in an era before antibiotics is attentive nursing. The care the mother would customarily provide, perhaps assisted by other family members or community women, is neither imagined nor acknowledged in any print accounts. Wound care after an injury this grave would have been exceedingly time consuming. Given the pain involved, it would also be emotionally difficult. Further, recovery does not end when bones knit, and tissues recover; we also have no details of how four-year-old A.J. learned to walk again after months in bed. We only read about the moment when he walked into the doctor's office to present him with a family heirloom. This act is written as a reflection of the family's gratitude, but it is also easy to interpret it as a show of pride in A.J.'s recovery and the family's ability to pay for the services rendered with a costly possession. We must imagine details of convalescence and rehabilitation, as well as the ultimately very personal meaning of the reward. But any critical engagement must consider the realities and contexts of family care, which were also noteworthy parts of managing accidental injury a century ago. And we draw new attention to a critical central character, who, despite her importance is not even given a name in previous narratives. We can now acknowledge the mother, Margaret, who went by "Maggie Pat." In part because of the doctor, but largely because of her, the boy would walk again.

CONCLUSION: ACCIDENTAL RISK AND REWARD

Looking back on this stunning event, the particular contexts that encouraged it and memorialized it, we see how the realities of rural living – particularly the threat of rural accidents – distributed the authoritative roles in surgical decision-making well beyond the clinician. It is critically important to explore holes in surgical stories that are preserved – like A.J. MacCormack's foot surgery – because otherwise, such tales overwhelm readers with the clinical gaze. Moving the central frame away from the doctor, we notice new details: how A.J.'s resulting disability, although it did not radically curtail his life, certainly shaped it. He went to college, found work as a teacher, walked to his schoolhouse for many years and then "farmed a bit" when his lameness became incapacitating. We learn that he lived to a ripe old age. This is not an unqualified happy ending, and reading between the lines we can see the cost of the mowing accident. We also see the lingering emotional impact on the family in A.J.'s sister's grief-stricken response a half century later, when a play about her brother's accident activates her own associated trauma. We can note how A.J. speaks of the event in ways that ensure no one in his family bears blame for the day he walked into a hay mower at the age of four. After thorough excavation of narrative accounts, we know more about the risk and rewards of kitchen-table surgery. We come to understand the ways these mattered to Dr Gus and A.J. MacCormack, and how clinician, family, and community all made sense of and responded to accidental happenings a century ago.

ACKNOWLEDGMENTS

Special thanks to my cousin George Mullally, who provided genealogical context and a tour through the house where the titular kitchen-table surgery took place. I am also indebted to the late Adele Townshend, whose work in the 1970s and '80s as a community historian provided a foundation for my work on PEI history, as well as the work of so many others. Finally, I wish to acknowledge the helpful comments and suggestions provided by three external reviewers and the tireless efforts and support of the volume editors, Geoff Hudson and Megan Davies.

NOTES

1 The potential and the limitations of small-scale mixed farming were commented on by many agricultural experts of the period. See Cumming, "Agriculture in the Maritime Provinces."

2 Oden, "Selling Safety." For the broader US context of mechanical threat from agricultural mechanization, see also Oden, *Harvest of Hazards.*

3 Lawrence describes how surgery rose from a relatively humble place in seventeenth-century life to being seen as one of the great achievements of late Victorian culture. But in so doing, it examines medical and surgical concepts of disease and their relation to the practice of surgery, including the social relations embedded in such concepts and the influence of particular historical settings to shape both. See particularly Lawrence, *Medical Theory, Surgical Practice*, chap.1. For more on "surgical optimism," see also Wangensteen and Wangensteen, *Rise of Surgery.* And, as Blake Brown has observed in his work on medical malpractice, as patients grew more optimistic about surgical success, they became more demanding and expected of good results from clinicians. See, for instance, Brown, "Canada's First Malpractice Crisis."

4 For a discussion of surgery and idea of modernity, see Lawrence and Brown, "Quintessentially Modern Heroes."

5 Some clinicians, however, resisted the germ theory and persisted with traditional empirical therapies to manage infection. See Greenwood, "Lawson Tait and Opposition to Germ Theory." For the reasons opposition persisted in the United States, see Breiger, "American Surgery and the Germ Theory of Disease."

6 These sites as "spaces of control" are explored thoroughly by Schlich in "Surgery, Science and Modernity."

7 The medical schools were tools of the empire, sending students into general practice, military service, the mission fields, high-class consultancies, and homeopathy in many lands, including Canada, where some taught at McGill and passed these ideas on to Augustine MacDonald when he was a student there at the turn of the century. Crowther and Dupree, *Medical Lives in the Age of Surgical Revolution.*

8 Hamilton, "Nineteenth Century Surgical Revolution."

9 As Williams has shown, paediatric surgery did not develop until after World War I, largely focused on the management and correction of congenital conditions. Williams, "Denis Browne and the Specialization of Paediatric Surgery"; see also Chang and Burrington, "Development of Paediatric Surgery."

10 Wangensteen and Smith discuss the history of amputation in "Some Highlights in the History of Amputation." As Shauna Devine argues, the American Civil War also advanced surgical practices as related to the management of traumatic injury, including the management of amputation and subsequent infection. See Devine, *Learning from the Wounded*; also Devine, "'To Make Something from the Dying in This War.'"

11 See, for instance, Wilde and Hirst, "Learning from Mistakes."

12 Schlich, "Risk and Medical Innovation," 2.

13 As cultural historians like Erin O'Connor have noted about industrial work, this focus on male productivity helped create an "industrial logic of disease," the dynamic that coupled pathology and production in Victorian thinking about cultural processes in general, both when considering disease and injury. Connor, *Raw Material*.

14 See Mullally, "Dr. Roddy, Dr. Gus, and the Golden Age of Medicine on Prince Edward Island."

15 Interview with Adele Townshend, 17 May 1994.

16 Ibid.

17 Anniversary Committee, *Souris*.

18 Townshend, *Ten Farms Become a Town*.

19 Ibid., 98–9.

20 Ibid., 98.

21 Ibid.

22 McQuaid, "A Biography of Dr. A.A. MacDonald," unpublished manuscript, quoted in Townshend, *Ten Farms*, 98n15.

23 Interview with Adele Townshend, 17 May 1994.

24 Ibid.

25 Ibid.

26 See Townshend, *Ten Farms*, chap. 1 and passim; O'Grady, *Exiles and Islanders*; O'Leary and Macdonald, *Memorial Volume, 1772–1922*. Catholic dominance in the eastern and western communities of the island are also discussed at several junctures in Edward MacDonald's *If You're Stronghearted*.

27 Townshend, "Brown Lustre Jug," 34–5.

28 Porter, "Accidents in the Eighteenth Century."

29 Coates, "Wind, Error, and Providence," in this volume.

30 Prince Edward Island farmers were by and large only one to two generations removed from tenant farming, a legacy of a famous land lottery that took place in 1767. Several classic surveys of changing land-tenure politics and the aftermath include Bolger, *Canada's Smallest Province*, esp. 37–134; Bumsted, "Origins of the Land Question"; Clark, *Three Centuries and the Island*. A well-cited broader perspective is offered in Sinclair, "From Peasants to Corporations."

31 The importance of agriculture to domestic economic markets is explored in Gerriets, "Agricultural Resources, Agricultural Production."

32 For a discussion of the large contribution of agriculture to income, see Inwood and Irwin, "Land, Income and Regional Inequality"; Inwood and Irwin, "Canadian Regional Commodity Income Differences."

33 Thornton, "Problem of Out-Migration from Atlantic Canada"; Otis, "Nouvelles perspectives sur le mouvement d'émigration des Maritimes vers les États-Unis." See also Brookes, "Outmigration from the Maritime Provinces."

34 Townshend, "Brown Lustre Jug," 35.

35 Townshend, *Ten Farms*, 99.

36 Borst, "Noblest Roman of Them All?"

37 Iconographic versions, whether produced by physicians themselves or biographers, tend to converge in celebration of country practice as honourable and fulfilling medical work, and function as recruitment narratives for increasingly underserved rural areas, as I argue in "Canadian Medical Life-Writing," 435–69.

38 For a discussion of domestic considerations that emerge from an analysis of casebooks, see the classic address by Leavitt, "'Worrying Profession.'"

39 Steven Stowe in *Doctoring the South* examines nineteenth-century "country modes" of medicine, and the importance of local folkways, community hierarchies and social patterns in shaping patterns of practice.

40 This term differentiates active heritage collectors from public and professional historians and can be seen as a textual antiquarian type common in small towns of the rural northeastern North America. See Batinski, *Pastkeepers in a Small Place*.

41 Neil Matheson, "Doctor Gus Beloved by Prince Edward Island," *Boston Sunday Globe*, 30 September 1962.

42 Ibid.

43 Neil A. Matheson, "Souris Doctor Visited Again," *Charlottetown Guardian*, 5 October 1962, 14.

44 Matheson, "Doctor Gus Beloved by Prince Edward Island."

45 Ibid.

46 Neil A. Matheson, "Kitchen Table Surgery Saved a Boy's Feet," *Medical Post*, 22 November 1966.

47 "Souris Doctor Is 90 Today," *Charlottetown Guardian*, 6 February 1964, 5.

48 Matheson, "Souris Doctor Visited Again," *Charlottetown Guardian*, 5 October 1962, 14.

49 Recorded operations at Charlottetown hospitals date only back to 1895, in which year the PEI hospital in Charlottetown saw five amputations: three mastectomies, and two leg amputations at the thigh. There was also a herniotomy, a hysterectomy, and a salpingo-oophorectomy. See "French Army Doctors Island Medical Pioneers; Medicine in Early Days Not Governed," *Charlottetown Guardian*, 31 August 1964, 6A.

50 Matheson, "Souris Doctor Visited Again," *Charlottetown Guardian*, 5 October 1962, 14.

51 Ibid. For a thorough discussion of how medical doctors replaced many other care attendants in childbirth, including midwives (as well as exceptions to this trend), see Mitchinson, *Childbirth in Canada*.

52 Ibid.

53 Anniversary Committee, *Souris*.
54 http://islandstories.ca/island_stories_viewer/cap:1376/Souris.
55 Anniversary Committee, *Souris*.
56 "Largely Attended Meeting Indorses [*sic*] New Hospital for Eastern Kings Co.,"
    Charlottetown Guardian, 20 March 1943, 11.
57 MacIsaac, *Lily Pond Memories*, 38.
58 Interview with Adele Townshend, 17 May 1994.
59 Ibid.
60 Ibid.
61 Hudson and Manitowabi, "Accidental History and Manitoulin Island," in this volume.
62 Brock, "Risk, Responsibility and Surgery."
63 Theriot, "Negotiating Illness."
64 See Wilde, *History of Surgery*; also Wilde, "Truth, Trust and Confidence in Surgery."
65 For thoughts on how the system of surgical referrals changed this relationship,
    see Wilde, "Elephants in the Doctor-Patient Relationship."

BIBLIOGRAPHY

Interviews

Interview with Adele Townshend, 17 May 1994.

Newspapers and Periodicals

Medical Post (Toronto)
Charlottetown Guardian
Boston Sunday Globe

Other Sources

Anniversary Committee, Souris, PEI. *1910–1980: A Profile of the Town, Town of
    Souris.* Souris, 1980.
Batinski, Michael. *Pastkeepers in a Small Place: Five Centuries in Deerfield,
    Massachusetts.* Amherst: University of Massachusetts Press, 2004.
Bolger, F.W.P., ed. *Canada's Smallest Province: A History of P.E.I.* Charlottetown:
    Prince Edward Island Centennial Commission, 1973.
Borst, Charlotte. "The Noblest Roman of Them All? Professional versus Popular
    Views of America's Country Doctors." *Journal of the History of Medicine and
    Allied Sciences* 76, no. 1 (January 2021): 78–100.
Breiger, Gert H. "American Surgery and the Germ Theory of Disease." *Bulletin
    of the History of Medicine* 40, no. 2 (1966): 135–45.

Brock, Claire. "Risk, Responsibility and Surgery in the 1890s and Early 1900s." *Medical History* 57, no. 3 (July 2013): 317–37.

Brookes, Alan A. "Outmigration from the Maritime Provinces, 1860–1900: Some Preliminary Considerations." *Acadiensis* 5, no. 2 (Spring 1976): 26–55.

Brown, R. Blake. "Canada's First Malpractice Crisis: Medical Negligence in the Late Nineteenth Century." *Osgoode Hall Law Journal* 54, no. 3 (2017): 777–804.

Bumsted, J.M. "The Origins of the Land Question on Prince Edward Island." *Acadiensis* 11, no. 1 (Autumn 1981): 43–56.

Chang, Jack H.T., and John D. Burrington. "The Development of Paediatric Surgery." *Clio Medica* 11, no. 3 (October 1976): 197–201.

Clark, Andrew Hill. *Three Centuries and the Island: A Historical Geography of Settlement and Agriculture in Prince Edward Island, Canada.* Toronto: University of Toronto Press, 1959.

Crowther, Anne, and Marguerite Dupree. *Medical Lives in the Age of Surgical Revolution.* London: Cambridge University Press, 2007.

Cumming, Melville. "Agriculture in the Maritime Provinces." In *Canada and Its Provinces*, edited by Adam Shortt and Arthur Doughty. Toronto: Glasgow, Brook, and Co., 1914.

Devine, Shauna. *Learning from the Wounded: The Civil War and the Rise of American Medical Science.* Chapel Hill: University of North Carolina Press, 2014.

– "'To Make Something from the Dying in This War': The Civil War and Rise of American Medical Science." *Journal of Civil War History* 6, no. 2 (June 2016): 149–63.

Gerriets, Marylin. "Agricultural Resources, Agricultural Production, and Settlement at Confederation." *Acadiensis* 31, no. 2 (Spring 2002): 129–56.

Greenwood, Anna. "Lawson Tait and Opposition to Germ Theory: Defining Science in Surgical Practice." *Journal of the History of Medicine and Allied Sciences* 53, no. 2 (April 1998): 99–131.

Hamilton, David. "The Nineteenth Century Surgical Revolution: Antisepsis or Better Nutrition?" *Bulletin of the History of Medicine* 56, no. 1 (Spring 1982): 30–40.

Inwood, Kris, and James Irwin, "Canadian Regional Commodity Income Differences at Confederation." In *Farm, Factory and Fortune: New Studies in the Economic Histories of the Maritime Provinces*, edited by Janes Inwood, 93–120. Fredericton: Acadiensis Press, 1993.

– "Land, Income and Regional Inequality." *Acadiensis* 31, no. 2 (Spring 2002): 157–84

Lawrence, Christopher. *Medical Theory, Surgical Practice: Studies in the History of Surgery.* London: Routledge, 1992.

Lawrence, Christopher, and Michael Brown. "Quintessentially Modern Heroes: Surgeons, Explorers and Empire, 1840–1914." *Journal of Social History* 50, no. 1 (Fall 2016): 148–78.

Leavitt, Judith Walzer. "'A Worrying Profession': The Domestic Environment of Medical Practice in Mid-19th Century America." *Bulletin of the History of Medicine* 69, no. 1 (Spring 1995): 1–25.

MacDonald, Edward. *If You're Stronghearted: Prince Edward Island in the Twentieth Century*. Charlottetown: Prince Edward Island Museum and Heritage Foundation, 2000.

MacIsaac, Kay. *Lily Pond Memories*. Charlottetown: Privately printed, 2003.

Mitchinson, Wendy. *Childbirth in Canada, 1900–1950*. Toronto: University of Toronto Press, 2000.

Mullally, Sasha. "Canadian Medical Life-Writing and the Historical Imagination: Unpacking a Cape Breton Country Doctor's Black Bag." In *Figuring the Social*, edited by Elspeth Heaman, Alison Li, and Shelley McKellar. Toronto: University of Toronto Press, 2008, 435–69.

– "Dr. Roddy, Dr. Gus and the Golden Age of Medicine on Prince Edward Island." Master's thesis, University of Ottawa, 1994.

O'Connor, Erin. *Raw Material: Producing Pathology in Victorian Culture*. Durham: Duke University Press, 2000.

O'Grady, Brendan. *Exiles and Islanders: The Irish Settlers of Prince Edward Island*. Montreal and Kingston: McGill-Queen's University Press, 2004.

O'Leary, Louis J., and Daniel B. Macdonald. *Memorial Volume, 1772–1922 – The Arrival of the First Scottish Catholic Emigrants in Prince Edward Island and After*. Summerside: Journal Publishing Co, 1922.

Oden, Derek S. *Harvest of Hazards: Family Farming, Accidents and Expertise in the Corn Belt, 1940–1975*. Iowa City: University of Iowa Press, 2017.

– "Selling Safety: The Farm Safety Movement's Emergence and Evolution from 1940–1975." *Agricultural History* 79, no. 4 (2005): 412–38.

Otis, Yves and Bruno Ramirez. "Nouvelles perspectives sur le mouvement d'émigration des Maritimes vers les États-Unis, 1906–1930." *Acadiensis* 38, no. 1 (Autumn 1998): 27–46.

Porter, Roy. "Accidents in the Eighteenth Century." In *Accidents in History: Injuries, Fatalities and Social Relations*, edited by Roger Cooter and Bill Luckin, 90–106. Amsterdam and Atlanta: Rodopi, 1997.

Schlich, Thomas. "Risk and Medical Innovation: A Historical Perspective." In *The Risk of Medical Innovation: Risk Perception and Assessment in Historical Context*, edited by Thomas Schlich and Urlich Tröhler, 1–17. New York: Routledge, 2006.

– "Surgery, Science and Modernity: Operating Rooms and Laboratories as Spaces of Control." *History of Science* 45, no. 3 (September 2007): 231–56.

Sinclair, Peter. "From Peasants to Corporations: The Development of Capitalist Agriculture in the Maritime Provinces." In *Contradictions in Canadian Society*, edited by John A. Fry. Toronto: University of Toronto Press, 1984.

Stowe, Steven. *Doctoring the South: Southern Physicians and Everyday Medicine in the Mid-19th Century*. Chapel Hill: University of North Carolina Press, 2004.

Theriot, Nancy M. "Negotiating Illness: Doctors, Patients, and Families in the Nineteenth Century." *Journal of the History of the Behavioral Sciences* 37 (2001): 349–68.

Thornton, Patricia. "The Problem of Out-Migration from Atlantic Canada, 1871–1921: A New Look." *Acadiensis* 15, no. 1 (Autumn 1985): 3–34.

Townshend, Adele. "The Brown Lustre Jug." *Atlantic Advocate* (July 1979), 34–5.

– *Ten Farms Become a Town: A History of Souris, Prince Edward Island, 1700–1920.* Souris: Town of Souris, 1986.

Wangensteen, Owen H., and Jacqueline Smith. "Some Highlights in the History of Amputation Reflecting Lessons in Wound Healing." *Bulletin of the History of Medicine* 41, no. 2 (March 1967): 97–131.

Wangensteen, Owen H., and Sarah D. Wangensteen. *The Rise of Surgery: From Empiric Craft to Scientific Discipline.* Minneapolis: University of Minnesota Press, 1979.

Wilde, Sally. "The Elephants in the Doctor-Patient Relationship: Patients' Clinical Interactions and the Changing Surgical Landscape of the 1890s." *Health and History* 9, no. 1 (2007): 2–27.

– "Truth, Trust and Confidence in Surgery, 1890–1910: Patient Autonomy, Communication and Consent." *Bulletin of the History of Medicine* 83, no. 2 (Summer 2009): 302–30.

– *The History of Surgery: Trust, Patient Autonomy, Medical Dominance and Australian Surgery, 1890–1940.* Byron Bay: Finesse Press, 2011.

Wilde, Sally, and Geoffrey Hirst. "Learning from Mistakes: Early Twentieth Century Century Surgical Practice." *Journal of the History of Medicine and Allied Sciences* 64, no. 1 (January 2009): 38–77.

Williams, David Innes. "Denis Browne and the Specialization of Paediatric Surgery." *Journal of Medical Biography* 7, no. 3 (1999): 145–50.

CONCLUSION

John Douglas Belshaw, Megan J. Davies,
Geoffrey L. Hudson, and Sasha Mullally

A popular superstition maintains that bad luck comes in threes. That may have been the case for the Hilborn family of Ten Mile Point in Victoria. In mid-November 1970, six-year-old Bobby Hilborn found himself alone in the family car. He released the handbrake, and the car began to roll. Attempting to escape the moving vehicle, he was crushed to death between the car and a tree.[1] Little Bobby's parents were still grieving his death when, around 1982, a car accident pitched another Hilborn son into a long-term coma. Two years later, the boys' father, William Hilborn, was shot dead by police in the midst of a violent emotional crisis.[2] The Hilborn family, from an ordinary middle-class suburb, appeared to be marked for misfortune.

What of accidents that end well? In 2002, former BC premier Mike Harcourt slipped off the wet deck of his waterfront home on Pender Island. He tumbled down the rocks below, landing in the ocean. Harcourt's accident garnered front-page attention; subsequently, the story emphasized the efficient emergency response, the rapid and effective action of surgeons, and Harcourt's gradual and near-complete recovery, not to mention his enormous good luck.

What do these events have in common? Superstitions about misfortune notwithstanding, accidents such as these, at least in hindsight, appear foreseeable. In both cases above, it is easy to believe in retrospect that precautions might have prevented these accidents. Child-proofing cars is possible, and Mike Harcourt's deck evidently did not meet provincial building codes. Both were private incidents that became public accidents, and both were subject to subsequent spin. The Hilborn family mishaps became part of local narratives and public news coverage that repeatedly returned to cautionary themes like the dangers of playing in cars, the risks attached to motor vehicles, and – in the case of William Hilborn – there-but-for-the-grace-of-God. Harcourt's public stature guaranteed sustained media attention and public engagement in many aspects of the story, which was spun as one of misfortune followed by a favourable outcome. These stories also say important things about equity. The Hilborn and Harcourt accidents happened in comfortably off, even well-known households. What we see in them is a framing of the narrative away from grim resignation in the face of accidental mortality to something like shock that accidents happen to middle-class entrepreneurs and politicians and their families.

The cases examined in this collection all consider what constitutes an "accident." In virtually every case, the key event – as with Bobby Hilborn and Mike Harcourt – was predictable, at least once the pieces started to move. This insight brings us full circle: ship traffic in Halifax Harbour was long a source of concern before the 1917 explosion; slash burning precipitated the Great Fire of Vancouver in 1886, and might predictably have done the same in the Ontario clay belt in 1918; nineteenth-century white railway workers refused to do the work that Chinese railway builders undertook in a racialized workplace precisely because it was too dangerous; engineer errors have led to injuries and mortalities since engineers first emerged and so could be expected on big construction sites; gales come annually to East and West Coast waters, and survival depends on ships' owners, captains, and crews making the right decisions; mechanically accelerating the speed of humans on the ground and then pitching them into the air is a risky enterprise. Nowhere in this litany do we find intent. Sloppiness, carelessness, irresponsibility, and even neglect, yes ... but intent, no.

Jessie Singer argues persuasively that the widespread public use of the word "accident" serves to mitigate responsibility, tends to blame the victim for error, and perpetuates structures of power and privilege that get in the way of substantial precautionary action; she advocates against the word's use. But what are we left with otherwise? "A foreseeable but unintended event arising from complex human errors"? That is a mouthful, and, from a historical perspective, it clogs the arteries of analysis. Historical studies are deeply concerned with the outcomes of those errors and the social and political structures that they reveal. A rural kitchen-table surgery is not really about a chance encounter with farming machinery: it is about the story that springs from those wounds, one that acts simultaneously as a heroic and a precautionary tale while defining the community in which that tradition is maintained.

The complex cultural, social, legal and economic ramifications of accidents mean that there are several ways in which the older literature on the subject is not helpful. For example, the 1990s studies by Cooter and Luckin and Green are not concerned with the multiple emotional effects and consequences of an accident or how a public accident lives in and serves collective memory. The oral histories of children who survived the Halifax explosion, for example, are bluntly factual yet oddly dreamy accounts of bloody limbs, vanished siblings, and miraculous rescues, lacking both ambiguity and sequence.[3] Narratives such as these and others explored here show how accident storylines evolve and are repurposed: they live on beyond the episode itself to become historical events in their own right.

In collecting and assembling the first anthology of articles on the theme of accidents in Canadian history, we see a clear path forward for this literature. The history of the accident in Canada needs to be broadened to include the experiences of racialized people and encompass the vast northern reaches of the country.[4] Fire histories, an expanding field in Canadian history, might be extended to include accidental fires, perhaps contextualized by emotion, age, and the immigrant experience.[5] We see the need for further close analysis of health and welfare policy formation regarding accidents at the provincial and municipal levels. We anticipate scholarship that uses insights from the field of disability studies to consider, for instance, accidents in institutions for vulnerable people where violence was often endemic. Similarly, the Mi'kmaq framework of Two-Eyed seeing could be extended to help us better understand settler and Indigenous experiences and the nature of colonialism. And greater attention to multi-generational experiences of accidents would lead to an enhanced understanding of historical change and continuity for individuals, families, and communities.

Currently, the prognosis for accident histories is good. That was not always the case. Writing in 1998, John Burnham speculated that the new field might not catch on because "historians hesitate to deal with events that are not within human control."[6] This position seems harder to sustain in 2024 as a pandemic, wars, and global climate change pile disaster atop disaster. The contributors to the current volume are convinced that interest in the history of the accident (including the study of prevention and precaution) has a future.

NOTES

1   *Vancouver Sun*, 14 November 1971, 31.
2   *Vancouver Sun*, 6 November 1984, A10.
3   Kitz, *Survivors*.
4   This gap is a problem in the historiography as a whole. Goodman is one exception, with a consideration in *Shifting the Blame* of how in minstrel and burlesque shows Black people were presented as accident victims.
5   Pyne, *Awful Splendour*; Tymstra, *Chinchaga Firestorm*; MacEachern, *Miramichi Fire*.
6   Burnham, "Review: Accidents in History," 242.

BIBLIOGRAPHY

Newspapers

Vancouver Sun

Other Sources

Burnham, John C. "Review: Accidents in History: Injuries, Fatalities and Social Relations by Roger Cooter and Bill Luckin." *Journal of Social History* 32, no. 2 (Winter 1998): 423–5.
Goodman, Nan. *Shifting the Blame: Literature, Law and the Theory of Accidents in Nineteenth-Century America*. New York: Routledge, 1998.
Kitz, Janet. *Survivors: Children of the Halifax Explosion*. Halifax, NS: Nimbus, 2000.
MacEachern, Alan. *The Miramichi Fire: A History*. Montreal and Kingston: McGill-Queen's University Press, 2020.
Pyne, Stephen. *Awful Splendour: A Fire History of Canada*. Vancouver: UBC Press, 2008.
Tymstra, Cordy. *The Chinchaga Firestorm: When the Moon and Sun Turned Blue*. Edmonton: University of Alberta Press, 2015.

CONTRIBUTORS

CEILIDH AUGER-DAY is a researcher and editor. Her doctoral research at the University of Saskatchewan focused on early twentieth-century Canadian health topics, particularly the shift towards statistical and insurance-based approaches to healthcare.

CAMERON BALDASSARRA's graduate studies at McMaster University focused on the deindustrialization of Algonquin Park. He teaches outdoor and experiential education in Toronto.

JOHN BELSHAW is the author of several scholarly books and three open textbooks dealing with Canadian and Indigenous histories. He is currently examining what cycling reveals of Vancouver in the past.

BLAKE BROWN is a professor in the Department of History at Saint Mary's University and is cross-appointed to the Atlantic Canada Studies program.

ANH-DAO BUI TRAN completed her PhD in 2023 at Sorbonne University in Paris. Her research interests include labour and imperial history and the history of medicine.

COLIN COATES, a specialist in the history of early French Canada, is a professor of Canadian Studies at Glendon College, York University.

MEGAN J. DAVIES is professor emerita at York University and an activist historian of health with scholarly publications and public projects relating to madness, old age, and everyday health.

GEOFFREY L. HUDSON, D.Phil. (Oxford), is an associate professor in the History of Medicine at the Northern Ontario School of Medicine University (Human Sciences Division). His areas of research include the social history of medicine, disability, and medical education.

DARREL MANITOWABI, PhD, is an associate professor in the Human Sciences Division at the Northern Ontario School of Medicine (NOSM) University, and the NOSM University-AMS Hannah Chair in the History of Indigenous Health and Indigenous Traditional Medicine.

JOHN R.H. MATCHIM holds a PhD from the University of New Brunswick's Department of History. His dissertation examines the International Grenfell Association of Newfoundland and Labrador and its hospital ship *Strathcona III*.

SASHA MULLALLY is a professor of history at the University of New Brunswick with a wide array of research and teaching interests. She has published widely in the field of health humanities and social science history.

TAMARA GENE MYERS is a professor of history at the University of British Columbia, specializing in the history of children and youth in Canada.

JOHN SANDLOS teaches history at Memorial University of Newfoundland. He is the co-author of *Mining Country: A History of Canada's Mines and Miners*, published with Lorimer Press in 2021.

SAMIRA SARAMO is a senior research fellow at the Migration Institute of Finland. Her current research project on mapping Finnish migrant-settler histories in Ontario is funded by the Kone Foundation.

INDEX

medical malpractice law, 93–4; and
medical mistakes and reputation, 90,
91, 93, 95, 96, 101–2; by mine unions,
75–7; of mining industry, 71–2, 78;
of mining safety violations, 73–5;
for shipwrecks (poor navigation),
259, 264, 265, 267; for shipwrecks
(weather), 260, 262, 264, 270
boat accidents, 282, 286–8, 290, 295,
297–8
Bourget, Bishop Ignace, 159, 160, 161
Bowell, John Moore, 116, 120
Boyce, Helen, 131
Braiden, Heather, 154, 157
Brassey, Thomas, 143, 147, 148, 150, 160
British Columbia Compensation Act: of
1903, 204, 206–7, 214; of 1917, 215
Bronstein, Jamie, 152, 161
Brooke, David, 160, 161
Brown, Audrey Alexandra, 329, 332, 333,
339
Burnett, Horace, 89, 94–107; death, 90–2
Burnham, John, 3, 8, 25n1, 26n23

Canadian Wheelmen's Association
(CWA), 141, 142, 165n22
canals, 159, 160
canoeing, 225, 228, 229, 232, 243–4; and
accidents, 232–4, 236, 241–2, 244; and
canoe tripping, 228, 231, 233, 245; and
capsizing response and prevention,
230–2; and national identity, 226
Cape Breton coast, dangers of, 262, 264
capitalism, 8, 10, 20, 36, 39, 40, 145,
217; and deindustrialization, 239;
and industry, 10–12, 16, 19. See also
industrialization
caregiving, 183, 351, 357–9, 362n51.
See also gender; maternal care
Catholic Church, 347–8, 354, 361n26
Charlevoix, Pierre-François-Xavier de,
259, 264
children and youth: accidents, 5, 9–11, 14,
17, 19, 23, 27n43; in British Columbia,
314–16, 318–19, 320–5, 326–33;

and connections through Finnish
newspaper, 37; and cycling accidents,
113, 118, 125–6, 129–30, 132–3, 135n95;
and exhibitionary culture, 316, 317,
321; and helio-sun-therapy, 327; on
Manitoulin Island, 282, 296, 299; in
narratives, 42–4; and physiotherapy,
325–7; on Prince Edward Island,
342–4, 345, 354, 356–7, 362n51; "public
child," 10, 17, 315–16; rehabilitation,
325–8
class, 10–13, 17–18, 171–2, 198, 211–13, 217;
and biking accidents, 116, 119, 120, 133;
and Finnish community accidents,
34, 39–40, 53; in relation to Victoria
Bridge, 150, 152, 159, 160
Cloutier, Tommy, 227, 240, 243, 244
Cobalt, ON, 65–6, 70
Coffey, Jim, 233, 243
colonialism, 13–14, 218, 258; and
Anglo-Saxon idealization, 198; on
Manitoulin Island, 281–9, 291–6,
298–303; and migrant settlerhood,
44, 54n2; and modern medicine, 173.
See also settler; settler colonialism
commissions, 201–2, 204–5, 211
Communist Party of Canada, 37
community supports, 33, 41, 48–53, 349,
354, 357–9; and community halls
(haali), 34, 38, 42; and fractures, 51–2;
and payment upon injury, 207; and
rural medical practice, 345, 347–8,
350, 352, 354–6, 359, 362n39
compensation, 159, 161, 197, 207
Cooter, Roger, 6–7, 14, 23, 26n18, 20, 62,
145, 146, 150, 151, 295, 306n76
Corkill, E.T., 66–7, 69, 80
coroners: and Coroners Act, Ontario,
94, 100, 106; Elie Cass, 94–5; and
mining accidents, Ontario, 71–2, 74,
77–9, 80; Morton Shulman, 89–107
Crespel, Emmanuel, Récollet, 259–61, 269
Crippled Children's Hospital,
Vancouver, 325, 332
Cross, Charles, 197